Creating a Modern Trauma Center

Selwyn O. Rogers, Jr
Editor

Creating a Modern Trauma Center

Springer

Editor
Selwyn O. Rogers, Jr
Medicine & Biological Sciences
University of Chicago
Chicago, IL, USA

ISBN 978-3-031-66523-3 ISBN 978-3-031-66524-0 (eBook)
https://doi.org/10.1007/978-3-031-66524-0

This Springer imprint is published by the registered company Springer Nature Switzerland AG
The registered company address is: Gewerbestrasse 11, 6330 Cham, Switzerland

I would like to dedicate this book to
my mother, Mrs. Lynette Simmonds Arson,
who served as my inspiration for my drive
and commitment to excellence.

Acknowledgments

We would like to acknowledge the trauma patients that the University of Chicago Medicine Trauma Center has served and continues to serve on the South Side of Chicago and beyond. We also recognize the activists who championed for an adult trauma center on the South Side over the decades.

Contents

Contributors

Gary An, MD, FACS Department of Surgery, University of Vermont Medical Center, Burlington, VT, USA

Fatima A. Aldarweesh Department of Pathology, Section of Transfusion, Hemostasis, and Apheresis (THAM), University of Chicago, Chicago, IL, USA

Debra Allen Independent Trauma Consultant, University of Chicago's Adult Level I Trauma Center, Chicago, IL, USA

John C. Alverdy Department of Surgery, University of Chicago, Pritzker School of Medicine, Chicago, IL, USA

Dr. Mark Anderson Dean of the Biological Sciences Division, Dean of the Pritzker School of Medicine, Executive Vice President for Medical Affairs, Paul and Allene Russell Professor, Department of Medicine, University of Chicago, Chicago, IL, USA

Peter Angelos MacLean Center for Clinical Medical Ethics and Department of Surgery, University of Chicago, Chicago, IL, USA

Andrew J. Benjamin Department of Surgery, University of Chicago, Chicago, IL, USA

University of Chicago Medicine, Section of Trauma and Acute Care Surgery, Chicago, IL, USA

Ira J. Blumen UCAN, UChicago Medicine, Chicago, IL, USA

Section of Emergency Medicine, Department of Medicine, University of Chicago, Chicago, IL, USA

Oloruntoba Bolaji Section of Trauma and Acute Care Surgery, Department of Surgery, University of Chicago Medicine, Chicago, IL, USA

Toba Bolaji Section of Trauma and Acute Care Surgery, Department of Surgery, University of Chicago Medicine, Chicago, IL, USA

Julian A. Bond Trauma Chaplain, Spiritual Care, UChicago Medicine, Chicago, IL, USA

Dana Branch Department of Physical Medicine & Rehabilitation, Shirley Ryan AbilityLab, Chicago, IL, USA

Kylie Callier MacLean Center for Clinical Medical Ethics and Department of Surgery, University of Chicago, Chicago, IL, USA

Mihir Chaudhary Section of Trauma and Acute Care Surgery, Department of Surgery, University of Chicago Medicine, Chicago, IL, USA

Julia Chavez Section of Trauma and Acute Care Surgery, Department of Surgery, University of Chicago, Chicago, IL, USA

Sophie Colt Urban Health Initiative, University of Chicago Medicine, Chicago, IL, USA

Jennifer Cone Department of Surgery, University of Chicago, Chicago, IL, USA

Franklin Cosey-Gay Urban Health Initiative, University of Chicago Medicine, Chicago, IL, USA

Section of Trauma and Acute Care Surgery, Department of Surgery, University of Chicago, Chicago, IL, USA

David Crump Urban Health Initiative, University of Chicago Medicine, Chicago, IL, USA

Jade Curless Urban Health Initiative, University of Chicago Medicine, Chicago, IL, USA

Kimora Custon Section of Trauma and Acute Care Surgery, Department of Surgery, University of Chicago, Chicago, IL, USA

Anthony Douglas II Department of Surgery, University of Chicago, Chicago, IL, USA

Tracey Fan Assistant Professor of Neurology, Neurocritical Care Section, Assistant Program Director Neurocritical Care Fellowship, University of Chicago, Chicago, IL, USA

Christine Goggins Urban Health Initiative, University of Chicago Medicine, Chicago, IL, USA

Section of Trauma and Acute Care Surgery, Department of Surgery, University of Chicago, Chicago, IL, USA

Fernando D. Goldenberg Professor of Neurology and Neurological Surgery, Neurocritical Care Section Chief, Medical Director Neuroscience ICU, Co-Director Comprehensive Stroke Center, University of Chicago, Chicago, IL, USA

Isaac Green Section of Trauma and Acute Care Surgery, Department of Surgery, University of Chicago, Chicago, IL, USA

Ameera Haamid Chicago South EMS System, Department of Medicine, Section of Emergency Medicine, University of Chicago Medicine, Chicago, IL, USA

David A. Hampton, MD Section of Trauma and Acute Care Surgery, Department of Surgery, University of Chicago Medicine, Chicago, IL, USA

Lea Hoefer University of Chicago Department of Surgery, Chicago, IL, USA

Marc D. Horton, MD FACS Swedish Medical Center General Surgery Residency Program, Seattle, WA, USA

Nicholas Jaszczak Section of Trauma and Acute Care Surgery, Department of Surgery, University of Chicago, Chicago, IL, USA

Dwayne E. Johnson Urban Health Initiative, University of Chicago Medicine, Chicago, IL, USA

Caitlin Kilcoyne UCAN, UChicago Medicine, Chicago, IL, USA

Stephen Leb Department of Physical Medicine & Rehabilitation, Shirley Ryan AbilityLab, Chicago, IL, USA

Jeffrey Leef, MD Loyola University Medical Center, Maywood, IL, USA

Jackquelin Loera Department of Surgery, University of Chicago, Chicago, IL, USA

Carly Loughran Section of Trauma and Acute Care Surgery, Department of Surgery, University of Chicago, Chicago, IL, USA

Ali Mansour Assistant Professor of Neurology and Neurological Surgery, Neurocritical Care Section, Chief Quality Officer, Department of Neurology, Medical Director of Informatics Neurosciences and Critical Care, Program Director Neurocritical Care Fellowship, University of Chicago, Chicago, IL, USA

Jeffrey B. Matthews Department of Surgery, The University of Chicago, Chicago, IL, USA

Michael McCartin UCAN, UChicago Medicine, Chicago, IL, USA

Section of Emergency Medicine, Department of Medicine, University of Chicago, Chicago, IL, USA

Mary Noory, MD Section of Trauma and Acute Care Surgery, Department of Surgery, University of Chicago Medicine, Chicago, IL, USA

Darlington Nwaudo, MD Department of Surgery, The University of Chicago Medicine, Chicago, IL, USA

Department of Orthopedic Surgery, The University of Chicago Medicine, Chicago, IL, USA

Michael O'Connor, MD Department of Anesthesia, University of Chicago Medicine, Chicago, IL, USA

Samuel E. Okum, BA Department of Surgery, The University of Chicago Medicine, Chicago, IL, USA

School of Medicine, Johns Hopkins University, Baltimore, MD, USA

Samuel Osei, MD Section of Trauma and Acute Care Surgery, Department of Surgery, University of Chicago Medicine, Chicago, IL, USA

Ernestina Perez Urban Health Initiative, University of Chicago Medicine, Chicago, IL, USA

Section of Trauma and Acute Care Surgery, Department of Surgery, University of Chicago, Chicago, IL, USA

Sharnae Phagan Section of Trauma and Acute Care Surgery, Department of Surgery, University of Chicago Medicine, Chicago, IL, USA

Rhea Pillai Section of Trauma and Acute Care Surgery, Department of Surgery, University of Chicago, Chicago, IL, USA

Timothy P. Plackett Section of Trauma and Acute Care Surgery, Department of Surgery, University of Chicago, Chicago, IL, USA

Priya S. Prakash University of Chicago Department of Surgery, Chicago, IL, USA

Carlos Robles Urban Health Initiative, University of Chicago Medicine, Chicago, IL, USA

Section of Trauma and Acute Care Surgery, Department of Surgery, University of Chicago, Chicago, IL, USA

Selwyn O. Rogers Jr, MD, MPH Section of Trauma and Acute Care Surgery, University of Chicago Medicine, Chicago, IL, USA

Urban Health Initiative, University of Chicago Medicine, Chicago, IL, USA

Department of Surgery, The University of Chicago Medicine, Chicago, IL, USA

William Roth Assistant Professor of Neurology, Neurocritical Care Section, University of Chicago, Chicago, IL, USA

Susan Rowell, MD, MBA Section of Trauma and Acute Care Surgery, Department of Surgery, University of Chicago Medicine, Chicago, IL, USA

Candice Schaper UCAN, UChicago Medicine, Chicago, IL, USA

Nisha Sen-Gupta Section of Trauma and Acute Care Surgery, Department of Surgery, University of Chicago, Chicago, IL, USA

Bruce Stamps Urban Health Initiative, University of Chicago Medicine, Chicago, IL, USA

Jason Strelzow Department of Orthopaedic Surgery, The University of Chicago, Chicago, IL, USA

Katie Tataris Chicago South EMS System, Department of Medicine, Section of Emergency Medicine, University of Chicago Medicine, Chicago, IL, USA

Elizabeth Tung Section of Trauma and Acute Care Surgery, Department of Surgery, University of Chicago, Chicago, IL, USA

Carly Uebel Urban Health Initiative, University of Chicago Medicine, Chicago, IL, USA

Dr. Randall P. White, PhD Professor at HEC Paris, Executive Development Group, LLC, and HEC Paris, Greensboro, NC, USA

Kenneth L. Wilson Section of Trauma and Acute Care Surgery, Department of Surgery, University of Chicago, Chicago, IL, USA

University of Chicago Medicine & Biologic Sciences, Chicago, IL, USA

Geoffrey D. Wool Department of Pathology, Section of Transfusion, Hemostasis, and Apheresis Medicine (THAM), Transfusion Medicine Fellowship Program, University of Chicago, Chicago, IL, USA

Tanya L. Zakrison Section of Trauma and Acute Care Surgery, Department of Surgery, University of Chicago, Chicago, IL, USA

Part I
Background

Prologue: A Journey of Cultural Transformation

Priya S. Prakash and Selwyn O. Rogers, Jr

As we embarked on our journey of standing up an adult Level 1 Trauma Center at the University of Chicago Medicine, we knew our work would extend well beyond the clinical care that we provided to the traumatically injured patient. We would have to be thought leaders and revolutionaries who challenged the existing status quo of an institution disconnected from the community's needs for almost three decades.

After closing its doors to adult trauma care in 1989, the relationship with the communities on the South Side of Chicago and the University of Chicago was deeply strained and fractured. Although the University of Chicago Medicine was an anchor institution as the only academic medical center on the South Side, the University of Chicago Medicine focused on mostly subspecialty care. Emergency services were limited. In this challenging context, the community clamored for an adult trauma center given the relative trauma desert, the extreme need for adult trauma services, and preponderance of firearm-related injuries. After a decade of protests and community advocacy, the University of Chicago Medicine acquiesced to re-open its doors to adult trauma care. The institution did not transform overnight but has evolved over the years that followed.

To successfully operationalize a system of trauma care that would also uplift clinical capacity for all patients, we led a cultural transformation across the institution. We focused on who we cared for and how we cared for them. This required a team of individuals dedicated to a common mission with a willingness to challenge

P. S. Prakash (✉)
University of Chicago Department of Surgery, Chicago, IL, USA
e-mail: pprakash@bsd.uchicago.edu

S. O. Rogers, Jr
Section of Trauma and Acute Care Surgery, University of Chicago Medicine, Chicago, IL, USA
e-mail: srogers@bsd.uchicago.edu

S. O. Rogers, Jr (ed.), *Creating a Modern Trauma Center*,
https://doi.org/10.1007/978-3-031-66524-0_1

the status quo. Our surgical team began with six recruits, including a visionary leader, a highly experienced military surgeon, and four energetic and idealistic young academic trauma surgeons. An experienced trauma program manager and a cadre of bright, young advanced practice providers rounded out the group. Although we came from various backgrounds from major trauma centers across the country, we coalesced to ultimately forge forward that we nicknamed the "UChicago Way". Initially seen as misfits, rebels, and troublemakers, the group emerged as meta-leaders. Our revolution was grounded in social justice and equity. We extended to advocate for improved access to care for all patients. Like a rising tide, we lifted all boats. The team would eventually grow to fifteen surgeon and twelve advanced practice providers in conjunction with all of the resources of an academic medical center. As our team evolved, our trauma program manager passed the torch of leadership to an experienced emergency medicine nurse. Our reach as an adult trauma center began to stretch beyond our local community to the rest of the country through education, research and advocacy.

The biggest challenge the group faced was resistance to change with concomitant protection of the status quo. Seemingly overnight, the institution was forced to embrace and care for a marginalized community suffering from the epidemic of gun violence. A massive overhaul of policy, procedure, and workflow took place as we continuously iterated and improved the systems of trauma care. Support for emergency services such as 24/7 in-house surgery attending presence and operating room capabilities emerged. Care for the critically ill was bolstered by evidence-based protocols and advanced methods for supportive care such as extracorporeal membrane oxygenation. Timely access to balanced blood product resuscitation for all patients was implemented. A unique collaboration between trauma surgeons and interventional radiologists pushed the boundaries on novel approaches to challenging trauma cases. This partnership led to the creation of an annual national conference appropriately entitled "How to Save a Life". All service lines throughout the hospital and all of the training programs were clinically strengthened by exposure to a diverse patient population with a spectrum of injuries. A robust quality and process improvement initiative shifted the culture on how care was rendered with a commitment to continuous quality improvement. Over time, the resistance to this movement weakened, and the identity of the institution and its approach to clinical care was transformed.

With firearm-related injuries as the leading mechanism of injury at our adult trauma center, it was paramount that efforts reached beyond just providing excellent clinical care. A hospital-based violence intervention program and a medical-legal partnership were implemented that provides wrap-around services, resources, and support for those who are violently injured as well as their families. We focused on decreasing re-injury rates and safe transitioning of individuals back into their communities. We engaged with community partners on the South Side of Chicago to connect patients with services to alter their life trajectory. The work continues to focus on eradicating violence and building safer communities. Discussing structural racism, social and political determinants of health, and access to care issues became embedded as part of our daily conversation, emphasizing their interplay with healthcare outcomes in marginalized communities. Research efforts have not only focused on clinical outcomes and basic science. We have committed to identifying the root causes of violence and developing innovative solutions with community partners. The institution has worked to rebuild its fractured relationship with the community through engagement, partnerships, and research.

This book will take you on the journey of a cultural transformation of a major academic institution through the creation of an adult Level 1 Trauma Center. It will highlight the invaluable contributions of the nurses, hospital staff, trainees, and subspecialty providers who joined the trauma team in a revolution that demanded access to equitable care for all people. It will tell the story of those willing to push boundaries, challenge the status quo, and take on the fraternities. It is the passion, commitment, and sacrifice of countless individuals over decades who advocated for an adult level one trauma center on the South Side of Chicago. Community advocacy has led to the success of the adult trauma center at the University of Chicago Medicine. Their continued efforts will allow for its evolution. Though there is still much more work to be done, the DNA of the institution has been transformed. With change comes progress. We must stay vigilant and face the challenges that is ushered in by change. In the end as we continue on this transformational journey, something great will emerge.

Creating an Oasis in a Trauma Desert: The South Side's Fight for an Adult Trauma Center at the University of Chicago Medicine

Anthony Douglas II, Mihir Chaudhary, and Selwyn O. Rogers, Jr

The Great Migration

Prior to recounting a history of the University of Chicago Medicine Trauma Center (UCMTC) and focusing on the community organizing that led to it, we begin with a broader historical contextualization of Chicago. Specifically, understanding the Great Migration during Jim Crow America and subsequent residential segregation in Chicago lays the historical groundwork for some of the deep racial health disparities on the South Side.

Following the formal and legal end of slavery at the end of the Civil War in 1865, millions of newly liberated slaves throughout the Southern United States found themselves living under a new political and social system of racism that was termed Jim Crow. Jim Crow consisted of state and local laws throughout the South that limited the political and legal rights of Black people and was undergirded by regimes of racial terror enforced by White supremacist civilian groups, such as the Ku Klux Klan. In response, beginning in 1910 and continuing into the 1940s almost six

A. Douglas II (✉)
University of Chicago Department of Surgery, Chicago, IL, USA
e-mail: anthony.douglas@uchicagomedicine.org

M. Chaudhary
Department of Surgery, Section of Trauma and Acute Care Surgery, University of Chicago Medicine, Chicago, IL, USA
e-mail: Mihir.Chaudhary@uchicagomedicine.org

S. O. Rogers, Jr
Section of Trauma and Acute Care Surgery, University of Chicago Medicine, Chicago, IL, USA
e-mail: srogers@bsd.uchicago.edu

S. O. Rogers, Jr (ed.), *Creating a Modern Trauma Center*,
https://doi.org/10.1007/978-3-031-66524-0_2

million African Americans migrated from the racism, lynchings, and plight of living in the South to seek sanctuary and opportunity in cities throughout the North and Midwestern regions, including the cities of Chicago, New York, Detroit, and Pittsburgh [1]. In the midst of war economies during World War I and II, many industrial positions were opened in these cities. Black people throughout the South migrated en masse for the economic opportunity that presented. Major corporations and the Chicago Defender, a Black owned newspaper, recruited African American families to flee oppression for what was hoped to be the promised land [2]. In reality, Black people migrating from the South found the same hostility and oppression in their new homes.

Residential Segregation

Historically and presently, Chicago is one of the most racially segregated cities in the United States. This is due to the response of White Americans, the government, and institutions to millions of African Americans seeking asylum in Chicago. "White Flight," describes the phenomenon of White people vacating the inner core of cities with growing Black populations for the distant suburbs to flee the integration of their neighborhoods [3]. The Federal government and institutions like the University of Chicago aided and abetted this racial separation. The Federal Housing Authority (FHA) upheld this through several racially discriminatory practices, such as restrictive covenants [3]. Restrictive covenants were obligations new owners of a property were bound to follow; these obligations disallowed renting or selling homes to Black people. Eventually, these restrictive covenants led to housing or community associations maintaining a racially homogenous community and making dwellers punishable in civil court for selling to Black people [3]. In Chicago, "by 1947, half of the city's residential areas outside its African American areas had such deed restrictions [3]." The FHA continued its support of residential segregation through their creation of redlining maps and favorable assignment of property value to houses and communities with clauses that prohibited Black settlement.

The University of Chicago's participation in residential segregation began at the end of the 1800s. Bronzeville, the original location of the university, was relocated to Hyde Park as the beginning of the Great Migration marked large influxes of Black Americans into the Bronzeville community [2]. Just a few decades later, the University of Chicago colluded with the FHA, Michael Reese Hospital, real estate moguls, the South East Chicago Commission, and the Chicago Land Clearance Commission to create a plan displacing Black Americans away from Bronzeville, the major landing pad for Black Americans fleeing the South [2]. This gentrification or urban renewal plan was intended to free up land for private ventures and rental apartments. This collusion led to the forced evacuation of Black Americans. Approximately 100 acres of land was decimated; 46 Black owned businesses and 4000 families were displaced [2]. The Black community referred to this period as the "Negro Removal." [4] Michael Reese Hospital and the Illinois Institute of Technology both joined in the planning and acquisition of this land. UChicago's motivation for supporting this urban renewal was clear: the "ghettos," or "slums," now inhabited by Black families were encroaching on the university, and this was unacceptable [5]. In order to prevent this from occurring, the areas referred to as the slums were replaced with upper- and middle-class housing. Those who once inhabited this area were replaced with White residents who could afford the new residential development [5]. The University of Chicago accomplished this not only for itself, but for 14 other major historic universities through lobbying for the Housing Act of 1959—an act that would allow universities to seek federal and private funds to support urban renewal projects [6]. This sort of land grabbing persisted until the 1980s. By that time, the University of Chicago created a barrier creating two Kenwood's, North Kenwood near the Negro slums of Bronzeville, and Kenwood, Hyde Parks' Black-free neighbor [5].

This history reverberates to this day, as many of Chicago's community members opposed the initial decision to build Obama's Presidential Library on the South Side [6]. This history is also how Chicago has become notorious for being one of America's most segregated cities. Segregated not only by geography, Chicago's segregation extends to differential distribution of investment, education, quality housing, and even food. Ultimately, this intentional policy led to destitute communities plagued by firearm violence. Certain tragic deaths and victims of this firearm violence were critical to the creation of a mass movement to eventually produce a more equitable landscape of trauma care in Chicago.

Benjamin "Benji" Wilson Jr.

Ben "Benji" Wilson was born March 18th, 1967, and raised on the South Side of Chicago. Benji was a 6′8″ gentle slender giant whose personality and basketball game captivated the attention of Magic Johnson, Isaiah Thomas, and all those who had the opportunity to meet him [7]. At the highlight of his career as a junior in high school, Benji was recruited by the NBA and honored as the #1 High School basketball player in the nation. Benji attended Simeon High School, located at 8147 S Vincennes Ave in Chatham, Chicago. On November 21st, 1984, just one day before his senior year basketball season, blocks away from his school, Benji was shot twice [7]. He was taken to St. Bernard Hospital, a community hospital without a trauma center approximately 2.5 miles away from where he was injured. He allegedly arrived at St. Bernard Hospital at approximately 1:20 pm and underwent surgery almost 2 h later [8]. Benji succumbed to his injuries on November 21st. His death garnished national attention and shook the South Side community. His death also led to the formation of the first trauma center network in Chicago in 1985 [9]. At that time there were reportedly 378 firearm-related homicides in the city [10]. With the passing of the trauma center network ordinance, nine hospitals were called on to build infrastructures for trauma services. This included six city and three suburban hospitals, including Cook County, University of Chicago, Northwestern, Michael Reese, Illinois Masonic, Louis Weiss Memorial, Advocate Christ Hospital, Lutheran General, and Loyola University [9]. In response to the untimely and unspecialized care that Benji received, the "Benji rule," was created, requiring all injured patients to be transported to the nearest trauma center staffed with the personnel to care for trauma victims.

Trauma Centers Withdraw from Network

The nine-center trauma network was not long lived. The University of Chicago opened its doors in 1986 to trauma patients. Two years later the university would become the second hospital to withdraw from the trauma network [11]. In May of 1988, the University of Chicago officially closed its adult trauma services, citing significant financial strain [12]. However, Michael Reese Hospital remained open and serviced the South Side community. That is, until February 1990, when Michael Reese would also withdraw from the network thus leaving the Near South Side of Chicago without an adult trauma center [9]. In the end, six trauma centers would remain after the withdrawals from the network: Advocate Illinois Masonic, Cook County, Mount Sinai, Northwestern, Advocate Christ, and Advocate Lutheran hospitals [9]. While the Far South Side of Chicago could rely on Advocate Christ for their trauma services, Near South Chicago became a trauma desert. Twenty-seven years would go by before this trauma desert would be addressed. After countless untold injuries and deaths in the Near South Side, one death, in particular, would spark widespread outrage and mass mobilization.

Damian Turner

Damian Turner, an 18-year-old teenager, had a dream of advocating for a trauma center to be reopened in the Near South Chicagoland area [13]. Wise beyond his age, Damian dedicated his time and energy to community activism. He co-founded two grassroot organizations, Fearless Leading by the Youth (FLY) and the youth division of Southside Together Organizing for Power (STOP). Family members of Damian said he lived for activism and had a strong passion for people. His infectious charisma mobilized young people on the South Side to organize for space and resources that were largely controlled by the University of Chicago. Damian's future was bright, but just weeks prior to his 19th birthday, on August 15th, 2010, his life was snatched [9]. Damian was struck in his back by a bullet on the corner of 61st and Cottage Grove, 4 blocks or 1 min by car from UCMTC. He stumbled into and collapsed onto the floor of his sister Jasmine's home in nearby Grove Park Apartments, at which point 911 was called.

When EMS arrived, instead of going to the University of Chicago Medicine, one minute away, he was transported to Northwestern University [9, 13]. Per the Benji rule, Northwestern was the nearest trauma center to the location where Damian was shot, a 10-mile transport to preserve his life. This ambulance ride took 10-min and Damian was pronounced dead after arrival to Northwestern, less than 90 min from the time of being shot. While no one will ever know whether Damian would have survived had the University of Chicago had a trauma center, his ability to ambulate from the scene and initial period of survival suggests that immediate hospital level interventions could have potentially saved his life. Damian's story is one of many, but his death sparked a social movement and created, to our knowledge, the first adult trauma center to be established on the grounds of community organizing. It sets a unique historical example for mobilizing resources to address urban trauma disparities. The political history undergirding its creation serves as a valuable lesson for what may be possible in other similar urban settings. It is a powerful narrative of Black resistance to state and institutional abandonment to garner the resources necessary for community survival.

The Movement

Between 2010 and 2015, following the aftermath of the death of Damian Turner and building off of the preventable violent deaths of many other Black residents of the South Side of Chicago, a massive social mobilization took place. Specifically, a Trauma Care Coalition (TCC) cohered community-organizing groups, including Southside Together Organizing for Power (STOP), Fearless Leading by the Youth (FLY), and Strong Humbled Empowered (SHE) with local politicians, churches, University of Chicago students and faculty, to build a movement that culminated in the eventual re-opening of the adult trauma center on May 1st, 2018.

Organizing for Survival

The death of Damian Turner was a tipping point that mobilized marginalized Black communities on the South Side to organize a campaign for an adult trauma center at the University of Chicago. Such organizing can be seen in the long historical arc of transformative political action by Black communities to survive structural racism in the United States. The movement began on September 28th, 2010, when Damian Turner's mother—Sheila Rush—staged a protest march on what would have been his 19th birthday [14]. This protest drew dozens of friends and neighbors and revealed the contradiction between the University of Chicago's stated values of equity and its lack of an adult trauma center to serve those nearby marginalized neighborhoods most affected by violence. The poignancy of this protest and the seeming disproportionate strength and power of the University of Chicago relative to a small group of nearby community members actually garnered significant media coverage including an article by the New York Times [15]. The community's critique of a lack of an adult trauma desert on the South Side, sitting under the shadow of a large, well-resourced academic medical center, presaged future empirical demonstrations inversely correlating trauma center distance and survival after injury in Chicago that would be used to support the movement for an adult trauma center at the University of Chicago.

Following the initial neighborhood level organizing by Sheila Rush, a period of sustained coalition building and direct action ensued by Black residents on Chicago's South Side [15].

A few months following Rush's initial protest in grief of the loss of her son Damian, STOP and FLY began mobilizing further actions. These actions were notable for being led by the young people on the South Side most intimately affected by the violence—and the associated institutional neglect—they faced. On November 12, 2010, 50 FLY and STOP protestors staged a "die-in" laying near the UCMTC on the concrete after performatively having been shot wearing "blood" stained T-shirts [16]. This die-in tactic became the most frequent tactic used by Black South Side youth to directly demonstrate to the public the contradiction of so many life-saving services at the University of Chicago Medicine adjacent to such a magnitude of racialized death. On January 25, 2011, a few months following this "die-in", Jasmine Harris, Darrius Lightfoot, and Toussaint Losier—all youth activists and community organizers with STOP and FLY—staged a mock funeral. About 25 FLY protestors lay in makeshift caskets as local news agencies, including CBS and the university newspaper, covered the event. This action, like many others, directly interrupted a major University event—in this case a MLK commemoration—to garner visibility and counter the historical neglect of the institution [17]. The University of Chicago responded to this initial period with a statement that the formation of an adult trauma center required specific equipment and staffing that would detract from its other health care services.

Mobilizing University and Community Partners

In the second phase of organizing, young activists from STOP and FLY demonstrated their community leadership abilities by forming broad based coalitions. They also established an "inside" and "outside" strategy to community organizing—mobilizing students and faculty at the University of Chicago—to exert internal pressure, while simultaneously activating community organizations and the media to exert external pressure.

The broadening of the movement was evidenced by an April 21, 2011, action that brought together 150 protestors from Kenwood Oakland community organizations, Grand Boulevard's chapter of CeaseFire, in addition to FLY and STOP youth [18]. The protestors marched into the University's Surgery Brain Research Pavilions and blocked traffic. The action led to a meeting with University of Chicago community relations who continued to cite concerns around costs and the detraction from other health services if an adult trauma center were opened.

Such visible political actions did eventually enter the consciousness of physicians working at the UCMTC and led to a forum at the University on May 11, 2011. The forum was co-hosted by the American Medical Students Association and the Emergency Medical Interest Group at the medical school. At the event, Carolyn Wilson the Chief Operating Officer of UCMTC, Linda Druelinger MD, an emergency medicine physician and Co-Chief of Emergency Medicine, discussed the absence of an adult trauma center at UCMTC with John Easton, a UCMTC spokesperson. Easton repeated prior arguments that an adult trauma center would take funding away from other services and detract from the mission to educate medical students and conduct research. Easton argued that "Illinois has the best access to trauma care of any Midwestern state and Chicago has more level-one trauma centers than any other region of Illinois—four for adults and four for children." [19] What he omitted was the relative racial and spatial disparity in these trauma centers—an argument that gained traction later in the movement. This town hall style event initially appeased many students' concerns though, as will be seen, did not co-opt University of Chicago students and faculty from joining STOP and FLY. Importantly, the community was not invited to this forum.

The next action organized by STOP and FLY occurred August 14–15, 2011, as FLY's two primary leaders, Darrius Lightfoot and Toussaint Losier, marked the 1-year anniversary of Turner's death by occupying the front of one of the University of Chicago's hospital entrances. This was a symbolic act of reclamation of space and resources that would have potentially saved the life of Damian. Activists chanted "How can you ignore – we're dying at your door?", asserting their humanity in front of institutional apathy [20]. All major Chicago news outlets covered the event—a sign of growing recognition of the campaign. Importantly, UCMTC countered that it provided $200 million in charity care, a figure contested by STOP and FLY, using Center for Budget and Tax Accountability data showing that UCMC only utilized $10 million in charity care, while receiving $58 million in non-profit tax breaks [20]. The contradiction between UCMTC resources and its negligence to provide trauma care deepened as protestors pointed out the plan to create a $700 million hospital expansion—the Center for Care and Delivery. The protestors directly addressed this contradiction on September 28th, 2011, with 75 protestors marching into the construction area for the UChicago Medicine expansion [14]. Religious leaders also attended this protest in Hyde Park and spoke at the event. This protest received national attention. It also captured the state public health department's attention who committed to gather data to determine if a trauma center was indeed needed.

The movement was reaching a critical mass with youth activists and religious leaders getting involved. By the time of the next action—another "die-in" on October 31, 2011—University of Chicago student activists were joining. Community and student activists "die" in large numbers as FLY and SHE protestors rose the dead accompanied to Michael Jackson's "Thriller" [21]. The youth demonstrated their resilience and ability to find joy even as they fought for their community's survival. The University responded to this more widespread protest and the emergence of University of Chicago student resistance with an open forum 10 days later. At this forum, a FLY activist—Veronica Morris-Moore—demanded a feasibility study [22]. Following this forum, the community coalition that had been built over the prior 15 months since Damian Turner's death entered a period of quiescence for nearly 6 months as it strategized about additional targets to organize around.

After a relative period of silence, FLY and SHE organized with community, faith-based groups and UCMTC faculty to organize a march for a trauma center on May 12, 2012. This event was used as a building point to organize the next large, and perhaps most pivotal action, months later in January. On January 27, 2012, 50 protestors from the STOP and FLY coalitions marched into the newly built, yet to be opened, Center for Care and Discovery and demonstrated in the lobby. While four protestors committed to remaining inside, the others were asked to leave by security. The University of Chicago police got involved forcing protestors to exit using their batons and forcibly pushing protestors towards the door—many protestors fell to the floor [23]. A University officer also struck the camera out of the hand of the group's reporter and knocked out his headphones, prior to handcuffing him on the ground. Four protestors, including an University student, were arrested, and the broad coalition rallied around them until released by the police [24]. The use of university police force to suppress peaceful dissent, including the use of plainclothes officers disguised as protestors, was widely reported by the media and galvanized young people and broader public to be involved in the movement [25].

Broadening of the Movement

The January 27th, 2013, protest was the largest that the movement had organized and the most direct confrontation with the University of Chicago's police force. Following this action, local clergy leaders began weekly prayers for a trauma center outside of UCMTC, while the graduate student union held its own vigil in support for those affected by police brutality in the January 27th action. SHE and FLY leaders strategically invited candidates in the 2nd congressional district to attend a meeting to discuss the trauma center of which only one candidate—Alderman Anthony Beale—showed and promised to fight for a trauma center [26]. Following this, on the day of the opening of the Center for Care and Discovery, a UChicago Medicine representative claimed to not have resources to build a trauma center. Seventy movement activists delivered petitions. FLY activist Veronica Morris-Moore stated "We were here 4 weeks ago to do a sit-in at the $700M research facility and we were basically attacked and brutalized by the police when we came here." [27]

The movement also began to attract other local academic faculty support. A professor of trauma surgery at Northwestern, Mary Crandall, published a paper in April

2013 in the American Journal of Public Health demonstrating that distance from a trauma center correlated with likelihood of mortality. She used Chicago to demonstrate that those suffering gunshot wounds more than 5 miles from a trauma center were more likely to die [28]. Activists with FLY used this paper to demonstrate what they were trying to voice to institutions for years and was now academically validated with Crandall's paper.

Following Crandall's paper, a regular stream of protest activities, vigils, and group prayers continued to exert pressure on UChicago Medicine and the movement for the adult trauma center used the empirical force of her paper throughout media outlets. The University attempted to respond with its prior argument as the former dean of the medical school—Dean Polonsky—said "we are at 100 percent capacity in our emergency room and our in-patient services. So, if we were to become a Level 1 trauma center, it's not 'in addition to': it's 'instead of.'" [29]

At this point, the movement even broadened itself to higher levels of government. In July 2013, a United States congressional representative from Illinois, Bobby Rush, introduced legislation to fund trauma centers in so-called trauma deserts with a $100 million fund. This legislation is in response to another possibly preventable death of a young Black man—Kevin Ambrose [30]. Following this, in November 2013, Illinois State Senator Mattie Hunter held a hearing on trauma deserts. The result of Senator Hunter's hearing was a call to the Illinois Department of Public Health to perform a feasibility study on a new trauma center on the South Side and to identify where this may be located [31]. This was followed by a large action by 200 activists leaving mock coffins outside UChicago Medicine. Mary Drs. Crandall from Northwestern and Philip Verhoef, clinical faculty from UChicago Medicine, spoke out during this action [31].

Aiming at Key Interests: The Obama Presidential Library and Certificate of Need

In the final phase of organizing prior to UChicago Medicine committed to re-establishing a level 1 adult trauma center, the coalition began to strategically target key interests. Yet another contradiction emerged as the University of Chicago Medicine released a report to promote itself as the best site to build the new Obama Presidential Library, while continuing to deny the South Side a level 1 adult trauma center [32]. The coalition for the adult trauma center began a "Week of Action" with protestors chaining themselves to the entrance of the UChicago Medicine parking garage, blocking its entrance, and requiring forcible removal by the police. This direct action followed in the movement's central tactic of interrupting the quotidian functions of the medical center. It was followed by the creation of a "tent city" outside the hospital's administration building, a candlelight vigil, and marches to President Zimmer's house [33]. These events grew support for the movement and inspired UChicago Medicine's physicians Dr. Evan Lyon and Dr. Philip Verhoef to raise concerns of contradictory university priorities at hearings for the Obama Presidential Library. USA Today and the Huffington Post, amongst numerous local and state news media sources, covered these actions broadly [32, 33].

The next central institutional interest that the movement focused on was the UChicago Medicine's pursuit of a "Certificate of Need" to establish expanded services worth $120 million in their new Center for Care and Discovery. In Illinois, healthcare institutions are required to demonstrate a compelling public need for services and obtain a "Certificate of Need," (CON) before major capital expenditures. The movement for the adult trauma center contested UCMC's pursuit of a CON claiming a "certificate of greed"—FLY's Victoria Crider stated "(UCMC) wants to spend over $120 million to replace perfectly good hospital rooms with luxury suites with private bathrooms and showers, while people who get shot are taken over 10 miles away because the U of C doesn't care enough to open a trauma center" [9].

The University of Chicago's "Reformist" Response

In response to mounting public pressure to establish a trauma center, UCMC attempted to co-opt the movement by offering certain reforms or smaller projects. In September 2014, the Bronzeville Dream Center, a trauma-counseling center for South Side communities struggling with violence, was founded [34]. The protestors contested the press conference opening the center, at which the mayor and Dean Polonsky spoke, by gathering protestors and clergy to pray for an adult trauma center.

At this point, media and community pressure continued to push the UCMC for an adult trauma center. In December 2014, the UCMC offered another reform-based measure and promised to seek state permission to raise the pediatric trauma age from 15 to include 16- and 17-year-old children [35]. Following this announcement in December, the UCMC began a feasibility study about expanding such services. While trauma center activists saw this as a partial victory, the coalition still believed that the ultimate goal remained for an adult level 1 trauma center at UCMC.

In January 2015, the Illinois Department of Public Health (IDPH) released its previously promised feasibility study for the establishment of an adult trauma center on the South Side. The IDPH report, which surveyed and studied the feasibility of a trauma center in various hospital systems bordering the South Side, concluded: "There were no hospitals among those surveyed in Chicago that have sufficient resources to meet the Level I designation with the exception of the University of Chicago Medical Center which expressed no interest in an adult Level I or Level II trauma center." [36]

Escalating Tactics and Campaign Victory

The Spring, Summer, and Fall of 2015 represented a series of escalating tactics by Trauma Care Coalition activists to finally secure an University promise to establish a level 1 adult trauma center.

Beginning in March 2015, nine trauma center activists chained themselves together across Michigan Avenue, a major thoroughfare in the city, interrupting a large Capital Campaign fundraiser for the University of Chicago. This event was widely covered in the wake of the prior feasibility study and now massive public support for an adult trauma center on the South Side [37].

In June 2015, nine Trauma Care Coalition protestors barricaded themselves in the main administrative building, which housed the office of the University president. Firefighters cut through bike locks to forcibly remove the students [38].

In September 2015, UCMC agreed to collaborate with another local healthcare system, Sinai Health, to establish an adult trauma center at Sinai's Holy Cross Hospital. However, given the relative cost constraints, UCMC eventually decided to establish its own independent adult trauma center in December 2015 [39].

The First Trauma Center Established by Community Organizing

About two and a half years following the initial announcement, the University of Chicago level 1 adult trauma center officially opened its doors on May 1, 2018. In addition to its clinical services, the adult trauma center also established a Violence Recovery Program—a hospital-based violence intervention program to reduce rates of violent re-injury by employing credible community members to engage with violently injured patients and connect them with relevant services [40].

Since its inception, the trauma center at the University of Chicago has cared for an estimated 21,700 patients—an average of over 4000 patients per year. About 40% of these patients suffer penetrating injuries, such as gunshot wounds or stab wounds. The majority of these patients are injured on the South Side of Chicago, with about half coming from the 12 zip codes surrounding the hospital on the South Side [40]. In addition to the wraparound services provided by the violence recovery program, the University of Chicago Medicine has developed a medical-legal partnership—Recovery Legal Aid—to connect violently injured patients with lawyers to assist in obtaining public benefits, criminal record expungement, and state crime victim compensation [41].

In an affirmation of the extended, broad-based community organizing by South Side youth, the establishment of an adult trauma center near the South Side has saved thousands of lives and has become a national leader in advocacy and trauma care (Fig. 1).

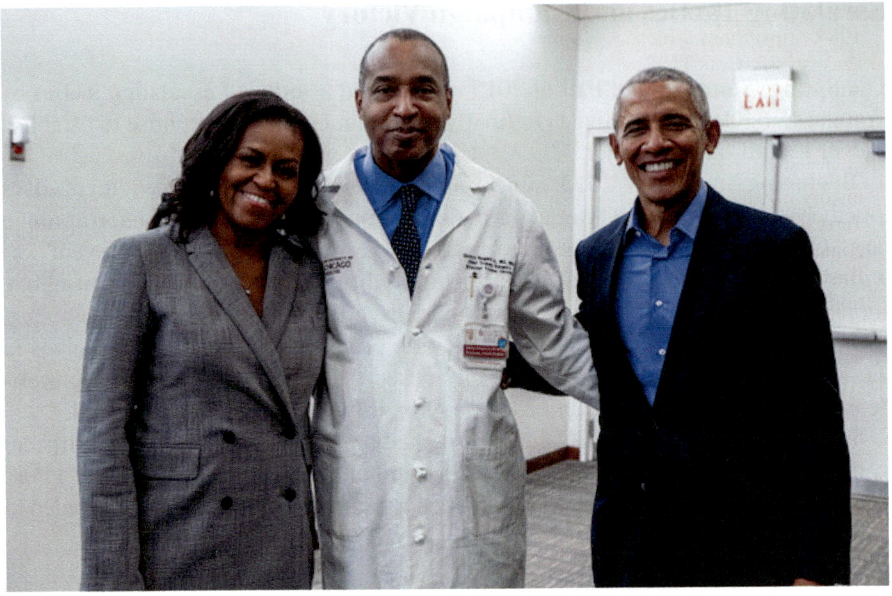

Fig. 1 Former President Barack Obama and First Lady Michelle Obama visit the University of Chicago Medicine Trauma Center, posing with Dr. Selwyn Rogers, James E. Bowman Jr. Professor and Founding Director of the UCMTC.

References

1. The Great Migration. African American Heritage. National Archives. 2021. https://www.archives.gov/research/african-americans/migrations/great-migration
2. Williams L. King David and Boss Daley: the Black Disciples, Mayor Daley and Chicago on the Edge. Prometheus Books; 2022.
3. Rothstein R. The color of law: a forgotten history of how our government segregated America. Liveright Publishing Corporation; 2017. https://doi.org/10.1111/puar.13119.
4. Rast J. The attack on the slums. In: The origins of the dual city: housing, race, and redevelopment in twentieth-century Chicago. University of Chicago Press; 2019. Chicago Scholarship Online, 2020. https://doi.org/10.7208/chicago/9780226661612.003.0006.
5. McClory R. The plot to destroy North Kenwood. Chicago Reader. 1993. https://chicagoreader.com/news-politics/the-plot-to-destroy-north-kenwood/
6. Schneider B. The Obama Center: caught in an old David vs. Goliath Drama. Bloomberg. 2018. https://www.bloomberg.com/news/articles/2018-06-08/obama-center-vs-south-side-chicago-caught-in-history
7. YouTube. 25: the ben Wilson story—full documentary. YouTube. 2014, November 12. https://www.youtube.com/watch?v=gUl47fZJGGg
8. Akouris ET. Flashback: in 1984, prep basketball phenom Ben Wilson's star was rising. Then two bullets destroyed everything. Chicago Tribune. 2019. https://www.chicagotribune.com/opinion/commentary/ct-opinion-flashback-ben-wilson-shooting-anniversary-20191115-suusnml73vdulj4vgoipdf46we-story.html
9. Trauma: timeline of protests. The University of Chicago Medicine. 2015, May.

10. Washington H, Rice F. Statistical summary 1985. City of Chicago, Chicago Police Department. 1985. https://home.chicagopolice.org/wp-content/uploads/2014/12/1985-Annual-Report.pdf
11. Prakash SP, ConeTJ. Trauma on the south side: the origins of a new trauma center. The American Association for the Surgery of Trauma. 2022. https://www.aast.org/disaster-detail/acs-highlight-trauma-on-south-side-origins-of-new-
12. Vega K. History of trauma center closing: UCMC adult level I trauma center operated 1986–1988. Chicago Maroon. 2015. https://chicagomaroon.com/20121/news/history-of-trauma-center-closing/
13. Terry, D. A death sparks a demand for care. The New York Times. 2010. https://www.nytimes.com/2010/10/03/us/03cnchospitals.html
14. Bushy C. The Rumble and the Reversal. 2016. https://www.chicagobusiness.com/static/section/trauma-protest.html. Accessed 13 Nov 2023.
15. Terry D. A death sparks a demand for care. 2010. https://www.nytimes.com/2010/10/03/us/03cnchospitals.html. Accessed 12 Nov 2023.
16. ABC 7. 'Die in' calls for South Side trauma center. 2010. https://abc7news.com/archive/7786457/. Accessed 13 Nov 2023.
17. Bob Roberts. Protestors ask U of C hospitals to reopen trauma center. 2011. https://www.cbsnews.com/chicago/news/protesters-ask-u-of-c-hospitals-to-reopen-trauma-center/. Accessed 13 Nov 2023.
18. Sailappan D, Lalljee J. Rallies, sit-ins, and padlocks: the history of trauma center activism. 2018. https://chicagomaroon.com/25853/news/rallies-sit-ins-padlocks-history-trauma-activism/. Accessed 13 Nov 2023.
19. Cao S. Officials defend lack of trauma center, tout UCMC's offerings. 2011. https://chicagomaroon.com/7168/news/officials-defend-lack-of-trauma-center-tout-ucmc-s-offerings/. Accessed 13 Nov 2023.
20. ABC7. Protestors call for South Side adult trauma center. 2011. https://abc7news.com/archive/8308041/. Accessed 13 Nov 2023.
21. CBS 2. Halloween protest demands trauma center at U of C. 2011. https://www.cbsnews.com/chicago/news/halloween-protest-demands-trauma-center-at-u-of-c/. Accessed 13 Nov 2023.
22. Hayes K. Community shout out: women who build movements. 2015. https://transformativespaces.org/2015/03/08/community-shout-out-women-who-build-movements/. Accessed 13 Nov 2023.
23. Hirst E. 4 protestors demanding trauma center at U. of C. arrested. 2013. https://www.chicagotribune.com/news/breaking/chi-protesters-arrested-at-u-of-c-20130127-story.html. Accessed 10 Nov 2023.
24. Huffpost. University of Chicago police officer on leave for going undercover at trauma care protest. 2013. https://www.huffpost.com/entry/university-of-chicago-pol_n_2812388. Accessed 10 Nov 2023.
25. Srikantha M. Undercover UCPD detective infiltrates protest. 2013. https://chicagomaroon.com/16801/news/undercover-ucpd-detective-infiltrates-protest/. Accessed 13 Nov 2023.
26. Bendaas H. Southsiders face off in 2nd district primary. The Chicago Maroon; 2013.
27. CBS2. Protesters March for adult trauma center at U of C. 2013. https://www.cbsnews.com/chicago/news/protesters-march-for-adult-trauma-center-at-u-of-c/. Accessed 10 Nov 2023.
28. Crandall M, Sharp D, Unger E. Trauma deserts: distance from a trauma center, transport times, and mortality from gunshot wounds in Chicago. Am J Public Health. 2013;103(6):1103–9.
29. Jain A. SHE, FLY reject trauma care argument. 2013. https://chicagomaroon.com/17470/news/she-fly-reject-trauma-care-argument/. Accessed 10 Nov 2023.
30. HuffPost. Rep. Bobby Rush wants $100 million to fund new trauma centers serving South Side. 2013. https://www.huffpost.com/entry/bobby-rush-trauma-centers_n_3639649. Accessed 9 Nov 2023.
31. ABC7. South Side 'trauma center desert' subject of state hearing. 2013. https://abc7chicago.com/archive/9334263/. Accessed 9 Nov 2023.

32. Stafford Z. Obama library not the urgent care Chicago needs as protests overshadow 'final campaign'. 2015. https://www.theguardian.com/us-news/2015/jun/08/obama-library-university-chicago-trauma-center-protests. Accessed 10 Nov 2023.
33. Kwan N. Trauma center protestors plan Friday tent city. 2014. https://www.nbcchicago.com/news/local/trauma-center-protestors-plan-friday-tent-city/70294/. Accessed 10 Nov 2023.
34. Venteicher W. Trauma counseling center proposed for South Side. 2014. https://www.chicagotribune.com/news/ct-trauma-counseling-met-0919-20140918-story.html. Accessed 10 Nov 2023.
35. UChicago News. University of Chicago Medicine seeks to expand pediatric trauma care. 2014. https://news.uchicago.edu/story/university-chicago-medicine-seeks-expand-pediatric-trauma-care. Accessed 13 Nov 2023.
36. Hasbrouck L. State of Illinois trauma center feasibility study. 2015. https://dph.illinois.gov/content/dam/soi/en/web/idph/files/publications/trauma-center-feasibility-study.pdf. Accessed 13 Nov 2023.
37. Trauma News. Trauma center protestors crash Chicago fundraiser. 2015. https://trauma-news.com/2015/03/trauma-center-protestors-crash-chicago-fundraiser/. Accessed 10 Nov 2023.
38. Esposito S. Trauma center protestors arrested at University of Chicago. 2015. https://chicago.suntimes.com/2015/6/4/18430522/trauma-center-protesters-arrested-at-university-of-chicago. Accessed 13 Nov 2023.
39. Glanton D, Bowean L. In about-face, U. of C. Medicine to build an adult trauma center on Hyde Park campus. 2015. https://www.chicagotribune.com/news/ct-university-of-chicago-trauma-center-hyde-park-campus-20151217-story.html. Accessed 13 Nov 2023.
40. Wang J. Five years after launching Level 1 adult trauma center, UChicago Medicine set to exceed 18,800 adult trauma patients. 2023. https://www.uchicagomedicine.org/forefront/trauma-articles/adult-trauma-center-set-to-exceed-18800-adult-patients. Accessed Nov 13 2023.
41. Carlton K. UChicago Medicine, Legal Aid Chicago launch bedside program to provide in-hospital legal support for trauma patients injured by violence. 2022. https://www.uchicagomedicine.org/forefront/news/uchicago-medicine-legal-aid-chicago-launch-bedside-program. Accessed Nov 13 2023.

Part II
Development of Trauma Ctr

Team Building: Who Am I? Who Are You? Who Are We? Where Are We Going?

Randall P. White

How was I going to get a group of type A personalities and high performers to work together for a common set of goals? Most of my core trauma faculty had succeeded to this work by their sheer dedication, brilliance, and hard work. I thought it would be a challenge for them to see bigger goals outside of their individual performances.

– Selwyn Rogers, MD

Contextual Leadership When the Context Is Resistant

Uncertainty is on your calendar every day—that's impossible enough—but Selwyn Rogers, MD was a leader in a second context: his team was not embraced by the larger institution.

A trauma center can be viewed as a "not in my backyard" necessity. And the University of Chicago Medical Center had managed to stick to its core hospital performance with excellence for 30 years since its original trauma center was disbanded. Some asked, why do we want trauma back?

"Because it's our #$%& job," is how Dr. Rogers explained it.

He was more eloquent than that as we discussed the task in the hospital parking deck after our first month or so of development work, but I knew that's what he meant. I started the conversation with my raw assessment: "They don't want you to succeed, do they?"

He conceded.

R. P. White (✉)
Executive Development Group, LLC, and HEC Paris, Greensboro, NC, USA
e-mail: randy@edgp.com

S. O. Rogers, Jr (ed.), *Creating a Modern Trauma Center*,
https://doi.org/10.1007/978-3-031-66524-0_3

"Yeah, I think that's accurate," said Selwyn. "But to be fair, if the organization had been hostile every time, I wouldn't be sitting here. That would have been intolerable. So, every good conversation helped to balance the bad conversations."

Selwyn's conviction was that the mission of the hospital was not being met until the South Side community started treating gun violence as a disease.

"One thing specifically about the trauma center at University of Chicago is that there are not that many trauma centers that have a social justice framing, or a leader who doesn't just talk the talk, but lives in this way," Selwyn told me. "And I personally think this is a compelling aspect of what all adult Level 1 trauma centers should be doing in their communities."

This was going to not only push the hospital into the twenty-first century, but it was going to push them into confronting clientele that were scary to them. They didn't know what would happen when gang members and (mostly) black and brown patients came. Lots of different people get shot—not just the ones with the guns, but innocent people from all walks of life. And so, there was a clear social justice imperative with the new trauma center.

Selwyn calls himself a pathological optimist. He faces conflict head-on with resolve and persistence.

This helped a lot, because I knew that I had a loyal and enthusiastic sponsor—even a physically larger sponsor in our Mutt and Jeff duo who was running interference on the politics. I was able to focus on building a much-needed team of "learning leaders."

Selwyn: "Given the community's need for an adult trauma center, failure was not an option. I needed to do everything at my disposal to tip the scales in my favor. Randy pictured prominently in this."

I walked in blindly, expecting to be treated as I've been treated at other medical facilities where I've done similar kinds of work, but I heard the hospital's subtle messages directed at Selwyn. And since I was there because of Selwyn, I felt the pressure, too.

I was there to do my thing—to facilitate leadership—but I was surprised, shocked really, that they didn't want Selwyn to succeed. How could this be?

I committed myself to be Switzerland: the neutral actor. And we started with the four basic questions that are the baseline for any senior level intervention: Who am I? Who are you? Who are we? Where are we going?

Everyone Had to Become a Leader

Selwyn's mission was to establish a trauma surgery service that was first rate in the socially and politically charged South Side of Chicago.

But in trying to get his own small group working and doing the things they were supposed to be doing—and valuing one another while they're doing it as fast as they can—Selwyn didn't have a lot of time or bandwidth.

He told me, "In the past, I would just overpower whatever is in front of me. But I knew that was not going to work. Not for this."

I will say he had courage, but did he want to expend whatever political capital he had on trying to create this space where they weren't more openly accepted?

Those challenges were on Selwyn's plate. My sole job was to teach a crash course in leadership development, dealing with leadership in behavioral terms: how each person saw leadership.

Because in the operating room everybody's a leader in one way or another: giving care, in management, and all that comes with trauma response. The leadership is passed around. It is in constant motion amidst the action of the trauma setting.

A Very Specialized, and Very Special, Team

"I recruited type A personalities," Selwyn told me.

"I wanted people who could stand toe to toe with me. That has its drawbacks, and has lots of upsides, but I would do the same again. I would ride to my death with these people, but they're tough people to lead."

I'll add that they are special people. Not just for the lifesaving work, but I say they're special because they're continually inventing things: new solutions, work-arounds, improvisation. It's constant learning in the face of limited time and resources.

I've worked with colleagues who don't consider medical doctors the best clients. They say that medical doctors dislike developing leadership and teamwork and can be difficult to teach. This has not been my experience.

My experience, as with one of my longest client relationships—a physician—is that doctors want to learn and grow. I've worked with many others in any number of other famous medical centers who love this stuff.

The University of Chicago trauma center team was like this, and they came together to advance the mission by growing as leaders.

Selwyn also felt that it wasn't just for his trauma people, so we opened this up to the larger group that needed to support the trauma people, which was a really good idea.

This would help to build some bridges and establish better relationships between the trauma team—the individual trauma surgeons—and the various services that they would work with.

Creating a Safe Space in a Trauma Environment

The intensity of trauma surgery and the bruising political context aside, our leadership development process was no different from what we do in the corporate world of nine-to-five and more predictable routines.

At the University of Chicago, we needed to have an extended conversation about what leadership looks like and what people see leadership as being in this kind of intense environment. Also, we had a lot of conversations about each person's strengths and weaknesses. What did each individual bring to this leadership enterprise? How would the team fit together? Then, how did it fit into the larger system of the hospital?

As a trauma surgeon, you need to lead every day, whether you're good at it or not. When you're in the trauma bay, when you're in the operating room, when you're on the floor, when you're in ICU, you're leading. People are looking to you and you are never a neutral actor in your exhausted state. Sometimes, your greatest behavioral strengths can be overused and can have negative behavioral consequences. That's not something that people would necessarily keep top of mind—especially when patient care is what matters most.

This was compounded by the underlying political resistance. Thus, Selwyn's role as leader required empathy, but also occasionally his very direct counsel:

"I would tell them all the time, every time you yell at someone, you are hurting the mission, because you're reinforcing that this will not work. Every time you want to wig out, every time you want to not toe the line, not do the thing you're supposed to, not be in the place you're supposed to be, you're hurting the mission."

Because this was the first "real job" for many in this kind of extremely demanding and occasionally hostile environment, my job was to create a safe space, so we could talk about those negative behavioral responses and decisions that worked against good teamwork.

High Performers Don't Always Work Well Together

Working with smart, highly trained, intensely focused people doing lifesaving work, my job had nothing to do with their technical expertise, but everything to do with their human interactions. In all organizational settings, we can disagree over how to solve a problem, but understanding how to convince someone or influence someone to see the world the way you do, and to be open to approaches other than your own, is essential to leadership. Most people need to learn this over and over.

"Differences" is a keyword here. How to communicate and deal with differences is the core of any leadership program.

We also learned that leaders must be versatile. You can't do the same thing with every person all the time.

For example, if you're traumatized and tired, and you're just trying to take care of your patients there are times when you'd like to push an autopilot button, and just act the way you've always acted. After all, it is what "got you here."

Effective leadership calls for you to be very personable, across people and situations, and that may not be easy for you when you're exhausted, not feeling very accepted, or you just had to reconstruct some part of a person in an almost impossible surgery. Any number of variables have an impact on your ability to lead effectively.

This is why we had to create a supportive framework for people to help one another to continue to hone their craft, and to learn how to deal with one another without becoming dismissive of a person's quirks.

And everybody in trauma had a quirk. Expand that to the other support groups and there were plenty of quirks to go around. We all learned to "speak quirk."

Building a Stage Where Everyone Excels

As a leader, you set out to create an environment where everyone can maximize their potential. In the O.R. they're trying to create an environment where everyone can do high performing surgical teamwork.

When you're coming out of that and handing off to a colleague, you have got to get that person invested in your treatment plan and your way of going forward. But if your colleague doesn't buy into your treatment plan, you've got a problem. If you're tired, you may even end up screaming at that person, because you're so pissed off that they won't do what you want them to do…and you've just spent hours using extraordinary measures to keep a child alive.

In our sessions we talked about a strategy for dealing with that next person on duty who had to lead.

Would you call this "shared leadership"? Not exactly. It's what I call "serial leadership"—I'm in charge, and then I hand the patient off to you, so now you're in charge. Everyone ends up leading and following, like passing a baton.

Standard Approach, Remarkable Team

Above, I noted the team's remarkable ability to adapt and invent. We had to take that ability and apply it to interpersonal relationships.

I brought my classroom to them and used assessments to gather a lot of data; we had long and deep leadership conversations on interpersonal relationships; we used case studies; we video recorded people working together. We did the same kinds of things we would do in my MBA classroom or corporate leadership development program.

Things would happen in real life between the sessions and sometimes they would be discussed one-on-one, or in larger groups, or back in our classroom. All interaction was live and could be brought back to class for discussion. In addition, we augmented this with team exercises designed to produce either conflict or cooperation as direct outcomes.

To baseline strengths and weaknesses and give continual feedback, we gathered data from several instruments. Among those were the Leadership Versatility Index, the Hogan Development Survey (the Darkside of Leadership), FIRO-B, and even the Myers Briggs Type Indicator Step II (mainly because everyone was already familiar with MBTI).

The group was conversant with the concept of identifying their strengths. However, they were not as conversant with the idea that under stress, your greatest strengths can be your undoing—and they were constantly under stress.

One critical point where everyone needed work was dealing with difference. We honed in on this.

Differences such as how they treated patients. Differences in how they attack problems, and how they approached problem solving. Their training had often focused on getting the right answer. Depending on where they trained, they may have been exposed to a very command-and-control approach of getting the one answer that was the preferred solution by their teacher.

We held discussions about this. We looked at various models of decision making. And we covered different styles of leadership. Individually, we asked the question, "What sorts of behaviors do I exhibit?" Then we explored how those behaviors have a positive or negative impact on others.

When you've been up half the night and you're trying to do things quickly, you move into a zone of doing things by rote and doing things the way you know to do them. The job is to work under stress. You don't want to try to appreciate difference. What you really want to say is, "Just do it, dammit!"

Selwyn saw this as something to address: "Former military guys can be all about command-and-control—telling me what to do, or I'll tell someone what to do, and they'll do it. Turns out, people are more complicated than that. And the problems that we encounter in trauma are so diverse, unscheduled, and unrehearsed. A pure command-and-control model fails horrifically, because if you've got to wait for someone to tell you what to do, you'll have a lot of dead human beings.

"So, it requires innovation, and it requires creativity. Inquiry is a part. It requires agility."

In this setting reading one another and considering difference takes on a slightly different tone, or a different way of doing things. It requires you to be very studied and even more intentional than what we ask of others in a civilian, less stressed context.

It's not easy to learn to be intentional when you're not at your best. When you're trying to handoff to a colleague so you can get some sleep and your colleague is somebody that needs all the detail, you might not feel like giving this person all the detail.

However, through our work with the personality instruments and all the discussions, you realize this person is someone who needs all the detail and you're better prepared to give it, because you're aware of how it affects the mission.

And it's got to work both ways: the colleague on the receiving end needs to understand that this person has come through this experience and is tired and maybe isn't at their best.

All this was to help each team member be more versatile and to have a wider band of patience in their ability to deal with difference.

And—hooray!—we had success. It's been encouraging to hear these high performers asking, "Have I changed any? Have I advanced?"

It's a continuing story. As people transition in and out of the group, there's a need for more intervention. And it keeps coming back around to: "Who am I? Who are you? Who are we? Where are we going?"

Kodachrome or Black and White?

This was a tough assignment for me, for the team, and mostly for Selwyn, our pathological optimist. Some participants welcomed seeing the value of self-awareness-based leadership development, others were dubious or maybe even suspicious. And again, not everyone wanted us to be there.

Looking back on the initial leadership engagement with the University of Chicago, I kept hearing the Paul Simon song, "Kodachrome," because one way to write the story is to make it all pretty, like the song's Kodachrome film. But the black and white facts were, there were as many unresolved conflicts as there were bright moments of breakthrough. We didn't know *exactly* what we were doing in this context, we just applied a methodology that had worked in other medical centers.

It started the way most of my regular engagements begin: Selwyn needed something to make his team and the larger supporting crew have a shot at working well together. He knew that they weren't going to be easily accepted and this was a way to break down some barriers.

It was true uncertainty. He had no idea for sure that it would help, but I think he was saying, "It can't hurt."

Diversity, Empathy, and Healing

In most surgical units in most cities, you see white men in charge. However, this new trauma center is diverse—composed of men and women, people of color, and military veterans. It's a fascinating collection of talent, personalities, and life experiences. It is one of the most diverse professional groups by demographics that I have ever had a chance to work with. Perhaps the *most* diverse.

In South Side this is not a DEI box to check. It's a commitment to be less detached from the patients and the crisis they face. Selwyn wants you to be dispassionately precise as a surgeon AND he wants you to *care deeply*. Getting to know Selwyn, he described himself as Dr. Inside Out. His team in Chicago is sort of inside out, and very good at what it does.

"To be honest, I didn't fully understand the complexity of the problem," Selwyn explained. "I naively viewed the development and launch of the adult trauma center as a change management problem. Given all the 'cheese that would need to be moved,' I envisioned that there would be resistance to change."

When Selwyn asked me to contribute to this book, I said, "What's to write about? You know, we did this, we did this, we did this, and we did this. We had some modest success."

But then the other piece is, it's this fascinating group. By their own performance, they've changed a hospital system. They're beginning to change the community and they're getting attention because they are providing first-rate healthcare to black and brown women, men, and children in South Side.

They are in the process of becoming the highest performing trauma team out there, where the target for excellence is ever evolving and they are pushing the curve.

Implementation Operating Room Preparation and Trauma

Kenneth L. Wilson

History

Gun violence remains endemic to Chicago, and GSWs account for the overwhelming majority of homicides within the city. The proximity to a trauma center has a positive effect on survival outcomes for GSW victims [1]. Half of all hypotensive trauma patients that are transferred directly from the emergency department to an operating room are for hemorrhage control [2]. To facilitate early hemorrhage control, numerous regulatory and verifying bodies have mandated the immediate availability of an operating room for acutely injured patients [3]. A mature trauma systems stands at the ready in anticipation of receiving an unstable patient from the emergency department.

The trauma center at the University of Chicago was not a pillar of the university hospital system for almost 30 years. The designation as a Level I trauma center was more than a wish list for the young men and women of the Southside, it was a moral imperative. The vectors for victims of penetrating trauma in the Southside pointed away from the closest treatment facility, the University of Chicago. In the absence of a trauma center on the Southside of Chicago for 30 years, the race against time was a sprint to hospitals not located within the perimeter of the zip codes of the Southside blocks most notoriously known for intention violence. A patient with a gunshot wound to the chest in immediate proximity to the University of Chicago would take the evacuation route downtown to Northwestern Hospital via picturesque Lake Shore Drive. A scoop and run by friends and families to a local community hospital would prove to be agonizing. Instead of stabilization and rushing into an available operating room, help would seldom arrive. They are left stuck

K. L. Wilson (✉)
Department of Surgery, Section of Trauma and Acute Care Surgery, University of Chicago, Chicago, IL, USA
e-mail: kwilson9@surgery.bsd.uchicago.edu; kwilson9@bsd.uchicago.edu

S. O. Rogers, Jr (ed.), *Creating a Modern Trauma Center*,
https://doi.org/10.1007/978-3-031-66524-0_4

watching a love one fade and eventually bleed to death. These examples are not hypothetical, but highlight the events of two actual occurrences that took place on the Southside with resultant deaths of a local basketball icon and a young community activist [4, 5]. Both deaths well chronicled because of their illustrious contributions to sports and community activism heaved heavily on the spirit of the Southside of Chicago because despite their fame and good standing they could not save themselves from gun violence. There was not a trauma center in proximity to make valiant attempts to return them alive to their families.

Operating Room Space

Prior to opening of the level I trauma center in May 2018, the hospital system was completely devoid of a stocked operating room available to receive trauma patients from the surrounding neighborhoods. A new trauma center would not coincide with a new operating suite. This meant crowding out a service line for the operating space and time. An argument to not become a trauma center was that an urban trauma at University of Chicago would be a repeat of a money losing trauma system. Financially, it did not make sense to reduce revenue for the University of Chicago Hospital system by removing surgical services that were already prestigious and financially solvent for the reanimation of a trauma service that failed miserably 30 years prior.

The University of Chicago has 28 active operating rooms in the Center for Care and Discovery primarily situated to support Adult Inpatient and Elective needs. The operative procedures performed range from microscopic surgery, minimally invasive surgery to entire organs being transplanted inside the chest and the abdomen and the skull being removed to eradicate brain tumors. At the commencement of planning activities there were 22 active operating rooms allocated at 90% to Elective and Semi-Elective procedural volume. In short, the "inn was full" at the University of Chicago and there was no operating space to surrender once the announcement of the impending trauma center was made public. The culture of surgery is to request more operative time, not relinquish operative time. The idea of forcing a surgical service out of an operating room meant risking immediate alienation by our surgical peers. A creative approach would be required to unlock operative space and to assure that a busy operating center did not spiral into chaos.

CCD-OR Proposed Block Schedule

It was believed that during the planning phases of the trauma center that penetrating trauma would represent a significant operative volume for the University of Chicago. Other significant contributors to the overall trauma volume would include motor vehicle collisions and elderly falls. In order to best support the development of the trauma center, the orthopedic service would need to request more operative time. An orthopedic trauma team was specifically hired just to meet the newly anticipated demands on the orthopedic service that had dealt with more elderly falls and bone metastasis than open book pelvic fractures and ballistic injuries. The orthopedic service would also enter the struggle to find operative time and a location devoted strictly to orthopedic trauma.

The surgical system was mostly elective with the nighttime reserved for cardiac transplant and the general transplant at night which was primarily supported by on call teams that required at least a 60 minute notice to activate and mobilize. The acute care surgery service, known formerly as the Resident Acute Care Surgery (RACS) service, did not do many general surgery catastrophes at night. The surgical set up did not anticipate what was already known by most trauma systems that urban trauma is a nighttime thing occurring at its peak during the weekend [6, 7]. Orthopedic surgery secured an operative Monday through Friday elective block ahead of the trauma service. In addition, they were also granted an additional room for three days as well in anticipation of an increase in orthopedic trauma volume. Discussions around modeling were critical to understand what the impact of a level 1 trauma center would have on the capacity and growth over the first 3 fiscal years after opening. This exercise included assumptions based on publically reported data from facilities that were situated in a similar urban setting. Upon review, we modeled a range of activation activity from 2600 to 3800 annually with 35% of activations requiring a surgical intervention and each of those patients needing surgery would have 1.4 surgeries during their inpatient stay. This exercise accounted for trauma distribution across all services and estimated a minimum need of 2.5 incremental rooms (~25 hours allocated during normal business operations) to accommodate the increase in volume. This represented a wide range of possibilities, with the goal of not being precise, but to ensure there was enough capacity planned. Under resourcing would hinder our ability to course correct quickly and set us down the same path as our first level 1 trauma attempt 30 years prior.

Level I trauma centers have dedicated operating rooms set aside to receive trauma patients. This was not the case for our new level I trauma center at The University of Chicago. The carve out for trauma was intended to designate a "floating" operating room for emergency procedures (essentially a first out methodology) and not a 24-hour operating room strictly devoted to injured patients. Trauma patients would not be distinguished separately from other patients needing emergency procedures. Any patient having a "*condition that is life-threatening takes precedence over any other case*." The designation meant that there would not be a specific carve out for trauma or the potentially substantial volume being projected that required a space to operate in with little to no notice; creating a new clamoring for any surgical section to interpret what they considered "Life threatening" and potentially place a trauma patient in a queue.

A hypothetical example that was debated but fortuitously never arose was a 12-hour combined service with reconstruction following cancer where a delicate microvascular anastomosis (under the microscope) was created, and the pulse became absent in the surgical intensive care unit. This is deemed an emergency that would require restoration of blood flow before negating the protracted efforts of combined services and leaving the patient with a failed procedure. This is not exsanguination but or life-threatening but stands to alter a surgical outcome if not addressed immediately.

A more theoretical reality could have been what to do when an elective procedure returning to the operating room with postoperative bleeding needs to happen, while there is a simultaneously arriving patient with a gunshot wound to the femoral artery being temporized with an applied tourniquet. It is a scenario where active bleeding trumps ischemia, but the scenario is still suboptimal for the trauma patient, which is the primary concern of the newly arriving trauma team advocating for equitable care. The surge of mass shootings in America highlight the need for a robust trauma response all hours of the day. There is no compelling argument to jump the line by an avarice attending wanting an operating room. Trauma is a social disease that require its own operating room with all the adjuncts needed toward patient salvage immediately available.

Case Classes

As the newest surgical section, we were searching for a way to free up operating room space for trauma patients without division, however we needed an operating room for the acutely injured patient. We were not demanding exclusive rights to a roped-off mausoleum that could only be entered when a trauma patient arrived. We were asking that an operating room needed to be available anywhere and immediately after a brief period of stabilization in the emergency department.

Pre-level 1 trauma, timing expectations for surgical interventions not planned in advance of the day of surgery were broad and did not provide enough specificity to account for the variability we would see. In order to create equity for entry into an available operating room, new criteria needed to be established for cases that were not elective. A case classification system was developed to insure that trauma patients were given proper access to the system and not placed inappropriately in a queue system. A classification system ranging A-D was created. "Class A" being designation would represent the most serious operative emergency, meaning that after notifying the operating room, the patient would enter the operating room within 30 minutes. It was requested that every surgical service submit a rank list from A-D signifying the full breadth of their emergency cases. The submission of a rank list was simple for the trauma service because our patients were entering the trauma system by EMS for lifesaving interventions. The list submitted by trauma essentially had most thoracic, abdominal and extremity vascular injuries listed as Class-A procedures.

If a trauma patient required consultation from other service lines in the emergency department, and the trauma service did not operate, the consulting service needed to assign their own case classification. The Trauma service does not do bones or brains, therefore, if a trauma patient sustained a broken femur or a traumatic brain injury, the orthopedic service or the neurosurgery service would assign a case class for their respective procedures.

Once the operating room was breached with a Class A trauma patient then a consultant service could enter the operating room to do complete the appropriate procedure after temporary vascular shunt placement (TVS) or definitive revascularization. In the case of the brachial artery laceration with the humerus fracture, the brachial artery produced the Class-A entry into the operating room. However, if the orthopedic service decided to delay the repair of the humerus, they would re-class the repair for another day. Since there is no such thing a "bone emergency," the subsequent return on another day would not meet a Class-A designation but more than likely a less emergent designation when deemed appropriate such as a Class D. The clinical operations team was empowered to monitor classification usage across all of the services to help curb mis-classification.

Damage Control

As we anticipated, penetrating trauma would become the number one mechanism of injury presenting to the University of Chicago. The presentation of penetrating trauma, specifically from gunshot wounds, lends to patients being unstable on arrival and completing a partial and truncated operation to avoid operating beyond the physiologic reserve of the patient. This is termed "damage control" with a brief stent in the surgical intensive care unit after the operation with a return to the operating room for definitive repairs. The case class for the index damage control procedure by design meets the Class-A designation, but they return operation could range from an Class-A to a Class-D, depending upon the nature of the injuries. Even with the presence of an open abdomen from a damage control procedure, we attempted to be judicious with returns to the operating room by not abusing the Class-A trauma designation. However, not all services were equally judicious, and would attempt to top load numerous procedures as Class-A procedures when in fact they were not emergent at all. The trauma service chose not to abuse the privilege of having mostly Class-A procedures, and often were operating late in the evening or at night as cases were continually post ahead of damaged control procedures. The classing system was not perfect for trauma patients, but at a minimum it reserved access to the operating room for the sickest trauma patients. The class system did not fade into non-existent but still stands as the booking into the operating room for all other cases.

Trauma One Operating Room (TOOR)

The trauma service ultimately ended up with OR #17 as "the fixed trauma room." The classing system did not need further clarification for trauma patients. We endeavored to never abuse our luxury of having trauma patients become Class-A patients with immediate access to OR #17. The claiming of OR #17, Trauma One Operating ROOM (TOOR) stocked with supplies and replete with rapid infusers was as much of a victory for trauma as it was for anesthesia. TOOR is located immediately across from the main nursing/command station and the huddle location for the anesthesiologist and nurse anesthetist. The blood refrigerators were just outside the door. A " yellow phone" was installed in the trauma bay that only rang at the OR command station, immediately alerting the operating room about incoming trauma patients and the suspected injuries. A script was posted next to the yellow phone in the trauma bay and at the command center allowing a conversation to plan ahead for which combination of operating room trays needed to be available in the operating room. The anesthesia resident or nurse anesthetist responded to the trauma bay for all level one activations and communicate anticipated anesthesia needs to the command center. TOOR was reserved for Class-A notifications via the yellow phone, and the room had to be available within 30 minutes. In reality, once the call was made, the room is available to receive a patient in 4–6 minutes with a robust resuscitation response. After 5+ years in operation, it is clear that employing the fixed trauma room was the only path to take. In hindsight, having a room ready and available within minutes of notification was not possible any other way. With a place for our first trauma, the next logical question to answer was what if another trauma patient requires a surgical intervention after the TOOR is occupied?

Room After First Trauma (RAFT)

The summer months translate into more opportunities for gatherings where multiple individuals are wounded. The TOOR is equipped to handle all operative emergencies. However, when multiple patients require surgical interventions, the additional flow of patient means entering another operating room immediately, and there is inadequate time to clean the TOOR and another operating room needs to be selected. We seldom go on trauma bypass, which includes 5 separate locations for anesthesia (not transplant which has their own team) such as cases in the children's hospital (Comer), interventional radiology, trauma or the Class-A or Class-B emergencies. We are more capable of expanding quickly at night but limited by a bolus of 5 trauma cases when the elective day has begun. Once OR#17 is offline, we expand into the Room after First Trauma (RAFT). If all operating rooms are occupied, every reasonable effort is made to have an operating room available with staff and equipment within 30 minutes of a Class A trauma notification. The preferred RAFT room is on either side of TOOR, per anesthesia to maintain easy access to blood frigs and easier coordination with the command desk.

The initial introduction of RAFT was somewhat controversial— the relinquishing of operative time is not preferable by any surgeon. If the RAFT room was always flanking OR #17, repeatedly delaying the fixed occupants of these rooms during the daytime, the trauma service would quickly produce an inequity in the system and a tremendous backlash from the surgeons being incessantly delayed. The concept of the RAFT room developed by the operating room leadership essentially created an unbiased approach as to which service line would have to donate their operating room as the RAFT room. The answer effectively was that every service line would have to be the RAFT room on a rotating basis with the frequency of assignment tied to the services footprint in the schedule. The schedule was set on a grid well in advance so that in theory the surgical service impacted could plan accordingly for their time designation as the RAFT room. The clout of the surgeon, the prestige of the service line did not matter. We never polled the surgeons for like or dislike of the RAFT room, but it was equitable and whether or not there was a strong dislike, the burden was shared equally. Limiting cases to short durations allowed for more predictable breaks in the RAFT room in case the TOOR was taken off line. Some services elected to clear their schedule completely from the assigned RAFT room while others followed the recommendations for "short" cases only. Though not perfect, this allowed for the OR control desk to make reasonable assumptions as to where to place our next trauma patient if the need arises. If the RAFT was unavailable due to a 2nd trauma patient or the timing of case completion did not align, a third lever to pull was needed.

First Empty Room (FER)

The maelstrom to avoid is picking up the yellow phone and hearing that there is not an operating room available. The operating room during morning hours of Monday-Friday could indeed have all cases going simultaneously, which includes the TOOR occupied by trauma from a late-night trauma flowing into the daytime elective day. The RAFT room may have an ongoing case as well, and all operating rooms have appropriately started their cases on time. The least attractive option becomes to delay a case by entering the "First Empty Room (FER)." FER room purposely delays an elective case from starting in their assigned operating when TOOR and RAFT are not available. Every effort is made to avoid this situation unless there is truly an overwhelming number of patients arriving simultaneously. I do not recall every utilizing FER to complete a trauma case. We saw our need to support multiple trauma patients on day 1 as a level 1 trauma center (actually our first 2 patients requiring surgical intervention arrived less than 60 minutes apart), quickly validating the 18 months of thought that went into the development of the protocols. Over the years, adjustments have been made to the room triage system. The RAFT designation remains in place as the key to setting up the next trauma room; whether there are two patients, three patients, four patients requiring a trauma surgical intervention. The RAFT in operation is not meant to be a singular room in the paradigm, but always the next step to immediately follow once the "Yellow" phone rings. Essentially, the RAFT is always the FER and the FER is always the next RAFT in current state.

Trauma Support Teams

There are numerous resources and teams outside of Surgeon, Nursing, and Anesthesiologist that play an integral role in trauma operations. Ensuring that team like Sterile Processing, Environmental Services, and Equipment techs understand what trauma means and why it's unlike anything else we do is critical. Including those teams in the design and development helped administration understand the turnover needs for things like tray and room processing. Conversations with these teams lead us to build redundancy into our system to align with other resources (like anesthetizing locations). Without these teams engaged; trays are not ready, rooms are not cleaned, and RAFTs are not set up in time to care for the next patient. Engagement of these support teams has allowed us to have a notification to in room average of 16 minutes (quickest in room is 4 minutes from notification) for Class A cases and meet the needs of 6 class A emergencies (trauma and other services) over the course of hours on one summer day in the last 5 years.

Trauma Nursing

The trauma service from inception sought to be become good partners with all of the surgical services and to not cause disruptions in the daily operative stream. The operating room staff has accommodated the trauma service immensely well by keeping the emergency trauma case flowing into an awaiting operating room. We are fortunate at the University of Chicago to have numerous surgical specialties that have intervened as consultants when requested. It is not in the best interest of the institution of we disrupt elective cases and decrease patient satisfaction and frustrated the cadre of nurses that have worked diligently to improve trauma care in the operating room. We find that anesthesia equips OR #17 (TOOR) better than any of the other operating rooms and the operating room nurses are staunch defenders of keeping the TOOR sustained 24–7.

The nighttime hours are not a chip shots for the nursing staff as well. During trauma alley, the nighttime hours can cause bottlenecking when trauma, transplant and emergency general surgery are all clamoring for start times. Trauma rooms are run three at a time, stretching the sustainable limits of nursing and anesthesia staff. An additional strain occurs when an injured child requires an operation activating an additional team to become activated to join the trauma and transplant teams. It seems flawlessly done, but a tremendous amount of preparation and education went into both the day and night productions.

Nursing Education

Whenever there is a scramble for the TOOR, RAFT, FER, a transfer from the pediatric hospital, it is nursing that makes the playbook make sense. They calmly direct traffic to the appropriate operating room with assembling teams out of thin air. This ease with which a trauma blitz is handled both day and night took a tremendous amount of dedication and coordination.

There was a weeding out process and re-training effort that took place during the ramp up to becoming a trauma center. There were individuals who did not exhibit enthusiasm about the addition of a trauma service and thought trauma did not match the stature of the University of Chicago. Some found the potential of a hectic pace intimidating and opted to make their objections by leaving the institution all together. In-house responsibilities would change and multiple teams had to be added to avoid delays in nurses racing to the hospital. The massive transfusion retrieval from the blood bank had to be revamped. The Childrens hospital would need trays assembled and dashed across the street to assist a young child that was shot.

References

1. Crandall M, Sharp D, Unger E, Straus D, Brasel K, Hsia R, Esposito T. Trauma deserts: distance from a trauma center, transport times, and mortality from gunshot wounds in Chicago. Am J Public Health. 2013;103(6):1103.
2. Bjerke HS, Petersen SR, Bokhari FG. Prehospital hypotension as a valid indicator of trauma team activation – discussion. J Trauma Injury Infect Crit Care. 2000;48(6):1037–9.
3. Task Force of the Committee on Trauma, American College of Surgeons. Resources for optimal care of the injured patient: an update. Bull Am Coll Surg. 1990;75(9):20–9.
4. Wilbon M. In Streets and Stands, Chicago Mourns for a Favorite Son Sorrow for a Star Athlete, Slain at 17. The Washington Post, Dec 2, 1984.
5. Terry D. A death sparks a demand for care. The New York Times, Oct 2, 2010.
6. Vaziri K, Roland JC, Robinson L, Fakhry MS. Optimizing physician staffing and resource allocation: sine-wave variation in hourly trauma admission volume. J Trauma Injury Infect Crit Care. 2007;62(3):610–4.
7. Ryan K, Levit K, Davis PH. Characteristics of weekday and weekend hospital admissions: Statistical Brief #87. Healthcare Cost and Utilization Project (HCUP) statistical Briefs Agency for Healthcare Research and Quality (AHRQ), Rockville; 2006.

Creating Trauma Staff

Sharnae Phagan, Debra Allen, and David A. Hampton

Introduction

Trauma does not discriminate by race, age, or socioeconomic status. It is the leading cause of death for individuals less than 44 years old. More people die from traumatic injuries than from HIV, cancer, flu, or any other cause. Globally, for every one person that dies of a traumatic injury [1, 3], another 129 trauma victims are seen, treated, and discharged from a Trauma Center [2, 3]. A successful outcome is due to the highly trained staff specialized and equipped to treat severely injured patients [3, 4].

In 2014 the trauma planning committee reviewed the number and location of traumatically injured incidents transported by Chicago's Emergency Management Services (EMS) [5]. It was determined The University of Chicago (UChicago) Medicine would receive 3036 trauma activations a year. Approximately 1850 would be admitted and 1186 would be discharged from the ED. This significant volume indicated the need for extensive preparation and education of the nursing staff to ensure optional care of the trauma patient. While some UChicago nursing staff had previous experience treating patients with traumatic injuries, there was a paucity who were capable of addressing this new patient population. Identified gaps were lack of knowledge regarding accurate triage, resuscitation algorithms, using appropriate supplies and equipment, and the psychosocial aspects of handling complex traumatically injured patients. Emergency Medicine, Intensive Care, General

S. Phagan (✉) · D. A. Hampton
Department of Surgery, Section of Trauma and Acute Care Surgery, University of Chicago Medicine, Chicago, IL, USA
e-mail: Sharnae.phagan@uchicagomedicine.org; dhampton2@bsd.uchicago.edu

D. Allen
University of Chicago's Adult Level I Trauma Center, Independent Trauma Consultant, Chicago, IL, USA

S. O. Rogers, Jr (ed.), *Creating a Modern Trauma Center*,
https://doi.org/10.1007/978-3-031-66524-0_5

Surgical Floors, Operating Room, and Critical Care Transport nurses, along with other first line responders, are members of the multidisciplinary team needed to perform the resuscitation, assessment, and care of the trauma patient throughout their hospitalization [4, 5].

In anticipation of providing Level I trauma services to the community, leadership developed Strategic Imperatives, Strategic Objectives, and an Annual Operating Plan. These included but were not limited to increase the pace and trajectory of organization change; determine cross-functional work that impacts and requires coordination across multiple functional areas; identify areas that do not have a clear functional "home" and/or there is little or no existing infrastructure to accomplish the work. Once the strategic imperatives were identified, a Trauma Core Team was organized. This included leadership from Patient Care Services, Finance, Facility Operations, Security, Emergency Medicine, Communications, Legal/Regulatory, Staffing/Recruitment, Information Technology, Out-Patient Services, and the Trauma Medical Director, and Clinical Nursing Director.

Change Management

In addition to opening as an Adult IDPH Level I Trauma Center in the Spring of 2018, the hospital was in the process of opening a new ED in the Winter of 2017. These large changes had the potential to cause undue stress on the nursing staff; therefore, the Director of Organizational Change was added to the Trauma Core Team. Change Management is the practice by which leadership deliberately plans for and assist their staff through a large transition using common language processes and tools [6]. The goal was to develop an engaged workforce who are ready, willing, and able to work in new ways. Change happens at the individual level—it is about people's emotions and attitudes. It is necessary to be inclusive and help everyone impacted understand their role in the successful transition. This would be accomplished through ensuring excellent and frequent communication, obtaining the necessary training/required certifications, and guarantee staff readiness.

Communication

Immediately after the announcement to become a trauma center, consistent communication with the nursing staff began. Initially, it consisted of monthly trauma updates via the hospital's publication, "*At the Forefront*." The Chief Nursing Officer (CNO) supplemented these updates through her monthly newsletter, monthly in-person meetings with nursing managers, assistant managers, and ancillary staff mangers. The Clinical Director of Trauma also performed weekly GEMBA walks through the ICUs, medical floors, ED, and operating room [7]. A GEMBA walk, derived from the Japanese word, gembutsu, meaning the real place, is designed to observe and understand employees, understand their work flow, and acknowledge and respect the work performed.

In addition to the trauma nursing leaders providing frequent communication, the trauma surgeons did monthly "meet and greets" to various nursing units throughout the hospital. To further foster open communication, the newly hired trauma surgeons volunteered to become liaisons between trauma and various nursing areas. Along with the meet and greets and becoming liaisons, the newly hired trauma surgeons also agreed to provide monthly lectures to the nursing staff on pathophysiology, violence, and mental health issues as it related to the trauma patient. Organized as well as impromptu nursing unit in-services were a frequent occurrence.

State Requirements

In the state of Illinois, trauma centers are designated and regulated by the Illinois Department of Public Health (IDPH) [1]. The IDPH oversees 200 programs governed by laws passed by the Illinois General Assembly and signed by the Governor. The trauma-specific Sections outline the educational certifications needed for emergency room nursing staff [8]. Prior to 2018, EDs were required to have a minimum of one nurse per shift certified as a Trauma Nurse Specialist (TNS). The TNS certification mandates nurses to participate and complete a standardized program facilitated by TNS Course Coordinators (TNSCCs). This Graduate-level program focuses on resuscitation of trauma patients, encompassing care in the prehospital, perioperative, and intensive care phases with a strong emphasis on pathophysiology and multidisciplinary coordination.

Currently, IDPH has modified it's certification requirements allows ED nurses the option of receiving a Trauma Certified Registered Nurse (TCRN), Advanced Trauma Certified Nurse (ATCN), Trauma Nursing Core Course (TNCC), or TNS certification [1]. However at the time of UChicago Medicine's designation, IDPH only accepted TNS certifications. Over 90% of the ED nurses did not have the required TNS certification. To address this requirement, UChicago Medicine worked in collaboration with IDPH and a TNSCC to present a course tailored to meet the nurses' needs whilst complying with TNS certification requirements. Selection for the TNS course was based on previous trauma experience as well as their interest in becoming a highly skilled trauma nurse. Upon successful completion, this cohort was named the "Trauma Champions." A Trauma Champion committee, consisting of nurses and emergency technicians, was formed and met weekly with the Clinical Director of Trauma. Their role was to ensure open communication between ED staff and the Section of Trauma, identify areas of concern, ensure state requirements were met, and to provide mentorship for future in-house nurses.

In addition to IDPH's requirements, it was determined that all nurses assigned to the trauma bays would have at least one year of emergency room experience, complete and pass the Emergency Nurse Association's (ENA) TNCC and have a TNS available to them for questions and guidance. Since there were limited TNCC nurses, multiple TNCC courses were provided prior to opening, ensuring a comprehensive core of trauma nurses [9]. IDPH's only requirements for ICU nurses is one Registered Nurse per shift with 2 years of ICU or critical care experience and the nurse has completed 4 hours of trauma-related critical care continuing education per year [1]. IDPH does not have specific educational requirements for general floor, OR, PACU, or rotor-winged nurses.

Needs Assessment

To assess the nursing staff's current level of clinical knowledge and skills when caring for trauma patients, a needs assessment was performed. This involved reviewing the staff's professional certifications, occupational histories, and personal experiences [3, 10]. Additionally, considering the historical context in which the center was established, we addressed personal feelings and biases relating to caring for Chicago's South Side, a traditionally marginalized population who exhibit a significant distrust of the healthcare system. These conscious and unconscious biases posed a barrier to performing professional duties and treatment to our patients (see Chap. 35).

Triage

One of the initial challenges was to ensure patients were correctly triaged. At the scene, EMS determines if the patient meets pre-hospital trauma criteria established by IDPH [1]. However, trauma centers have internal criteria which activate the trauma team and may differ from EMS trauma criteria. Internally, two activation levels, Level 1 and 2, were developed which would trigger the trauma team to respond to the ED. The activation criteria were accomplished by reviewing the guidelines set forth by the American College of Surgeons (ACS) with consensus amongst the trauma surgeons. These standards are based on physiologic and some anatomic criteria [11]. Level I activations are the most severely injured patients. They require an immediate response by the entire trauma team. The Trauma Surgeon is required to respond within 15 minutes of patient arrival. Level II activations, are less severely injured patients requiring the team to respond within 30 minutes of being activated.

Emergency Communications Registered Nurses (ECRN) are specifically trained to manage incoming calls from the field medics, and to determine which activation criteria the patient meets. Subsequently ECRN would page the trauma team directly through the electronic medical record. Understanding the difference between EMS trauma criteria and the newly developed internal trauma team activation criteria was imperative. Whilst over-triage may not harm the patient, it leads to unnecessary mobilization of resources and can result in costly care [12]. Under-triage is the failure to identify significant injuries causing a delay in diagnoses and treatment and is associated with increased mortality [13]. Due to the complexity and significance of understanding how to correctly activate the trauma team, intensive didactic lectures with corresponding written material and testing were completed prior to opening.

Trauma Specific Skills

In collaboration with the Department of Nursing Education, the CNO, Nurse Directors, Nurse Managers, and bedside nurses, specific educational priorities were outlined for individual units. A Trauma Work Plan was developed to itemize the list of educational needs for specific units. This included the emergency department, operating room, central lab, blood bank, inpatient units, spiritual care, security, and outpatient services. The spreadsheet consisted of 25 pages separated into nursing units. The items on the sheet were identified from IDPH requirements, the needs assessment, GEMBA rounds with direct input with staff nurses, question and answer forums, and unit nurse managers and assistant managers.

In the Emergency Department, a multidisciplinary team composed of Board-Certified Surgeons, General Surgery Residents, Trauma RNs, respiratory therapists, and ED technologists provided didactic as well as hands-on education. Five months prior to opening, an intense training curriculum was created. Developed and lead by the Clinical Director of Trauma and a Trauma Surgeon, 1-hour classes were conducted 3 days per week at 7 am. Morning shift change was selected to maximize staff availability and participation. The training was provided for nurses, ED technologist, respiratory therapist, ED residents and Attendings. Based on ACS recommendations and requirements the initial team of trauma surgeons, along with the Clinical Director of Trauma, outlined the personnel, their placement, and clinical obligations during a trauma activation [14]. The nursing training curriculum covered:

- Trauma activation job descriptions
- Moving a patient from the Emergency Medical System gurney to the hospital cart
- Placement of cardiovascular monitors
- Obtaining a manual blood pressure
- How to place nasal cannula
- How to place a cervical collar and maintain cervical spine precautions
- Appropriately turning a patient to assess their back
- Placing a pelvic binder
- Placing a lower extremity splint

- Moving a patient to the Computer Tomography scanner table
- How to use a rapid fluid infusion system
- An introduction to basic surgical instruments
- How to establish an arterial line monitoring system
- How to prepare a PleuroVac for a chest tube (Thoracostomy tube)

This training initially included running through scenarios with high-fidelity simulation mannequins and subsequently with hospital personnel acting as trauma patients. Once these core skills were mastered, the training focused on patient transportation from the Trauma-bays to the OR and Interventional Radiology (IR). This training consisted of:

- Wayfinding—ED to OR; ED to IR
- OR room preparation
- Appropriate verbal sign-out to the OR and IR Anesthesia Staff
- Removing monitoring equipment and returning the ED supplies

The trauma nurses were then challenged by executing multiple mock mass casualty scenarios. This higher-level training involved integration of the entire Trauma Surgery Team and ED staff. The pre-inaugural day preparation enabled the team to understand trauma activation flow, anticipate members' movement and responsibilities, and work as a coordinated unit. This higher level of planning, preparation, and coordination led to the development of an integrated multidisciplinary team [15].

Our training program culminated in a comprehensive 8-hour lecture and skills class entitled "Traumapalooza". All available surgical disciplines provided supplemental education that included:

- Orthopedic injuries and pelvic binding
- Primary and Secondary Survey
- Chest tube set-up and care
- Trauma documentation with the electronic medical record (EMR)
- Rehearsing the correct pathways to the operating room (OR) and blood bank
- Skill in using the rapid fluid warmer

Day-in-the-Life

Whilst the required education and training were underway, anticipated patient flows were outlined. Several months prior to opening an adult trauma center, day-in-the-life (DITL) scenarios were completed. Completing DITL scenarios allowed us to study the complex workflow of trauma patients arriving via EMS, presenting to the waiting area, helicopter, or inter-facility transfers (See Fig. 1) [16]. This involved following the "patient" through the system, observing the workflow thereby allowing us to identify issues and gridlocks. These were addressed immediately thus preventing major issues prior to opening the doors on May 1.

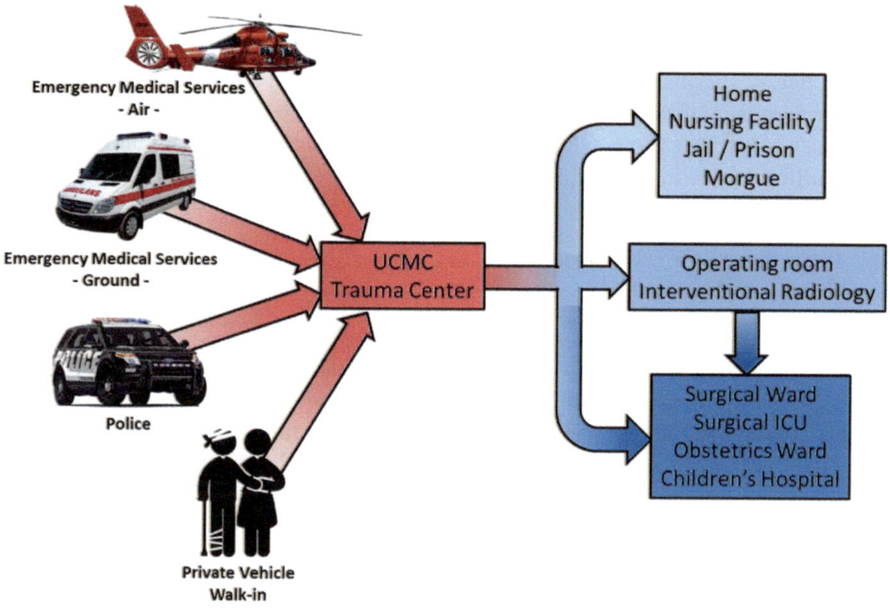

Fig. 1 Patient throughput—Injured patients enter the trauma system by multiple mechanisms. After the appropriate care within the trauma bays they are discharge or triaged to higher level care

Specialty Areas

Operating Room

Based upon prior analysis, we anticipated a high level of operative penetrating trauma. This necessitated a complete change in the structure and staffing of the OR as discussed in Chap. 3. Setting up the trauma room, acquiring new equipment and instruments, and ensuring readiness to receive a trauma patient within minutes of notification became an imperative. The transit time from the ED trauma bay to the OR is 4 minutes, underscoring the importance of readiness and education.

To facilitate the notification process direct communication from the trauma bay to the operating room nurse's station was established. A protected phone was programmed to automatically call the operating room enabling the trauma team to provide the operating room nurse with information. In conjunction with OR nurse leaders, the Department of Education, and trauma nurse leaders the operating room nurses received the following education:

- Trauma alert phone etiquette
- Learning new trays and instruments

- EPIC trauma patient documentation
- Pathophysiology, mechanism of injury and injury patterns
- Practice scenarios—random 5-minute warnings to open a room, prepare the instruments, and start documentation
- Processing crime scene evidence—ensuring proper chain of command
- Handling Police investigations
- Notifying County Coroner

ICU and Surgical Floors

The skill level of the nurses handling critical care patients prior to opening of the trauma center was exceptional. Their longevity with complex transplants and neurological patients provided a highly developed knowledge base. However, the nursing staff's experience was augmented with the following trauma specific education:

- Trauma Care After Resuscitation (TCAR) classes (nationally recognized program providing continuing education to in-patient units) [17]
- In-depth hands-on education for new equipment—provided by vendors and the nursing education department
- EPIC documentation
- Order-sets
- Post-mortem care—notifying the County Coroner
- Contacting Sexual Nurse Examiners
- Collecting Driving Under the Influence specimens
- Releasing Medical Information to Law Enforcement
- Trauma Informed Care

Documentation

Trauma resuscitations requires accurate and complete documentation. It serves as a legal document, but is also used for performance (PI) and quality improvement (QI) projects [18]. The ED nurses, in conjunction with the Information Technology team, created a novel electronic medical record application, called a "Trauma Navigator". This application was designed to capture a patient's hospital intake, physical examination findings, and trauma-specific orders to include laboratory work, x-rays, and computed tomography (CT) scans [1]. The trauma narrator was designed to follow the ACS ATLS primary and secondary assessments [14]. Due to our patient population, in addition to patient documentation, the nurses were educated on crime scene evidence chain of custody and documentation, recording rapid neurologic assessments, and recording invasive trauma procedures such as thoracotomies or manual cardiac massage.

Creating an Orientation

After the successful Trauma Center opening, the "Trauma Champions" created and proctored a new core curriculum encompassing the Section of Trauma and hospital policies. UChicago Medicine Trauma Center is a quaternary referral center, receives a diverse range of trauma injuries, necessitating our nursing staff to possess a broad oversight and skillset in the care of multisystem injured patients. The new curriculum's clinical foundation was the ACS ATLS course.

To further streamline their education, a Nursing Trauma Orientation Manual was created. The manual encapsulated critical information and procedures necessary to be successful in the trauma bay. It includes learning objectives and a skill set checklist (Appendix A). Understanding ENA TNCC and ACS ATLS guidelines, as well as familiarity with trauma bay equipment are emphasized during the first week of training. Some of the other skills and processes taught during trauma orientation include:

- Activation criteria for a level I and level II trauma
- Trauma activation paging process
- Trauma nurse documentation
- Laboratory and radiology order entry
- Understanding frequently used medications and their dosages
- Process for using the Blood Refrigerator
- Location of blood products
- How to initiate and execute a Massive Transfusion Protocol (6 units of PRBC and 6 units of FFP) and a Pediatric packs (2 units of PRBC's and 2 units of FFP)
- Understanding the American Burn Association resuscitation algorithm and the care of burn patients
- Basic ventilator set-up and management
- Legal process such as DUI (driving under the influence) kits
- How to appropriately interview a minor
- Care of the deceased patient, proper documentation, and process for viewing and removal of the decedent
- Familiarization with the Trauma Service Protocols.

Future of Nursing Education

The COVID era has led to an increase in on-line educational opportunities, but it has also resulted in a lack of bedside clinical experiences. Integrating hands-on clinical training into the educational curriculum has become a priority. Additionally, due to the reduced patient-provider interactions, UChicago Medicine has begun a structured mentorship program with critical feedback sessions. The aim is to address educational deficits while providing the highest level of care. Furthermore, considering our patient population and the potential for numerous adverse psychological experiences, we have adopted a trauma informed care approach—a holistic methodology to addressing physical and psychological experiences—that has become the standard of care. Nursing care involves a continuum of experiences. Tailoring nursing education and practice to suit the patient population will result in the best physical and psychological outcomes.

Appendix A

Nurse Trauma Competencies/Skills List

Registered Nurse must have one year of Emergency Department experience, completed ED checklist and a current TNCC, TNS, TCRN, or ATCN certification to precept in the resuscitation bay. Successful completion of orientation includes: all education and activation(s) requirements are met and checklist is completed and signed off by employee, Preceptor, Trauma Program Manager, and ED leadership.
*extension of orientation is case by case basis and discussed with employee, Preceptor, ED Educator, Trauma Program Manager, and ED leadership

Employee Name/Title ____________________ Start Date: ____________

Orientation End Date: ____________________ Dept. /Unit: CCD ED

Date (week 1)	Preceptor Initials	Date (week 2)	Preceptor Initials	Date (week 3)	Preceptor Initials
(Day 1)		(Day 4)		(Day 7)	
(Day 2)		(Day 5)		(Day 8)	
(Day 3)		(Day 6)		(Day 9)	

Date (week 4)	Preceptor Initials	Extension*	Precepto r Initials	Extension*	Preceptor Initials
(Day 10)		(Day 13)		(Day 16)	
(Day 11)		(Day 14)		(Day 17)	
(Day 12)		(Day 15)		(Day 18)	

Trauma Orientee Meetings	Day 0 (Date & Initial Required)	1 week (Date & Initial Required)	2 week (Date & Initial Required)	3 week (Date & Initial Required)	4 week (Date & Initial Required)
• Pre orientation meeting (Receive binder, checklist and meet with a mentor)					
• 1 week meeting (Trauma orientation progress report w/mentor & educator)					
• 2 week meeting (Trauma orientation progress report w/mentor & educator)					
• 3 week meeting (Trauma orientation progress report w/mentor & educator)					
• 4 week meeting (Trauma orientation progress report w/mentor & educator)					

Continuing Education Recommendations/Offerings (Not required to complete Orientation)	Dates (*approximate dates)
TraumaCon	End of March (yearly)
UCAN	Late Spring/Early Summer (yearly)
Advocate Trauma Symposium	Mid-November (yearly)
Region 6 Trauma Symposium	Date varies (yearly)
APP Education	Bi-weekly, Thursday at 2 pm
UCM Trauma/ IR Conference	Fall (yearly)

Trauma/Critical Care Skills & Rationale	Verbal Review (Date & Initial by Preceptor)	Return Demonstration (Date & Initial by Preceptor)	Observed (Date & Initial by Preceptor)	Competent (Date & Initial by Preceptor)
	Day 0			
Trauma Skills (Role play trauma activation, C-collar placement, c-spine stabilization, log roll from left to right)				
Epic Downtime/Forms (location and use)				
Trauma Paging (script and Walk-in algorithm)				
Art Line Setup				
Measurement for Abdominal Compartment Syndrome				
Blood/Whole Blood/MTP Protocols and Policy				
Burn/Depth/Rule of 9's				
EVD/Bolt setup (competency not required to complete orientation)				
IO				
Pelvic Binder/Sheets & Clamps				
Chest Tube Drainage System (Pleuravac)				
Rapid Infuser (Level 1)				
Sam Splints				
Trauma Nurse Role (Stick Figure)				
Trauma Room Set-up				

Computer Technology	Verbal Review (Date & Initial by Preceptor)	Return Demonstration (Date & Initial by Preceptor)	Observed (Date & Initial by Preceptor)	Competent (Date & Initial by Preceptor)
	Day 0			
Documenting required information in Trauma Narrator completely and accurately				
• Trauma Transfers (Scribe enters order set 6700)				
• Trauma Activations ○ Treatment PTA ○ Mechanism of Injury (MOI) ○ Staff Arrival ○ Trauma Start/End ○ Primary and Secondary Survey ○ Trauma Documentation End				
• CTA Poly Trauma (Order Set #7033)				
• Required documentation ○ Beta HCG (females under 55yo) ○ Temperature within 30 minutes of patient arrival				
• Expiration Documentation in Epic ("Disposition" tab) ○ Nursing--GOH (1-800-5454438) ○ Physician--Medical Examiner (1-312-666-0200)				
Position Specific Skills & Competencies	**Verbal Review (Initial & Date by Preceptor)**	**Return Demonstration (Date & Initial by Preceptor)**	**Observed (Date & Initial by Preceptor)**	**Competent (Date & Initial by Preceptor)**
	Day 0			
ENSURES THE TRAUMA BAY IS PREPARED APPROPRIATELY BEFORE PATIENT ARRIVAL				
Objective 1: Performs a systematic assessment of seriously injured patients, including special populations following TNCC principles				
• Use knowledge of MOI to focus on predictable injuries/bay setup				
• Facilitates assessing the patient for respiratory, circulatory and neurological status, exposes and warms patient (Primary Survey: ABCD and E)				
• Facilitates evaluation of patient pupillary status, head/face, neck and thorax, abdomen, genitourinary region, extremities and skin (Secondary Survey: FGHI)				

Position Specific Skills & Competencies	Verbal Review (Initial & Date by Preceptor)	Return Demonstration (Date & Initial by Preceptor)	Observed (Date & Initial by Preceptor)	Competent (Date & Initial by Preceptor)
	Day 0			
Objective 2: Assumes overall nursing responsibility for the patient. Directs and supervises nursing and ancillary staff activities.				
• Be familiar with Stick Man diagram/roles (RN1, RN2, ERT, etc.) and who is doing primary/secondary assessment.				
• Promote an organized and calm environment in the trauma bay, including crowd control				
• Communicate directly with Lab/Blood Bank, Radiology (CT, X-ray, ICU staff, etc.)				
• Confirm that labs are obtained and sent to Lab and documented in chart				
• Ensure that patient ID band is secured on patient and belongings labeled with patient sticker				
• Verify patient name and DOB and ensure chaplain and/or VRP verifies NOK and patient ID with nurse prior to notifying Trauma attending of family presence in the ED.				
Objective 3: Assures protection of the neck and spine based on MOI				
• Knowledge of appropriate size and correct application of both Philly and Aspen collar and when to use Aspen vs. Philly				
• Log rolls patient while maintaining proper c-spine alignment				
• Identifies endpoint for removal of protective devices (c-collar) and notifies trauma service				
• Documents placement and removal of protective devices				

Position Specific Skills & Competencies	Verbal Review (Initial & Date by Preceptor)	Return Demonstration (Date & Initial by Preceptor)	Observed (Date & Initial by Preceptor)	Competent (Date & Initial by Preceptor)
	Day 0			
Objective 4: Accurately documents trauma clinical assessment and interventions				
• Documentation accurately reflects patient condition based on TNCC, TNS, TCRN, ATCN principles (arrival note-AVPU, MOI, pertinent info and narrative from EMS/CFD/UCAN)				
• Sequential times of clinical care observations and interventions to capture care flow				
• GCS accurately documented (Primary & Vitals/Trauma score)				
• Assess, co-manages pain and identifies indication for pain medication				
• Documentation and verification of all wounds and injuries				
• Enters all orders for imaging, medications and Lab add-ons (bHCG for all females under 55)				
• Notification, response and presence of MDs are documented as to time of arrival *(Necessary Staff arrival documented: RN scribe & Trauma attending/chief resident present)*				
• Information from police/detectives (RD number, Beat, Star)				
• Patient belongings and security of valuables are documented in patient chart (cash/valuables given to security to put in safe)				
Objective 5: Demonstrates familiarity with trauma equipment/supplies and protocols				
• Knowledge of location of all stock and equipment in the trauma bay, supply carts and trauma supply room				
• Completes trauma bay set-up and ensures all bays are stocked appropriately				
• Accesses and reviews Trauma Protocols (See Trauma Binder):				
○ Level 1 and Level 2 criteria				
○ Trauma & Pregnancy (Dr. Stork activation vs OB consult)				
○ MTP, Emergent and Whole blood protocol				

Position Specific Skills & Competencies	Verbal Review (Initial & Date by Preceptor)	Return Demonstration (Date & Initial by Preceptor)	Observed (Date & Initial by Preceptor)	Competent (Date & Initial by Preceptor)
	Day 0			
o Pediatric Trauma (overview)				
o Burn Care Management (Notify Burn ICU)				
o Care of Cervical, Thoracic, Lumbar, Sacral or SCI				
o Disclosure of PHI and Verification of immediate family/NOK				
o Notification/documentation for GOH and ME				
o Family viewing of expired patient (Chaplain & Security)				
o Post-mortem care (ME, Allied and Epic Expiration record)				
Objective 6: Demonstrates expertise with advanced clinical procedures and protocols				
• Location and set-up of equipment for advanced procedures:				
o Chest Drainage Management				
o ICP monitoring devices				
o Emergent Thoracotomy				
o Emergent Cricothyrotomy				
o Bovie				
o Pelvic Binder/Sheet & Clamps				
o Hare Traction/ Sam splint				
o Central Line Set-up & Management				
• Conscious sedation procedure/charting (Formal conscious sedation w/consent, use Sedation Narrator)				
• Documents procedures performed for time sequence and clinical response				

Position Specific Skills & Competencies	Verbal Review (Initial & Date by Preceptor)	Return Demonstration (Date & Initial by Preceptor)	Observed (Date & Initial by Preceptor)	Competent (Date & Initial by Preceptor)
	Day 0			
Objective 7: Applies special considerations for Pediatric, Geriatric and Burn patients				
• Locates the Broselow tape, pediatric code cart, and isolette and describes its application in pediatric nursing care: IV, drug dosages, size of equipment, etc.				
• Under 18 years can speak to CPD or other law enforcement as a victim, without a parent/guardian present				
• Describes the potential for unique injuries and complications related to the patient age, MOI and pre-existing conditions of patient.				
Objective 8: Demonstrates correct collection, preservation, security and documentation of forensic evidence.				
• Identifies and secures all types of evidence properly (PAPER BAG = EXPIRED PATIENTS)				
• Documents chain of possession of items in patient chart (hand off to HOA #7500)				
• Describes injuries in a concise and objective manner				
• Documents statements made by patient and others related in a manner consistent with legal principles				
• Documents, enters Surgical Pathology order, completes Chain of Custody form, and appropriately sends specimen for analysis (contact HOA #7500)				
• Proper collection and documentation of DUI kit				

Position Specific Skills & Competencies	Verbal Review (Initial & Date by Preceptor)	Return Demonstration (Date & Initial by Preceptor)	Observed (Date & Initial by Preceptor)	Competent (Date & Initial by Preceptor)
	Day 0			
Objective 9: Performs tasks associated with the admission, discharge and transfer of the trauma patient and expired patients				
• Establishes "60 seconds of silence" for EMS to provide report upon patient arrival to trauma bay				
• Accurately completes documentation to include ○ MOI ○ Verified NOK name and contact information ○ Any barriers present (language barrier, safety concern) ○ Updates patient name in Epic when appropriate and at appropriate time				
• Identifies injury risk prone behaviors in all patients at time of initial contact (non-use of protective devices, ETOH/Drug use, fall hx, combative/restraints etc.)				
• Provides appropriate discharge education, referred to and included in discharge instructions (up to and including f/u appointments, wound care, proper use of devices/immobilizer)				
• Completes Body Release Form/Allied Services and files in appropriate binder for all EXPIRED patients ○ Copy of Body Release Form ○ Copy of Allied Services employee badge ○ Copy of ME form (1/2 sheet) from Allied ○ Notify Medical Records of Name change and Body Release form sent ○ Print Facesheet and Patient chart to send with body				
• Document paperwork completed, disbursed to appropriate departments/parties and time body left the department in the patient chart				
• EXPIRED PATIENTS—PAPER BAGS ONLY and remain with the body				

Employee: ______________________ Date: ______________

Preceptor: ______________________ Date: ______________

Preceptor: ______________________ Date: ______________

Preceptor: ______________________ Date: ______________

Preceptor: ______________________ Date: ______________

Preceptor: ______________________ Date: ______________

Trauma Program Manager: ______________________ Date: ______________

ED Leadership: ______________________ Date: ______________

COMMENTS/ FEEDBACK:

Employee Name: ______________________________

Trauma Activation Participation Log					
	Level 1 (MOI)	Date/Preceptor Initial		Level 2 (MOI)	Date/Preceptor Initial
1			1		
2			2		
3			3		
4			4		
5			5		
6			6		
7			7		
8			8		
9			9		
10			10		

References

1. Health IDoP. Section 515.2030 Level I Trauma Center Designation Criteria. 2022. https://www.ilga.gov/commission/jcar/admincode/077/077005150H20300R.html
2. Prevention CfDCa. WISQARS™—Web-based Injury Statistics Query and Reporting System. 2023. https://www.cdc.gov/injury/wisqars/index.html
3. Ding M, Metcalfe H, Gallagher O, Hamdorf JM. Evaluating trauma nursing education: an integrative literature review. Nurse Educ Today. 2016;44:33–42. https://doi.org/10.1016/j.nedt.2016.05.002.
4. Choi J, Carlos G, Nassar AK, Knowlton LM, Spain DA. The impact of trauma systems on patient outcomes. Curr Probl Surg. 2021;58(1):100840. https://doi.org/10.1016/j.cpsurg.2020.100840.
5. Williams A. Shooting hotspots and relative distances to level 1 trauma centers in Chicago. November 2014. https://via.library.depaul.edu/mom/18/
6. Coursera. What is change management? How to use it effectively. Coursera. https://www.coursera.org/articles/change-management#Principles%20of%20Change%20Management
7. Tarlengco J. Gemba walk: meaning, process, and examples. https://safetyculture.com/topics/gemba-walk/
8. Health IDoP. Title 77: Public Health, Chapter I: Department of Public Health, Subchapter F: Emergency Services and Highway Safety, Part 515 Emergency Medical Services, Trauma Center, Comprehensive Stroke Center, Primary Stroke Center and Acute Stroke Ready Hospital Code. Illinois Department of Public Health. https://www.ilga.gov/commission/jcar/admincode/077/07700515sections.html
9. Association EN. Trauma Nursing Core Course (TNCC). ENA University. https://www.ena.org/enau/educational-offerings/tncc
10. Pilcher J. Learning needs assessment: not only for continuing education. J Nurses Prof Dev. 2016;32(4):122–9. https://doi.org/10.1097/NND.0000000000000245.
11. Surgeons ACo. Resources for optimal care of the injured patient. Chicago: American College of Surgeons; 2014.
12. Cook CH, Muscarella P, Praba AC, Melvin WS, Martin LC. Reducing overtriage without compromising outcomes in trauma patients. Arch Surg. 2001;136(7):752–6. https://doi.org/10.1001/archsurg.136.7.752.
13. Jeppesen E, Cuevas-Ostrem M, Gram-Knutsen C, Uleberg O. Undertriage in trauma: an ignored quality indicator? Scand J Trauma Resusc Emerg Med. 2020;28(1):34. https://doi.org/10.1186/s13049-020-00729-6.
14. Surgeons ACo. ATLS student course manual: advanced trauma life support. American College of Surgeons; 2018.
15. Litzinger TL, Cohen TN, Cabrera JS, et al. A data-driven approach to team training for nurses in a level II trauma Center. J Trauma Nurs. 2019;26(3):134–40. https://doi.org/10.1097/JTN.0000000000000438.
16. Cigniti. Day-in-the-life testing: why is it important for enterprise customers. https://www.cigniti.com/blog/day-in-the-life-testing-ditl/
17. Visionem. TCAR Education Programs. https://tcarprograms.visionem.org/
18. Montagna S, Croatti A, Ricci A, Agnoletti V, Albarello V, Gamberini E. Real-time tracking and documentation in trauma management. Health Informatics J. 2020;26(1):328–41. https://doi.org/10.1177/1460458219825507.

The Violence Recovery Program: The Development and Implementation of a Hospital-Based Violence Intervention Program in a Level One Trauma Center on the South Side of Chicago

Franklin Cosey-Gay, Sophie Colt, Dwayne E. Johnson, Christine Goggins, Ernestina Perez, Carly Uebel, Jade Curless, David Crump, Carlos Robles, Bruce Stamps, and Selwyn O. Rogers, Jr

Introduction

Violence is plaguing our nation. If we look at the deaths, injuries, and harm caused by gun violence, it is clear that we are in the midst of a persistent public health crisis. However, violence is not solely a problem of individual people. Instead, primarily due to the intergenerational harm caused by oppressive systems, and in the context of Chicago, for African Americans, this systemic violence has existed for over a century. Addressing root causes of violence has become a famous phrase as an emerging public health approach to violence prevention. However, seldom are the processes explicitly described to help uncover how these root causes shape factors that act as barriers to promoting healthy, violent-free communities.

This chapter will begin by outlining specific historical events that have weakened the financial, physical, and social well-being of African American individuals and communities in Chicago over multiple generations. Structural harms have led to significant rates of community violence in Chicago, particularly on the South and West sides. This chapter argues for a public health approach to addressing these structural inequalities that serves survivors of violence in a hospital setting, as well as the families and communities impacted.

F. Cosey-Gay (✉) · S. Colt · D. E. Johnson · C. Goggins · E. Perez · C. Uebel · J. Curless · D. Crump · C. Robles · B. Stamps · S. O. Rogers, Jr
Urban Health Initiative, University of Chicago Medicine, Chicago, IL, USA
e-mail: fgay@uchicago.edu; sophie.colt@uchicagomedicine.org; dwayne.johnson2@uchicagomedicine.org; christine.goggins@uchicagomedicine.org; ernestina.perez@uchicagomedicine.org; jade.curless@uchicagomedicine.org; David.Crump@hhchealth.org; carlos.robles@uchicagomedicine.org; srogers@bsd.uchicago.edu

S. O. Rogers, Jr (ed.), *Creating a Modern Trauma Center*,
https://doi.org/10.1007/978-3-031-66524-0_6

The authors of this chapter tell the story of how they developed and implemented the Violence Recovery Program (VRP) a hospital-based violence interruption program, in the spring of 2018, at the University of Chicago Medicine (UCM). Over the past five years, VRP has engaged over 9000 patients through October 2023. Of those engaged, approximately:

- 70% suffered a gunshot wound
- 81% were male
- 96% were African American
- 86% were harmed by community violence
- 60% were between the ages of 22–40

The story of the Violence Recovery Program sheds light on the power of community activism, the urgency to name structural inequalities, and the importance of collaboration to create a multi-disciplinary intervention that addresses violence through the lens of public health and to one day achieve true justice. The chapter also describes the effect of the COVID-19 pandemic on the program and the communities served by VRP. The end of the chapter offers strategies for expanding the program to further address structural harms, as well future steps to sustain, grow, and evaluate the program's impact on individuals and communities.

Structural Roots of Community Violence in Chicago

Violence in Chicago has been durably high in black and brown communities for the past 50 years, specifically in the early 1970s, followed by the early 1990s, and the height of the COVID-19 pandemic in 2021, which represented homicide counts above 800. Furthermore, violent rates have been highly concentrated in Black communities on Chicago's South Side. In 1986, Chicago and state of Illinois government officials created a Trauma-Care Network that designated nine adult Level I trauma centers as members, including six within Chicago and three in the city's surrounding suburbs [1]. Two network members were on the South Side of Chicago: The University of Chicago Medical Center (UCMC) and Michael Reese Hospital and Medical Center (MRHMC). Although UCMC would keep its children's trauma center open, in 1988, UCMC dropped out of the Adult Trauma Center Network, leaving MRHMC as the only Level 1 trauma adult trauma center on the South Side of Chicago. In 1991, MRHMC would also close its trauma center, leaving the South Side of Chicago residents with no Level 1 trauma center until UCM reopened its trauma center in 2018.

Despite 1992 representing the second highest homicide level in Chicago's history as well as levels hovering above 800 homicides a year for the first five years of this decade, South Side hospitals were not in the business of providing care for adult South Side residents with most serious injuries. With a population density surrounding these two institutions consisting of over 80% African American residents, many community stakeholders and activists considered the abandonment and neglect of proximate health care and access to trauma care as structural racism. Unfortunately, this story of abandoning Black and Brown communities and the consequential neglect of their basic needs is typical of Chicago's style of structural racism.

The origin story of private and public practices to oppress African Americans began over a century ago, soon after the worst incident of mass violence in Chicago's history, the 1919 Chicago Race Riots. This week-long series of violent attacks and terrorism used to restrict African American movement in housing, labor and recreation space resulted in 38 individuals killed, 537 injured, and 1000 left homeless [2]. In the decades that followed this brutal violence, Black Chicagoans experienced a series of government-sanctioned policies and practices that formally excluded, contained, and isolated Black Chicagoans, by implementing restrictive covenants, urban renewal programs, and redlining.

Government-backed Federal Housing Authority loans allowed white Chicagoans to build equity, and thus generational wealth, through home ownership and denied the same opportunity for Blacks in Chicago. Redlining created a predatory market in Chicago known as "Contract Selling" [3]. Land speculators exploited Black home-buyers who were unable to secure mortgages due to redlining practices by selling them counterfeit mortgages. The fake mortgages allowed the predatory contractors to keep the deed to the property and to withhold actual ownership from the African American who believed that they had bought their home. This predatory arrangement included inflated down payment costs, unregulated high interest rates, the risk of eviction, and forfeiture of investment on the home if a payment to the seller was missed [4].

Predatory contracts impacted between 75% and 95% of homes sold to Black Chicago residents during the 1950s and 1960s, and has contributed to a present-day 3–4 billion dollar wealth gap between Black and white Chicagoans [4]. This present-day wealth gap makes Chicago look and feel like two cities within one. One city is comprised of communities on the South and West Sides where violence and public safety dominate its narrative despite the persistent economic divestment and isolation from equitable access to economic, housing, and social resources. The other city is a well-resourced web of communities that is largely perceived as safe, on the North Side.

Chicago Style Activism and the Opening of a South Side Trauma Center and HVIP

Despite the structural mechanisms that weaken community-level protective factors, like social support, community cohesion, and informal social control, African American communities are steeped in a vibrant, culturally rich heritage and history, and possess deep social bonds that are anchored by vital community and faith-based organizations. Dynamic resistance and resilience contribute to this vitality and yet they are often missing from the dominant narratives about African American communities in Chicago. In the late 1960s, over 500 victims of redlining and predatory housing contracts banded together to create The Chicago Contract Buyers League [5]. Through this collective action, victims of exploitative contracts used protests, lawyers, and media to raise awareness to end the predatory practice. Nearly 50 years later, this same activism was critical to not only the launching of the reopening of a South Side trauma center after 27 years, but also the implementation of the Violence Recovery Program at UCM.

On August 15th, 2010, Damian Turner, an 18-year-old African American male, was a victim of a stray bullet less than four blocks from the University of Chicago Medical Center. UCM's trauma center was still closed in 2010, and the nearest Level 1 care facility was 10 miles away on the city's North Side. Damien died on the way to the hospital. Community residents, close friends, and loved ones strongly believe that Damien would have survived his injuries if he had not traveled nearly 10 miles in an ambulance.

Community stakeholders were well aware of the cruel irony that Damian was a youth community organizer. Damian protested Chicago's twenty-first-century style of structural violence such as the demolition of public housing, closing schools, and mental health clinics on the South and West sides, which live in infamy as the most significant instances of public divestments in United States history. Damian's death catalyzed new activism, which would include a diverse group of friends, family, University of Chicago undergraduate and graduate students, medical students, faculty, and staff. This activism was bolstered by a 2013 research study correlating increased risk of death when trauma centers are more than 5 miles away from the location of the violent incident [6]. Collective action and coordination contributed to consistent daily and weekly protests, sit-ins, and vigils rallied against the UCM tagline, "At the Forefront of Medicine," through their slogan, "You cannot be at the Forefront of Medicine while taking a backseat to trauma!" It was activism that increased the political will to open a trauma center. The next step before opening a trauma center was attracting a chief trauma surgeon. This chief would be Dr. Selwyn Rogers. Dr. Rogers would not agree to lead the trauma center without an accompanying Hospital-based Violence Intervention Program (HVIP).

Securing HVIP Leadership and Support

A significant predictor of violent injury is having a previous violent injury [7]. The director and chief of trauma knew that launching a Level 1 Trauma Center after multiple decades of dormancy needed to be accompanied by an HVIP with credible messengers who possessed lived experience and knowledge of how to engage survivors of violence in a healing centered way, and connect them to resources that would support recovery and help prevent re-injury [8].

The HVIP program at UCM was inspired by the collaboration between a street outreach worker, David "Mecca" Crump, and a trauma surgeon, Dr. Selwyn Rogers, in Boston who worked around the clock responding to violence. Through their parallel support of survivors of violence and bereaved families in the community and the emergency room, they realized that they were more similar than different. Dr. Rogers admired that Mr. Crump was embedded in highly tense situations in the community following violent victimization, aiming to mediate conflict, manage non-aggression agreements, and provide connection to victim services. Mr. Crump admired Dr. Roger's humility that trauma surgery was just a component of recovery and understood community-based violence interventions were an equally important component not only to recovery, but also to preventing re-injury. Late at night, while Mr. Crump was in the community and Dr. Rogers was in the procedure room, they would call each for support with hip hop artist Public Enemy's song "Fight the Power" blasting in the background. This friendship was forged by their relentless pursuit of justice, love, and support. When the University of Chicago Medicine wanted to open a new trauma center and asked Dr. Rogers to lead it, he said yes on the condition that it be accompanied by an HVIP and that Mr. Crump would lead it with a line item of operational support from the hospital for his position.

Mr. Crump moved from his role in Boston to become the manager of the first hospital-based violence intervention to accompany the opening of the adult Level 1 trauma center at the University of Chicago Medicine. One of the first steps was to connect this Mr. Crump with the community affairs team at the hospital's Urban Health Initiative (UHI). UHI, led by Brenda Battle, is UCM's public health arm and oversees UCM's health equity and community benefits strategy.

UHI facilitates and coordinates efforts to address residents' complex public health and social needs in the 28 neighborhoods across 12 zip codes that make up the South Side of Chicago. UHI does this by:

- Bringing a culturally competent, community-based participatory approach to the health and social needs of patients and the broader community.
- Increasing access to high-quality and culturally competent educational programs, financial and healthcare resources that empower community members to live their healthiest lives.
- Generating goodwill and social capital needed to create new services and programs that improve the health and wellbeing of communities served by UCM.
- Serving as a bridge to communities to facilitate training and research opportunities.
- Acting as a platform for amplifying community-based collaborations.
- Serving as UCM's community conscience, enabling UHI to listen to communities and communicate their needs and wants back to UCM leadership, and serve as an honest broker when needed.

UHI core activities include:

- Administering a community health needs assessment (CHNA) every three years,
- An annual community health benefit report,
- Administering community benefit grants to community-based organizations
- Community health program implementation to address needs, and
- Ensuring equitable access to quality health care.

Violence Prevention was identified as a top health need priority in the UHI's 2015–16 Community Benefit report. In 2016, Mr. Crump, the new HVIP manager and the UHI community affairs coordinator, Dwayne Johnson, began a two-year process of listening sessions with community stakeholders, community-based organizations, churches, police, alderman, street outreach organizations, and residents. These sessions were centered on the vision for a HVIP, assessing the needs of the community, and soliciting recommendations for additional resources, as well as determining what was available to support the implementation and evaluation of the program. These community-level feedback sessions informed hospital leadership on the specific needs of community partners. Some highlights included prioritizing staff demographics to reflect the community most impacted by violence and establishing MOUs with community partners.

Another vital external relationship included a site visit to the University of California at San Francisco's (UCSF) HVIP, The Wraparound Project, to learn about the development, implementation, and evaluation of UCSF's HVIP. This experience provided further insight into how to develop a new HVIP while leveraging existing community partners, internal service lines and programs within within UCM to create a comparable model. This experience, plus recommendations from the National Network of Hospital-Based Violence Intervention Programs (renamed the Health Alliance of Violence Intervention (HAVI) in 2019) and the Center for Nonviolence and Social Justice at Drexel University, helped to inform the design the HVIP at UCM.

Returning from UCSF, the need to foster more external partners and manage collaborative relationships within existing service lines within the adult and children's trauma centers was paramount. Service lines like Spiritual Care, Social Work, Child Life, and programs like Healing Hurt People-Chicago had specific missions at UCM before the launch of the proposed HVIP. Two years of internal meetings and collaboration helped these departments and programs maintain their service delivery identities while dedicating staff to design a HVIP program at UCM. The services of VRP would be carried out by the HVIP staff, called Violence Recovery Specialists (VRS) who would engage victims of violence beginning the moment they enter the emergency department. VRSs would continue to support survivors of violence who became admitted to the hospital by coordinating care and services with the entire multi-disciplinary team at UCM to promote comprehensive recovery and reduce the risk of re-injury post-discharge.

HVIP Implementation

May 1, 2018 marked the launching of the Violence Recovery Program (VRP) at UCM, which began modestly with two full-time dedicated HVIP staff. The former UHI community affairs coordinator, Mr. Dwayne E. Johnson served as the full-time Violence Recovery Specialist (VRS), and the other staff member, Mr. Mark Ortman, served as the clinical manager. The specialist's workflow begins with the VRS receiving notifications through the Emergency Medical Systems alerts connected to the UCM trauma paging system, which provides information about incoming trauma patients and their injuries. The specialist only responds to trauma activations resulting from intentional violence, including traumatic arrests and injuries from gunshot wounds, stab wounds, and assault. The VRP model for responding to intentional violence requires that specialists arrive at the emergency room and wait for the patient's arrival with the trauma clinical staff. VRSs also respond to pages, consults, and requests from trauma teams for Level 2 and non-trauma activations for cases such as graze wounds and assault disclosures.

When the patient enters the resuscitation bay, the VRS engages with Emergency Medical Staff, police officers, UCM hospital staff, and patients to collect the patient's medical record number, name, date of birth, and location of the incident, as well as establish whether family members or loved ones are enroute to the hospital, and begin assessing for safety risk. Trauma-responsive care is the framework for engagement with the patient. This style of engagement prioritizes only collecting information from the patient when they are willing and able to share. One of the primary goals is to establish the specialist's role as an advocate for the patient's recovery. Toward that aim, the VRS must respect the patient's autonomy while supporting the patient in regaining control. Thus, it is vital to only push for additional details when necessary, and to share information with non-UCM personnel only if requested by the patient.

Once the patient is medically stable, the team uses Psychological First Aid (PFA) to engage the patient. This process includes introducing self and role to help advocate for the patient and making them as comfortable as by possible by providing physical and emotional comfort, addressing their immediate concerns, and offering practical assistance toward patients' needs, wants, and goals. As the VRS fosters a supportive connection with the patient, the VRS uses psychoeducation to help normalize any reactions to the traumatic experience of being victimized. This includes educating the patient on the prevalence and signs of trauma as well as coping strategies. The specialist also helps facilitate medical updates for patients' families, advocates for and assists with patient-family visitation, supports hospital wayfinding, supporting the patient's loved ones through medical updates, supports attending surgeons in the death intervention process, and refers patients and families to immediate mental health services.

VRSs serve as trauma-informed ambassadors with an overarching aim to prevent further harm. VRSs serve as victim advocates, and throughout the engagement with patients and their loved ones, the specialists work to prevent re-traumatization and criminalization in the hospital setting. The program's founding lead specialist's mantra, "You are having a normal response to an abnormal experience," not only helps guide the teams' introduction to psychoeducation to support patients and family members but also educates patients on their legal rights and options, including their Constitutional protections under the Fourth, Fifth, and Sixth Amendments. The founding and former lead specialist describes his experiences advocating for survivors of violence and defending trauma responsive engagement of patients and their families on the "opening night" of the program on May 1, 2018:

My first evening? Oh, What a Night! The assaults, gunshot wounds, and stab wound patients started rolling in. The incident that resonates with me most was when a young African American teen was admitted for a stab wound to the abdomen in a domestic dispute with his significant other. This teen was previously shot in the stomach in the community. During my initial engagement with him, he described his horrible experience in another medical institution. He stated that he felt like the staff at the institution did not care that he was shot. The patient's experience contributed not only to his lack of trust in the traditional medical model but also to predominately white institutions. This African American teen, like many before this patient, had an experience as a violence survivor where there was no consideration of a cultural or trauma-informed perspective to improve the quality of care, the patient experience, and best practices demonstrated.

While I accompanied this young patient in the trauma bay and eventually an exam room, waiting to be seen by a physician for the stab wound, I engaged with the patient to get him a phone charger and a blanket. While getting to know the patient and providing psychoeducation to normalize the patient's acute stressors, someone from the trauma team shared with the young man that his mother was misinformed that he was in surgery. His mother had been sent to the surgical floor and would be updated by a doctor upon completion of his surgery. However, he wasn't in surgery, and his mother was worried. It was a mistake. This was extremely re-traumatizing for this young man, and he began to exhibit heightened stressors related to anger and anxiety as a result of this experience. The young man was emotionally dysregulated. The young man was having a normal response to an abnormal experience he had recently experienced. Unfortunately, some team members perceived this as disrespectful and questioned, "What is wrong with this young man?" instead of framing the question as, "What happened to this young man? Having a trauma-informed lens especially during crisis was a massive part of my role. I began educating hospital staff on how to operate from a trauma-informed lens. Eventually, I was able to connect with the young man and his mother. The patient was eventually discharged against medical advice (AMA). About 30 minutes after the young man was discharged, his mother reached out to me via phone and shared that he had injured himself even more as a result of swiping at a fence out of anger and cutting his hand open. The mother asked me to walk to a nearby block to see if I could find her son. I walked into the community and located the patient, and I asked the young man for permission to work with him to get him access to the care he desperately needed. The young man agreed to return to the emergency room for further treatment.

However, my advocacy didn't end with the patient. Unfortunately, I needed to convince a hospital staffer to readmit the patient. I needed to overcome some hospital staff's anger with a "contentious" patient who left AMA. As I attempted to see the patient, a nurse refused services and summoned public safety. As this patient was bleeding profusely, I advocated for readmitting the patient to the nursing staff and public safety; I explained the acute stressors the patient was experiencing and restated our program goals as trauma-informed ambassadors tasked with supporting the patient's recovery. One nurse overheard the conversation and offered to readmit the young man. Fortunately, I would resolve the conflict and get the young man the services he deserved and desperately needed. Ultimately, through teamwork, the young man was able to get the care that he needed through trauma-responsive engagement. I escorted him to his room for the night, and he thanked all the staff for helping him. He was discharged the next day and assigned to my caseload to support his immediate goals for recovery. I was motivated by my first night, the program's first hours, because the most important things to me are justice, equity, and access to quality care in a culturally competent and trauma-informed manner to empower the black community that I so passionately love to serve.- Dwayne Arra Johnson SR, LCSW.

While the patients are hospitalized, the VRS conducts a risk and social services needs assessment to assess for risk of reinjury and retaliation, history of violent injury, social support and protective factors, and acute mental health needs. Patients admitted to the hospital from the emergency room are assigned to an inpatient VRS tasked with following patients to support recovery goals. When patients are discharged directly from the emergency room, they are then assigned a case manager. In this role, the specialist provides intensive long-term case management, including trust-building relationships through continued psychoeducation and conducting social service needs assessment to establish person-centered recovery needs and goals.

This person-centered approach is another vital theory of practice for VRSs that emphasizes three principles: genuine engagement, unconditional positive regard, and empathy [9]. Using this approach, the Violence Recovery Program resists the "teachable moments" notion. Instead, it foregrounds that individuals are the experts of their lives, and through trauma informed interventions, we aim to provide a safe space during this "golden moment" following a traumatic experience to support the patients' self-actualizing core characteristics, which include self-awareness, freedom, honesty, caring, trust and autonomy [9].

Through this approach, patient-centered needs typically are structural, including legal advocacy, housing stability, food security, employment and education status, transportation reliability, substance use support, crime victim compensation, and connecting patients to resources to address acute and ongoing mental health needs. VRSs work to mitigate barriers to care and provide a "warm hand-off" to other service providers by directly linking and personally connecting survivors with referral sources to ensure a successful transition of care. VRSs maintain meaningful, trusting, and open relationships with the survivors and, when necessary, make home visits for added follow-up support. Case management is tailored to the patient's individual needs and progress. This approach allows for intensive yet flexible support for clients with long-term or complex needs by helping them navigate and follow through with health and social service referrals.

After the first year of operation, VRP engaged 765 patients. Of the 765 patients,

- 85% of the patients admitted were male
- 69% of the patients admitted were between the ages of 22 and 50
- 23% were between 16 and 21, and 1% were under 16
- 90% of the patients engaged were victims of community violence
- 65% of the victims' injury type was gunshot wound
- 65% of the patients were admitted to the hospital
- Almost 9% of the patients died after their violent injuries.

Over the first few years of the program, UHI leadership secured funding from various donors including but not limited to the McCormick Foundation, Prince Charitable Trusts, Polk Bros. Foundation, Michael Reese Health Trusts, and private family donors to grow its capacity from two specialists to a team of eight VRS, two trauma chaplains, one VRP social worker, all embedded in the adult trauma center, and six Healing Hurt People Trauma Intervention Specialists who were dedicated to pediatric community violent injuries.

In 2019, to secure the sustainability of the program, UHI leadership received funding from the Block Hassenfeld Casdin Collaborative for Family Resilience to help fully integrate the Violence Recovery Program with Spiritual Care, Child Life, Social Work service lines, and the Healing Hurt People and REACT clinical programs. This collaboration for family resilience provided much-needed tertiary prevention structure and stability to implement a comprehensive model that included growing the program to increase essential staff to provide 24/7 coverage for 365 days a year. This growth included adding:

- Two Violence Recovery Specialists
- Four child life specialists to serve both children in the Comer Emergency Department and children of adult patients on the adult side
- Two Healing Hurt People-Chicago Trauma Intervention specialists
- Two postdoctoral scholars in psychology and psychiatry to provide clinical supervision
- A dedicated epidemiologist to oversee data collection, analysis, quality improvement, and evaluation.

This expansion in funding through the BHC collaborative for family resilience uniquely positioned VRP to become one of the most comprehensive HVIP models in the nation. This funding was not limited to tertiary prevention; recognizing the power of community-based local organizations' programming, the BHC issued primary prevention grant funding opportunities under the oversight of the UHI Community Advisory Council's Trauma Care and Violence Prevention. This investment was prescient and timely. As the capacity grew, unfortunately, so did the volume levels. By the end of the second year of operation, the number of patients the Violence Recovery Specialists engaged with increased by 58% to 1299 patients.

In addition to strengthening the program capacity and high-quality implementation, in 2020, VRP became a member of the national network, Health Alliance for Violence Intervention (HAVI). HAVI is a leader in promoting trauma-informed care to violently injured patients in hospital settings and after discharge, supporting their psycho-social healing when they are back in their communities. Strengthening VRP's operational capacity and serving in HAVI's national network makes UCM's VRP well-positioned to engage with national HVIPs, engage in policy, workforce development, mental health, and research and evaluation monthly workgroups, as well as present annually at HAVI's national conference.

In addition to strengthening our national network with HVIPs through HAVI, VRP leveraged its relationships with local Chicago hospitals through the Hospital Engagement Action and Leadership (HEAL) initiative [10]. Senator Dick Durbin of Illinois launched the HEAL initiative in October 2018 to urge healthcare providers on the city's South and West Sides to bolster their efforts to help reduce Violence and address healthcare needs associated with violence prevention and intervention. The Violence Recovery Program at UCM and the Trauma Recovery Center at Advocate Christ Medical Center used the relationships fostered through Senator Durbin's HEAL initiative to launch Southland RISE (Resilience Initiative to Strengthen and Empower). Recognizing that UCM and ACMC trauma centers serve most of the trauma patients from the greater Southland Chicago area, the Southland RISE initiative was launched to leverage collective expertise to coordinate equitable access to quality care, promote prevention programming, address structural racism in systems of health and healing, and building a network for healing justice advocacy and building a network of sustainable programs dedicated to healing justice advocacy and violence prevention.

On March 5, 2020 UCM and ACMC hosted a Southland RISE summit to highlight and explore innovative strategies and approaches that communities and multisector partners are using to promote recovery, build resilience, and decrease the effects of trauma on individual and community health. The summit also provided a platform for organized discussions about the strengths and gaps across partners, allowing the group to think about how it can create a "multiplier effect" through more strategic collective action. Through the Southland RISE community Violence Prevention Grant Program, 50 community-based organizations on the South Side have received over $650,000 in funding programs that try to keep youth and community members engaged and safe during the summer months that typically increase risk for exposure to violence in South Side communities. The funding for community-based programming included activities to support mental health, build trauma resiliency, youth mentorship, restorative justice, job readiness, youth literacy, dance education, homelessness support, and street outreach conflict mediation.

Just days after the Southland RISE summit, these collaborative prevention and intervention approaches were met with an altering structural challenge: the COVID-19 pandemic. The pandemic not only altered the operational structure of the VRP, but also weakened the tenuous support systems in many marginalized communities Chicago and across the nation. As a result, in 2021, VRP saw a 27% increase in violent incidents. Chicago homicide rates climbed to rival the second-highest number of homicides seen since the early 1990s.

The pandemic offered an opportunity to reimagine the VRP model. The heightened volume of violent activations was a barrier to meaningful community-based case management. As the world became closed to in-person social contacts, case management continued safely from home. However, admitted patients on caseloads were in the hospital and isolated from their loved ones who could not visit due to restrictions. Consequently, the VRS support, rapport and trust building process was deeply constrained by virtual engagement, compared to the standard bedside approach. There is no proxy for human-to-human interactions that involve listening to and supporting patients through their most vulnerable moments.

Fortunately, this virtual adaptation of engagement lasted for only for two months, and in-person engagement at bedside for returned. Furthermore, the social isolation required to prevent the spread of the COVID-19 virus weakened previously under-resourced and overused social support structures, especially in communities impacted by policies and practices that have eroded social networks and equitable access to resources over multiple generations.

The pandemic constraints provided an opportunity to revisit strengthening important collaborations with Community-based Violence Interruption (CVI) peacemakers with social, cultural, and human capital credibility. CVI frontline staff establish credibility with survivors of violence by sharing their personal experiences of navigating interpersonal and structural trauma as survivors of violence from the same community. To strengthen working relationships with CVI organizations, in 2021, VRP secured a Memorandum of Understanding (MOU) with Metropolitan

Family Services (MFS) Metropolitan Peace Initiative (MPI) to collaborate with its Communities Partnership 4 Peace (CP4P) initiative. CP4P provides a community-driven multi-sector response to reduce gun violence within 27 Chicago communities with the highest rates of gun violence. CP4P elevates the role of 13 community-based violence intervention organizations within these communities. CP4P aims to engage residents, community stakeholders, survivors of Violence, and bereaved families to participate in the solution to gun violence while forging closer partnerships with public agencies, hospitals, and the police department.

As partners in the CP4P initiative, VRP sent two Violence Recovery Specialists through two cohorts of the MFS MPI's Metropolitan Peace Academy (MPA). MPA is a 144-hour, 18-week public health model curriculum taught by street outreach, trauma, case management, and victim advocacy experts. The curriculum includes restorative justice, trauma-informed care, nonviolence principles, and hyper locality as the framework.

Membership in CP4P has allowed VRP to foster and expand existing relationships with the credible messengers who make up the 13 CVI organizations across 27 Chicago neighborhoods that have persistently high levels of violence. This HVIP-CVI relationship is critical to helping survivors of violence with a comprehensive recovery, as well as improving VRP's safe-discharge strategies through CVI's increased knowledge of community-based conflicts and coordinating with street outreach partners to develop plans to prevent re-injury. As CP4P collaborators, VRP leadership participates in the Mayor's Office of Violence Reduction Community Safety Coordinator Center (CSCC) and attends weekly, biweekly, and monthly meetings such as:

- Weekly citywide victim services meetings
- Chicago Police Department Area 1 and Area 2 violence response coordination calls with CVI partners
- South Side of Chicago High-Risk Intervention meetings
- CSCC biweekly leadership meetings

Through funding from the Illinois Department of Human Services Reimagine Public Safety and Violence Prevention initiative, VRP significantly expanded its program, creating an outpatient case management specialist embedded in the outpatient trauma clinic as part of the program's model. This funding allowed VRP to strengthen communication with CVI partners following a violent incident. The VRS outpatient teams meet with CVI partners weekly to conduct reviews of the CSCC's Crime Prevention and Information Center (CPIC) alerts, which summarize violent incidents by police district and beat, including the type of injury, age and gender of the victim, and hospital destination. These weekly sessions allow our collaborative violence response teams to evaluate our respective workflows, understand the community-level and hospital-based responses to incidents, help evaluate the risk for re-injury through the perspectives of our CVI partners, learn about their community-level mediation strategies, and exchange essential resources to contribute towards the path of comprehensive recovery.

The partnership between VRP and CVIs significantly contributed to the advancement of VRP's outreach efforts. Thanks to the framework created by our CVI leaders, VRP has successfully implemented text thread communications to provide real-time updates when someone is violently injured in these communities.

A notable testimony comes from our Street Outreach partner, Claretian Associates (C.A.), who highlighted that since this collaborative relationship began in 2022, C.A. saw an increase of referrals from less than 10% of survivors of Violence from our target communities on the South Side, to 70–80% connected into community-based services through UCM Violence Recovery Specialists. Open lines of communication and referrals between the organizations are essential to creating an ecosystem of support for survivors of violence that includes hospital-based and community-based violence interventions.

Survivors of violence are often impacted by recurring exposure to violence as well as the pernicious effects of structural violence. As a result, trust can be impacted at individual, relational, community, and institutional levels. Therefore, to help patients on the path of recovery, it is crucial to possess collaborations that reinforce patient-centered choice and agency. This sentiment is best captured by victim advocate partner from our CVI agency, CA:

> We are building more bridges and more channels…we need to be mindful about what trauma does to people in the moment…how they can't really express themselves…sometimes it takes a little time and sometimes it takes a different voice…they may open up in the hospital or later with hospital staff or sometimes there is more trust with a community-based violence intervention worker. How many people don't feel that a hospital is an extension of a prison and the police? Why? Because you are relegated, told what you can't do, you can't see your loved one, Zero Tolerance signs in the hospital… You have a loved one harmed and you are told you can't smoke, he can't get a walker and he wanted to get the hell up out of there…sometimes survivors don't want to be engaged with the hospital and being told what to do because of their personal trauma, seeing police around it rubs them the wrong way… sometimes there is more trust with a community-based violence intervention worker.

Understanding the Impact of the Violence Recovery Program

Chicago has over a century of racial injustices that no one program can tackle alone. Emerging public health practices investigate the root causes of violence at a structural level and engage in collaborative multi-disciplinary strategies, including on the policy level, to achieve an equitable and just society that prevent further violence from taking place. Although the VRP model has advanced dramatically over the past five years, the evaluation efforts have made modest advancements in understanding the program's impact. The program measures success and impact using mixed methods that incorporate frontline staff and patient voices through stories and experiences alongside quantitative measurements on the frequency and types of patient engagement over time. Our program's success and impact indicators are currently focused on process measures, including, number of engagements, interventions, and referrals during hospital stay and post-discharge. Our evaluation focuses on investigating:

1. What are the patient and family's immediate and long-term needs?
2. How were the patient and family's self-identified needs met (# of encounters, interventions, and referrals needed to meet said needs)?
3. What are individual-, hospital-, and community-level barriers and facilitators to meeting said needs?

Five years of running the Violence Recovery Program suggest that improving social and structural determinants of health is a vital component of healing and comprehensive recovery. Our data show that access to public benefits (e.g., SSI/SSA, TANF/AABD, SNAP, SSI, and CVC) and access to mental health services, housing, food security, employment, and criminal record expungement are high on the list of the immediate and long-term needs of patients. VRP also recognizes the importance of connecting patients to legal services to help address economic instability, access to public benefits and employee benefits, housing, and State victim compensation programs. Understanding the administrative burden and time-consuming process for VRS to address health-harming legal needs, the Lead Violence Recovery specialist, Christine Goggins, connected with a then-third year law student, Carly Loughran, to discuss how VRP could use lawyers to help overcome these barriers. Loughran secured a two-year Equal Justice Fellowship through Pfizer to expand the Violence Recovery Program to provide medical-legal services for adult VRP clients.

Thanks to the leadership of principal investigator and UCM trauma surgeon Dr. Tanya Zakrison, Loughran and her lawyer colleagues from Legal Aid Chicago, in 2022, this multi-disciplinary team of clinicians, lawyers, violence recovery specialist and coordinators collaborated to improve strategies to address social-structural determinants of health through legal intervention. This medical-legal partnership helps to address the health-harming legal needs by improving access to benefit programs designed for survivors but that are typically "hard and confusing…people either do not know about aid designated for them or are burdened by the application process" [11]. Zakrison and the team secured NIH funding to identify the types of legal needs patients have, develop a novel VRP-MLP intervention, examine the feasibility of this novel intervention at UCM, and ultimately conduct a randomized control trial to understand patient and family outcomes of the VRP-MLP intervention compared to VRP only intervention outcomes. Preliminary pilot phase data show that embedding an MLP within the VRP program is highly feasible and acceptable, with a high participation rate of 95% and 91.5%, respectively [12].

Next Steps

Interpersonal and community violence can be solved through collaborative and coordinated public health prevention and intervention programs. Hospital-based violence intervention programs like the Violence Recovery Program at The

University of Chicago Medicine are critical pieces to solving this complex puzzle. Hospitals are no longer a "sew and go" operation where violently injured patients are treated and released to the same violent context where they were harmed and be at high risk of re-injury, arrest, incarceration, and death [13]. Instead, now, survivors of violence at UCM are now discharged from the hospital with a safety plan and a recovery tool kit. Our Hospital-Based Violence Recovery Program uses multidisciplinary collaboration and coordination within the hospital and in the community to interrupt the dangerous cycle of violence and contribute to creating a path for comprehensive recovery [13].

In late 2023, our collaborative efforts will continue with the Southland Chicago area trauma center through the Southland RISE initiative. Southland RISE staff from VRP at UCM and TRC at Advocate Health Care teamed up with Metropolitan Family Services to curate-seven cohort cross-training workshop for 60 plus CVI-HVIP attendees. Each hospital response staff and CVI staff attended four-day workshops. Recognizing that HVIP and CVI programs play equally essential roles in the recovery process of survivors, the Southland RISE trainings are designed to enhance understanding of the respective workflows in crisis intervention, victim services, case management, and street outreach, as well as an opportunity to engage in developing strategies to strengthen collaboration and narrow the gap on existing challenges. In 2024, Southland RISE plans to reconvene a violence prevention summit, similar to the one held in March 2020.

It is widely known that the direct costs of gun violence exceed $14 Billion annually [14]. In addition to the physical costs of being injured from Violence, there is also a mental health toll. The trauma of violent victimization can leave survivors stuck in a state of flight, fight, freeze, or fawn mode. Ranging from carrying guns for protection, being easily aroused and defensive over what can be perceived by others as minor incidents, or being completely frozen and unable to cope or engage with anyone. This trauma can impact relationships, physical health, and the ability to contribute to society meaningfully. Although the VRP model provides outreach, support, and mental health support through a trauma intervention specialist, a clinical social worker, and a supervising psychiatrist within the Recovery and Empowerment After Community Trauma (REACT) Clinic, these resources have been limited to youth 20 years and younger. Thanks to expanded funding from the Illinois Department of Human Services, we can provide these services for adult survivors of Violence and their families.

Our program is also aiming to break down silos at the University of Chicago by strengthening existing relationships with the Crown School of Social Work with the aim of including the school as a component of an expanding Violence Recovery Model. Over the past five years, the program has served as a clinical field placement site for masters-level social work from Crown; four students joined the team full-time after graduating from the MSW program, including our current lead specialist, Christine Goggins who was inspired by her work with the Violence Recovery Program to obtain her second masters in clinical social work from Crown, and recently graduated. In addition, the program clinical manager, Carlos Robles, LCSW, has served as an adjunct lecturer at the school for the past four years.

Since November 2023, we have also leveraged support to secure a clinical therapist faculty member to provide trauma group consultation for our frontline staff. Many of our staff are not only exposed to vicarious trauma from their advocacy in the trauma bay, but Violence directly impacts some of them. The group consultations are brave space hybrid sessions exclusive to frontline specialists where staff can engage in candid conversations about their experiences, discuss self-care strategies, and engage in experiential learning without the presence of the leadership team.

In 2024, we aim to work with Crown faculty member Dr. Janelle Goodwill to offer free and accessible mental health treatment for young adult survivors of Violence in Chicago through a pilot study that will include a 3-month randomized control trial of a mindfulness-based intervention using Acceptance and Commitment Therapy. This funded study will provide funds to hire a full-time clinical social worker and a therapist to provide mental health counseling to see if clients randomized into VRP only vs. VRP plus counseling have significant outcome differences in post-traumatic growth, hope, PTSD symptoms, anxiety, and depression.

The program will continue to foreground opportunities to bust silos that exist between the University's hospital and the academic and social environment at the University. We aim to sustain practices that give staff respite from the trauma recovery work by building connections to the broader University, including securing gym memberships and library cards and accessing campus resources often dedicated to students but open to faculty and staff, including the University's gaming lab, the athletic center, the University library and lending privileges from one of the highest volume book holdings in the world, as well as University reading rooms, museums, and Rockefeller Chapel that conducts meditation courses, yoga classes, and the University's performing arts center.

In calendar year 2022, the Violence Recovery Program engaged 38% of all pediatric and adult trauma patients. Of patients engaged in our program since 2018, 2.1% have been re-injured and re-engaged with our program. While this re-injury rate outcome speaks to the power of the program's coordination and collaboration within the hospital and community partners, this re-injury rate is only at the program level. Although some research has found significantly lower injury re-injury rates among participants in an HVIP program than those in a control group [15, 16], no national re-injury rate statistic exists. However, thanks to Senator Durbin's Hospital Engagement Action and Leadership (HEAL) initiative, we are working to establish data-sharing agreements with the Chicago Department of Public Health along with nine other Chicago area Level One trauma centers and emergency rooms. In 2023, various HEAL working groups were established to discuss ways to help improve coordination with different departments within and across hospitals to build an infrastructure that would allow programs like ours to share data, standardize definitions for community violence, firearm injury, and HVIP eligibility criteria, to assess further our goals toward reducing re-injury and promoting recovery.

Finally, the Violence Recovery Program is aligning its operations to a list of eight standards and subsequent indicators released by HAVI in early 2023 that will serve as a basis for becoming an HAVI-accredited HVIP. We strongly believe these indicators will strengthen the model's success in program planning, high-quality implementation, and design to promote service delivery best practices, foster community partnerships, invest in staff development and self-care, support the monitoring of program delivery through evaluation, research, and participant engagement, secure funding to maintain and grow programs to address programming opportunities and promote hospital systems transformation.

Clinical Pearls

- Hospital-based violence intervention programs (HVIPs) are critical pieces to solving the complex public health puzzle of Gun Violence in the United States of America.
- HVIPs frontline staff should consist of trained paraprofessionals, many directly impacted by violence as survivors, who often come from the communities they serve, to be the first point of engagement as trauma-informed ambassadors.
- HVIPs must prioritize a multidisciplinary collaborative approach within the hospital and community to ensure comprehensive recovery and reduce re-injury after discharge.
- HVIP approaches must include strategies to target social and structural determinants of health as violence is not solely an interpersonal problem but largely structural.

References

1. Van J. City Sets Up Trauma-Care Network. Chicago Tribune; 1986, May 16th. Retrieved from https://www.chicagotribune.com/news/ct-xpm-1986-05-16-8602040340-story.html
2. Chicago Commission on Race Relations. The Negro in Chicago: a study of race relations and a race riot. University of Chicago Press; 1923.
3. Rothstein R. The color of law: a forgotten history of how our government segregated America. 1st ed. Liveright Publishing Corporation; 2017.
4. George S, Hendley A, Macnamara J, et al. The plunder of black wealth in Chicago: new findings on the lasting toll of predatory housing contracts. Durham: Samuel DuBois Cook Center on Social Equity at Duke University; 2019.
5. Finley ML. Inside the Contract Buyers League. Fighting Against Housing Discrimination. The Chicago Reporter; 2016, February 15. Retrieved from: https://www.chicagoreporter.com/inside-the-contract-buyers-leagues-fight-against-housing-discrimination/
6. Crandall M, Sharp D, Unger E, Straus D, Brasel K, Hsia R, Esposito T. Trauma deserts: distance from a trauma center, transport times, and mortality from gunshot wounds in Chicago. Am J Public Health. 2013;103(6):1103–9. https://doi.org/10.2105/AJPH.2013.301223. Epub 2013 Apr 18. PMID: 23597339; PMCID: PMC3698742
7. Purtle J, Rich JA, Fein JA, James T, Corbin TJ. Hospital-based violence prevention: progress and opportunities. Ann Intern Med. 2015;163(9):715–7. https://doi.org/10.7326/M15-0586. Epub 2015 Aug 25. PMID: 26301734

8. The Health Alliance for Violence Intervention. NNHVIP white paper: hospital-based violence intervention: practices and policies to end the cycle of violence; 2019. Retrieved from: https://static1.squarespace.com/static/5d6f61730a2b610001135b79/t/5d83c0d9056f4d4cbdb9acd9/1568915699707/NNHVIP+White+- Paper.pdf
9. Rogers CR. On becoming a person: a therapist's view of psychotherapy. 17th ed. Chicago: Houghton Mifflin; 1995.
10. Chicago HEAL Initiative Assisted by the University of Chicago Crime Lab and Civic Consulting Alliance An Action Plan from Chicago Hospitals & U.S. Senator Richard J. Durbin. Strengthening Neighborhood Engagement to Reduce Violence & Improve Health; 2018, October. https://www.durbin.senate.gov/imo/media/doc/Chicago%20HEAL%20Initiative%20FINAL.pdf
11. Desmond M, Graham D. Poverty, by America. Crown Publishing Group; 2023.
12. Pillai R, Tung EL, Zakrison T, Cosey-Gay F, Elgindy M, Goggins C, Green I, Loughran C, Muntz N, Perez E, Rogers S, Sen-Gupta N, Stolbach BC. National research conference for the prevention of firearm related harms, Chicago, Illinois, November 1, 2023. Feasibility of integrating a bedside medical-legal partnership into firearm violence recovery. The Recovery Legal Care.
13. The Health Alliance for Violence Intervention and National Alliance for Trauma Recovery Center. Keys to collaboration. Hospital-based violence intervention programs and trauma recovery centers; 2023. Retrieved from: https://static1.squarespace.com/static/5d6f61730a2b610001135b79/t/652fcfad06564c109da5ada4/1697632175139/Final_HVIP_TRC.pdf
14. Everytown Research and Policy. The economic cost of gun violence. Everytown Research and Policy; 2022. https://everytownresearch.org/report/the-economic-cost-of-gun-violence/
15. Bell TM, Gilyan D, Moore BA, Martin J, Ogbemudia B, McLaughlin BE, Moore R, Simons CJ, Zarzaur BL. Long-term evaluation of a hospital-based violence intervention program using a regional health information exchange. J Trauma Acute Care Surg. 2018;84(1):175–82. https://doi.org/10.1097/TA.0000000000001671.
16. Mueller KL, Cooper BP, Moran V, Lew D, Ancona R, Landman JM, Marguerite S, Marotta P, Liss DB, Mancini MA, Schuerer D, Ranney ME, Foraker RE. Incidence of and factors associated with recurrent firearm injury among patients presenting to St. Louis Trauma Centers, 2010 to 2019. A cohort study. Ann Intern Med. 2023;176:1163–71. https://doi.org/10.7326/M23-0069.

Part III
Departmental Contributions

Neurotrauma

Ali Mansour, Tracey Fan, William Roth, and Fernando D. Goldenberg

Definition and Scope

Neurotrauma, a pervasive cause of global morbidity and mortality, often represents an avoidable condition, notably exemplified in incidents such as road traffic accidents and assaults [1]. In the United States, the gravity of neurotrauma is underscored by staggering statistics: there were approximately 214,110 traumatic brain injury (TBI)-related hospitalizations in 2020, with 69,473 TBI-related deaths in 2021, equating to over 586 hospitalizations and 190 deaths per day [1, 2]. The impact extends beyond TBI, as around 190,000 individuals in the USA grapple with paralysis resulting from spinal cord injuries [3]. A concerning trend emerges from data spanning 1990 to 2016, revealing a significant rise in age-standardized incidence (3·6% [95% uncertainty interval 1·8–5·5]), prevalence (8·4% [7·7–9·2]), and years

A. Mansour
Neurology and Neurological Surgery, Neurocritical Care Section, Department of Neurology, Informatics Neurosciences and Critical Care, Neurocritical Care Fellowship, University of Chicago, Chicago, IL, USA
e-mail: Ali.Mansour1@bsd.uchicago.edu

T. Fan
Neurocritical Care Section, Neurocritical Care Fellowship, University of Chicago, Chicago, IL, USA
e-mail: Tracey.Fan@bsd.uchicago.edu

W. Roth
Neurocritical Care Section, University of Chicago, Chicago, IL, USA
e-mail: William.Roth@bsd.uchicago.edu

F. D. Goldenberg (✉)
Neurology and Neurological Surgery, Neurocritical Care, Neuroscience ICU, Comprehensive Stroke Center, University of Chicago, Chicago, IL, USA
e-mail: fgoldenb@bsd.uchicago.edu

S. O. Rogers, Jr (ed.), *Creating a Modern Trauma Center*,
https://doi.org/10.1007/978-3-031-66524-0_7

lived with disability (YLD) rates for TBI [3]. Although the rates for spinal cord injuries remained relatively stable during this period, the growing global population suggests an overall increase in the number of individuals living with such injuries [3].

Neurotrauma's impact extends far beyond the immediate physical toll, influencing societal dynamics and economic landscapes. Persons experiencing moderate to severe TBIs often require sustained care for recovery, profoundly affecting not only their lives but also placing significant burdens on their families and society at large. The repercussions are not merely clinical; the economic cost of TBIs, encompassing direct and indirect medical expenses, was estimated at a staggering $76.5 billion (in 2010 dollars) [2]. Fatal TBIs and those necessitating hospitalization contribute substantially, constituting approximately 90% of the total medical costs associated with TBIs [2]. As we delve into the intricacies of neurocritical care within trauma centers, it becomes imperative to acknowledge the profound societal and economic dimensions of neurotrauma, driving our pursuit of sophisticated and targeted clinical interventions.

Subspecialized Neurocritical Care (NCC) is associated with improved survival and functional outcomes for critically ill adults with brain and spine injury [4]. Cohorting patients under the guidance of a specialized multidisciplinary team, led by a neurointensivist and complemented by a specialized allied health team, has demonstrated promising results. The incorporation of advanced multimodal neuromonitoring and standardized NCC protocols further characterizes the evolution of NCC units. Notably, the outcomes of specific neurological conditions, such as subarachnoid hemorrhage (SAH) and traumatic brain injury (TBI), pose substantial challenges, underscoring the need for specialized care. Given the diverse etiology and management of acute brain injuries (ABIs), the introduction of NCC in trauma centers becomes paramount.

Early Engagement of Neurocritical Care and Neurosurgery

Early involvement of neurocritical and neurosurgical services in the management of severe (and often moderate) neurotrauma is essential for optimal multidisciplinary care in modern neurotrauma centers. Neurotrauma patients are at heightened risk following the primary injury for secondary CNS injury from various insults, including brainstem herniation from focal mass lesions or extra-axial intracranial hemorrhage, seizures and status epilepticus, cerebral or spinal cord edema, hypoxia, ischemia, inflammation and oxidative cell damage [5, 6]. As in other forms of acute CNS disease, early diagnostic evaluation and management by those with neurotrauma expertise is necessary for the prevention of further irreversible CNS injury.

Acquisition of a quick, formal neurological examination prior to initiation of sedation for management of extracranial injury or airway compromise, for example, is a vital element for any decision-making regarding advanced neuromonitoring, empiric management of suspected intracranial hypertension, or as an indication (or exclusion) for early neurosurgical management. Current evidence suggests that prehospital hypoxemia and hypotension may be the impactful known mediators of secondary CNS injury and mortality in patients with TBI [7]. Neuroscience clinicians can also guide appropriate use of seizure prophylaxis for the prevention of early post-traumatic or peri-operative seizures and advise on reversal of coagulopathies and use of empiric interventions for intracranial hypertension. Ideally, neuroscience clinicians work at bedside to ensure neuroprotective parameters are established based on evidence-based standards.

Neurotrauma patients frequently require advanced diagnostic evaluation beyond the initial trauma survey to guide interventions. These advanced diagnostics may include screening for traumatic cervical or intracranial vascular injury, electroencephalography to evaluate for seizures, specialized imaging for operative guidance, and follow up imaging to assess for lesion stability or expansion. Neuroscience clinicians must also collaboratively make determinations of eligibility for emergent neurosurgical interventions, such as need for invasive neuromonitoring, spinal decompression, intracranial hematoma evacuation, early debridment surgery on penetrating trauma, or decompressive craniectomy.

Coordination of Care

Patients with neurotrauma often sustain additional extracranial traumatic injuries requiring surgical intervention. Neurosurgical and neurocritical care clinicians provide vital insights into urgent prioritization of necessary interventions. Polytrauma patients often have concomitant life-threatening injuries which must be addressed in parallel or rapidly in sequence with CNS injury. Neuroscience clinicians are indispensable members of the multidisciplinary care team to assist in triage and timing of interventions. Additionally, the degree of extracranial injury typically influences fitness for neurosurgery, and rapid assessment of risks posed by extracranial factors are considered when making emergent planning for surgical or medical interventions. Oftentimes, advanced neuromonitoring with an invasive ICP monitor, for example, is necessary for optimal neurological intraoperative management of extracranial trauma.

One study analyzed the impact of extracranial surgical interventions on outcomes in patients with TBI [8]. Patients who suffer TBI and undergo early extracranial surgical procedures fared worse than those who did not. While this association may be accounted for by the overall severity of injury, other factors, including sedation, anesthesia induction, surgical blood loss, systemic inflammation and post-surgical complications may induce or exacerbate secondary brain injury. Patients may therefore benefit from involvement of acute neurological services in the careful consideration of benefits, risks, timing, and peri- and intraoperative management of extracranial procedures.

One additional benefit to early engagement of acute neurological service is improvement in the coordination of care between services in the trauma bay and the receiving critical care unit. Transitions in care, especially between geographically remote sites, represent an especially vulnerable timeframe for patients from lapses in care due to potentially insufficient neuromonitoring, inter-rater variability in the reporting of neurological examinations between services, and secondary CNS insults posed by patient transport [9–11]. In patients with polytrauma including CNS injury, appropriate ICU disposition may not always be clearly defined. Early discussion between trauma surgery, NCC, neurosurgery or dedicated neurotrauma providers is necessary to determine individualized needs of patients. In patients with isolated brain or spinal cord injury, neuroscience ICUs with expertise in neurotrauma may be best suited for targeted neuromonitoring, while those who also suffer life-threatening extracranial traumatic injury may be better observed and managed by non-neuroscience ICUs. Defining individual patient needs and triaging based on relative severity of these issues is common practice in modern neurotrauma centers. Adoption of protocols for inclusion or exclusion of polytrauma patients to specific ICUs with multidisciplinary involvement can help facilitate safer and more rapid transfers to the appropriate ICU environment.

Avoiding Futility and Nihilism/Early Prognostication

The process of crude acute neuroprognostication is often indispensable in guiding patients and surrogate decision-makers when faced with severe intracranial injuries. Current guidelines advise against formal early neuroprognostication in cases of neurotrauma and various acute neurological injuries [12–14], however neurological and neurosurgical clinicians often find themselves tasked with synthesizing available information shortly after the arrival of the patient to the emergency department. Their goal is to formulate a preliminary risk and benefit profile, aiding in the determination of patient suitability for invasive or otherwise risky interventions. Early involvement of neurocritical and neurosurgical expertise proves crucial, not only for managing the neurological injury itself but also for assessing the viability and timing of extracranial and systemic interventions.

During this early and critical timeframe, maintaining close communication with surrogate decision-makers is paramount. Often, prediction of neurological outcomes remains unclear early in the hospital course, requiring clinicians to guide proxies toward rapid decisions amid prognostic uncertainty. In addition to discussing the risks and benefits of potential lifesaving interventions, clinicians must also address and consider the impact of personal, cultural, and religious beliefs held by decision-makers and patients. To uphold patient autonomy, clinicians frequently advise surrogate decision-makers to consider the patient's known or hypothetical willingness to undergo these interventions. Those clinicians possessing the most expertise in understanding early prognostic indicators are best equipped to facilitate and guide these complex discussions.

Combatting Nihilism

The traditional view of aggressive treatment for severe traumatic CNS injury as a futile endeavor has been challenged in recent years, primarily due to a deeper understanding of biases, particularly the self-fulfilling prophecy bias, in earlier prognostication models [15]. Long-term outcomes from large prospective registries of patients with traumatic CNS injury, such as the Transforming Research and Clinical Knowledge in Traumatic Brain Injury Network (TRACK-TBI) have shown that those with severe TBI can often have favorable long-term outcomes when early clinical and radiographic indicators might suggest otherwise [16]. In those with traumatic SCI, more severe injury based on initial neurological exam and level of injury is predictive of long-term ambulation, bladder control, and other functional measures. Despite significant functional deficits in isolated traumatic SCI, long-term survival with a reasonable quality of life outcome is common [17–19]. The recovery timeline generally extends beyond the initial hospital period, posing challenges for providing specific prognostic guidance to patients and caretakers regarding functional outcomes.

Often patients presenting with severe TBI are concomitantly intoxicated with substances that depress CNS function or have received sedative medications at the initial hospital that receievd them. These circumstances can contribute to an apparent worse initial neurological exam but that is reversible.

Modern neurotrauma centers leverage available outcomes data to inform neuroprognostication, considering variables like admission Glasgow Coma Score, radiographic Marshall Classification, and ASIA score in traumatic SCI for early interventional decision-making. While these variables offer insight into the degree and possible trajectory of recovery, decisions regarding aggressive treatment should not hinge solely on the presence or absence of any single variable. Instead, patient-centered decision-making is essential, considering realistic outcomes and the range of potential results in early medical or surgical decision-making [20].

Penetrating Brain Injury Experience

Understanding Penetrating Trauma

Gun violence has become a pervasive and deeply rooted issue in urban areas, with Cook County, and particularly Chicago, experiencing a concerning surge in firearm-related homicides. In January 2022 alone, there were 1002 gun-related homicides in Cook County, a staggering increase of 121 compared to the previous year and twice the number reported in 2019. This surge in gun violence has led to a widening life expectancy gap between Black and non-Black residents in Chicago, increasing from 8.3 to 9.2 years [21]. Among the factors contributing to this gap, gun violence stands out, with homicide rates in Black communities reaching nine times that of non-Black communities.

The financial toll of gun violence is not only measured in lives lost but also in economic terms, with an estimated cost of $1.9 million for each injury, accumulating to an annual burden of approximately $5 billion. This alarming statistic highlights the urgent need for a comprehensive understanding of penetrating trauma, focusing on gunshot wounds and stab injuries, to address the unique challenges in diagnosis, treatment, and the pivotal role of surgery.

Penetrating brain injuries (PBI) refers to when a foreign body penetrates the skull and traverses through the dura into brain parenchyma causing focal damages, intracranial hemorrhage, cerebral edema and/or ischemia. The invasion of fast-moving projectile can lead to transient tissue cavitation, which further exacerbates injuries. Most common PBIs are gunshot wounds and stab injuries in civilian, which present unique challenges in comparison to blunt TBI. Differing from blunt TBI, which often results in axonal injury as a result of shearing forces, PBI necessitates precise evaluation of the projectile's trajectory and management of related secondary injuries. Rapid and precise initial interventions are crucial in minimizing secondary brain injury and improving overall neurologic outcome.

Gunshot Wounds and Stab Injuries

More than 40% of trauma injuries treated at the University of Chicago fall under the category of penetrating trauma. Notably, over 300 patients suffering from penetrating brain injuries, predominantly caused by gunshot wounds to the head, have been treated between May 2018–May 2023. However, the lack of uniformity in existing studies on penetrating brain and spine injuries poses a significant challenge. This variability extends to assessments, clinical examinations, imaging modalities, and management approaches, hindering the synthesis of data and the establishment of guiding principles for clinical and surgical care.

To address these challenges, it is imperative to delve into the causes, patterns, and consequences of penetrating trauma. Most cases at UChicago Medicine stem from gunshot wounds, emphasizing the pressing need for targeted interventions and research to improve outcomes for this patient population.

Gunshot wound (GSW) to head is the most lethal PBI among civilian with statistics describing up to 71% of patients dying at the scene, up to 90% dying before reaching hospital and less than 50% survival among those that reached the hospital [22, 23].The high velocity nature of bullets can cause extensive damage including cavitation and shockwaves. The high kinetic energy associated with ballistic injury can not only cause widespread diffuse neuronal cell death, axonal injury, compromised blood brain barrier, but also vasospasm, vessel occlusions, pseudoaneurysm formation, hyperemia, and cerebral edema [24]. The extent of brain injury, size of the cavitation and severity of neurologic damage also depends on the type of weapon used, proximity of the shot, bullet caliber, jacketing and velocity of the bullet. In addition to permanent cavity at the initial site of entry, deformation of the projectile after impacting hard tissues can causes an increase in the size of permanent cavity. After striking bone, fragmentation of the projectile and/or bone can result in the formation of numerous secondary projectiles each producing additional wounding potentials. Due to the severity of these GSW injuries, patients typically present in critical conditions including hemorrhagic shock, traumatic coagulopathy, and respiratory failure. Early aggressive resuscitation in the trauma bay, correction of hypoxemia, hypotension, and coagulopathy are important factors for improved survival in these patients [23]. Neurologic assessment and CT and CTA of the brain are essential in assessing the extent of injury and triaging these patients for appropriate next steps management including use of hyperosmolar therapy, invasive intracranial monitoring, and neurosurgical intervention.

Stab Injuries to the head caused by knives, arrows, nail guns, spears and other sharp objects often cause more localized damage compared to ballistic injury, however the depth and trajectory of the penetrating injury can vary. Advanced imaging such as CT and CTA of the brain will help evaluate depth, trajectory, and potential involvement of vascular and other vital structures.

Unique Challenges in Diagnosis and Treatment

The surge in penetrating trauma, particularly from intentional, interpersonal violence such as stabbings and shootings, presents unique challenges in both diagnosis and treatment. The trauma center at the University of Chicago, designated as a Level 1 Adult Trauma Center in 2018, has experienced an 82% increase in overall trauma presentations from 2019 to 2021. Penetrating traumas, accounting for 39–49% of all adult cases, place a considerable burden on the healthcare system.

Moreover, the lack of standardized data infrastructure around gun violence exacerbates the challenge of understanding and addressing this complex issue. Basic questions about the target population, acute management, surgical intervention, critical care, outcomes, long-term complications, rehabilitation, and reintegration strategies remain unanswered. This dearth of information impedes the development of effective programs and policies, contrasting starkly with the robust data systems in place for tracking motor vehicle-related deaths.

Additionally, the target population of gunshot wound victims often comprises young and otherwise healthy individuals. This demographic characteristic, coupled with the broader societal burden of violence and socioeconomic deprivation, introduces a unique challenge in family interactions during these situations. The inherent sensitivity required in managing families dealing with the aftermath of gunshot wounds further complicate the already intricate landscape of penetrating trauma. The emotional toll, coupled with potential long-term physical and psychological consequences, underscores the need for holistic and compassionate approaches in trauma care that extends beyond the immediate medical intervention. Addressing these multifaceted challenges is crucial for providing comprehensive and effective care to both the victims and their families in the aftermath of penetrating trauma.

Management and Gaps

In Cook County Hospital in Chicago (1983–1992) an aggressive surgical strategy was adopted in management of cranial gunshot wound victims. Of 480 patients with an overall mortality rate of 34%, 150 patients underwent craniotomy [25]; the study supported the premise that patients with severe neurological deficits and massive cerebral damage can benefit from aggressive treatment and make satisfactory recoveries. Additional data suggests that early aggressive resuscitation including aggressive management with blood products and hyperosmolar therapy is independently associated with survival in PBI [23]. More recent data suggests that a bundle of aggressive resuscitation and care including early neurosurgical intervention and intracranial pressure monitoring is associated with a mortality benefit in a population of moderate and severe predominantly isolated PBI [26, 27].

The neurocritical care unit at the University of Chicago is the primary facility for treating victims of gunshot wounds to the head and spine. Despite the grim outlook often associated with penetrating brain injuries, the neurocritical care team has observed an approximate 50% survival rate over the last 5 years while adopting an aggressive early involvement, resuscitation, and monitoring strategy. Most importantly, we recognize that traditional prognostic signs utilized in traumatic brain injury may not be always applicable to PBI. In addition, a multidisciplinary team approach that emphasizes avoidance of early prognostication is adopted early in care [28].

Considering the prevailing challenges and gaps in knowledge regarding penetrating trauma, the neurocritical care group at the university of Chicago in collaboration with Trauma Surgery and Neurosurgery launched the first of its kind symposium on penetrating brain injury on September of 2023. In parallel, the group is working diligently to put together the first Firearm Inflicted Brain Injury Data Commons to offer a promising avenue for developing a comprehensive understanding of this disease state. By building a consensus data dictionary, collecting and harmonizing data, and establishing a data commons infrastructure, this project aims to provide clinicians, policymakers, and researchers with the essential tools for advancing research goals and improving outcomes for individuals affected by penetrating brain trauma.

Difficult Family Interactions: Role of Violence Recovery

Traumatic brain and spinal cord injuries represent some of the most challenging medical conditions, not only for patients but also for their families. The road to recovery is often fraught with emotional and social challenges, and navigating through difficult family interactions becomes crucial. Here we delve into the emotional impact on families dealing with traumatic brain and spine injuries, exploring coping mechanisms, support systems, and the pivotal role of violence recovery programs in the journey toward healing.

Emotional Impact on Families

Coping with Trauma

Families confronted with traumatic brain and spinal cord injuries experience a profound emotional disturbance. The abruptness and severity of such incidents often plunge family members into a whirlwind of shock, fear, grief, and uncertainty. Navigating these intricate emotions necessitates the adoption of coping mechanisms. The impact on children, especially in cases of parental trauma, is particularly challenging. Young children, who lose a parent, may find themselves competing with the affected parent for attention from the healthy parent. Similarly, older children living away from home may grapple with conflicting loyalties between their own families and that of their parents. Families with several young children are particularly vulnerable, and when coupled with financial challenges and limited social support, the stress can reach levels that impede normal functioning. Moreover, conflicts with the medical team, comprising doctors, nurses, and therapists, further intensify the stressors. Traumatic brain injuries predominantly affect young adult men, consequently impacting young, burgeoning families, often with one or more young children, and exacerbating financial burdens [29]. The aftermath of traumatic brain injury introduces heightened stress, increased dysfunction, and a cascade of issues, leading to a vicious cycle of mounting stress, escalating conflict, and persistent challenges. Attempts to break this cycle often prove futile, amplifying the complexity of the situation.

Support Systems for Families

Establishing a robust support system is essential for families confronting traumatic brain and spinal cord injuries, both throughout and following the trauma. In the domain of neurocritical care, we underscore the imperative of delivering unwavering support to families right from the onset. This entails clear and early communication with family members or surrogates, guiding them through the intricacies of care steps and decisions, and initiating early involvement with social work and trauma recovery resources.

While various avenues are available, such as connecting with families who have encountered similar challenges to foster shared understanding and empathy, we particularly highlight the significance of commencing support early in the traumatic journey. This involves consistent, informative interactions with the family, ensuring they are kept abreast of care processes and decisions. Additionally, elucidating team roles and dynamics becomes crucial in averting family frustration and nurturing a collaborative healing environment. Furthermore, we extend our assistance to reach out to extended family members, explaining the patient's condition to alleviate the burden from the primary caregiver.

It is imperative to traverse this support framework with empathy, refraining from presumptions about shared experiences or claiming to completely comprehend a family member's emotional journey. Recognizing the distinct challenges each family faces and offering a compassionate understanding of their situation contributes to a more effective and considerate support system.

Support System for Team Members

Establishing a resilient support structure for the medical teams immersed in the acute care of neurotrauma patients is indispensable. Within the dynamic realm of neurocritical care, we underscore the crucial necessity of providing steadfast support to healthcare professionals right from the initiation of their involvement. This involves transparent communication, guiding team members through the complexities of care protocols and decisions, and fostering early engagement with additional support services and resources.

While various avenues are available, such as connecting with other medical teams who have confronted similar challenges, fostering shared understanding and empathy, we particularly emphasize the significance of initiating support early in the neurotrauma care journey. This includes consistent, informative check-ins with the medical team, ensuring they are adequately coping with the daily stress presented by their role, as well as provide resources and interventions early on to tackle any concerns that arise. Moreover, providing clarity on individual roles and team dynamics as well as clarifying available resources and escalation protocols is integral in preventing professional frustration and cultivating a collaborative healing environment.

In addition to these measures, we extend our support by actively checking in on care team members, recognizing the cumulative toll of trauma as they navigate patient after patient. Acknowledging and addressing the potential impact on their overall well-being is essential for sustaining a healthy and resilient medical team. We help in facilitating a supportive atmosphere, where healthcare professionals can openly discuss their experiences and seek guidance as needed. Recognizing the unique stressors each healthcare professional encounters and providing a compassionate understanding of their situation contributes to a more effective and considerate support system.

Role of Violence Recovery Programs

Early Engagement of Violence Recovery Team Members

The inclusion of Violence Recovery Program (VRP) team members in the support system for families grappling with violence-induced traumatic brain and spinal cord injuries is paramount to fostering positive family dynamics. Early engagement of

VRP ensures that families receive specialized assistance in navigating the emotional aftermath of violent incidents. VRP play a pivotal role in offering trauma-informed care, guiding family members through the complexities of their emotions, and facilitating communication within the family unit. Their involvement provides a tailored approach to addressing the unique challenges associated with violence-induced trauma, helping family members cope with grief, fear, and uncertainty. By initiating their support early in the traumatic journey, VRP members contribute to the prevention of potential conflicts within the family, promoting resilience, and aiding in breaking the cycle of mounting stress. Their expertise in violence recovery equips families with coping mechanisms and strategies to rebuild relationships, creating a more supportive and understanding environment. The favorable impact of their intervention extends beyond individual family members to the overall family dynamics, reinforcing the importance of incorporating specialized violence recovery support into the broader framework of care for those affected by traumatic brain and spinal cord injuries.

Community Outreach

Violence recovery programs play a pivotal role in helping families navigate the challenging aftermath of traumatic brain and spinal cord injuries. Community outreach initiatives can raise awareness about the impact of violence on families and provide resources for support. Educational programs within communities can help dispel myths and reduce the stigma associated with such injuries, fostering a more compassionate and understanding environment. Furthermore, education and awareness as well as working with community leaders to create opportunities for survivors of acute brain and spinal cord injury is of paramount importance to foster.

Mental Health Resources

Access to mental health resources is crucial for both patients and their families. Violence recovery programs should collaborate with mental health professionals to ensure that adequate support is available. This includes counseling services, therapy sessions, and educational programs to help families cope with the emotional challenges they may encounter during the recovery process.

Dealing with traumatic brain and spinal cord injuries is a multifaceted challenge that extends beyond the patient, their families and healthcare providers. Recognizing the emotional impact, establishing robust support systems, and integrating violence recovery programs are essential components in facilitating the healing process. Through a collective effort, communities can work towards creating a more compassionate and supportive environment for families facing these difficult circumstances.

Brain Death and Organ Donation

Definition of Brain Death

Medical Perspectives

Brain death (BD) or death by neurologic criteria (DNC) accounts for 2% of adult and 5% of pediatric in-hospital death in the United States [30]. The American Academy of Neurology (AAN) established practical parameters of brain death in 1995 that have been revised in 2010 and 2023 [31]. BD or DNC is defined as the complete and permanent loss of all functions of the entire brain, including the brainstem, resulting in coma, brainstem areflexia, and apnea in the setting of an adequate stimulus.

The Uniform Determination of Death Act provides a legal basis for BD diagnosis, equating death by circulatory-respiratory criteria and DNC. Embraced by five world federations and 30 international, national, and regional medical societies, this alignment was reinforced by the World Brain Death Project in 2020 [32]. The clinical diagnosis of BD necessitates demonstrating catastrophic and irreversible brain injury, absence of confounders, clinical coma with the loss of brainstem reflexes, loss of independent capacity to breathe, and absence of blood flow to the brain on ancillary tests if a full clinical evaluation is impeded.

Legal and Ethical Considerations

1. **Variability in Beliefs:** Diverse cultural, religious, and individual beliefs surround death.
2. **Global Legislation:** Varying global legislation and definitions of brain death pose challenges.
3. **Medicolegal Framework:** The legal framework for determining death raises implications for healthcare professionals. Despite growing acceptance, BD/DNC faces ongoing ethical and legal challenges, with certain ambiguity in definitions. For instance, the concept of BD in the US requires loss of whole brain function, differing from the United Kingdom's focus on brainstem function alone. Some variability exists in the number and qualification of examiners, mandatory waiting periods, and details of clinical evaluation and ancillary testing.

One approach to mitigate family objections is obtaining consent before evaluation, addressing ethical concerns such as autonomy, freedom of religion, and concerns about potential harm. However, the evaluation for death by circulatory-respiratory criteria does not require consent (unless otherwise stipulated by the institution's policy or state laws or regulations), emphasizing clinicians' non-negotiable role.

While state laws currently don't mandate consent to perform a BD evaluation, the AAN and the World Brain Death Project recommend notifying families before a BD evaluation.

Challenges

Navigating critical situations for surrogate decision-makers involves emotional responses, prognostic considerations, decisions about life support withdrawal, and respecting end-of-life wishes. Communicating brain death diagnoses to families requires cultural sensitivity and empathy, emphasizing the irreversible nature of brain death and its treatment implications. Conflicts may arise, particularly when grief, misunderstanding, distrust, or religious differences contribute to disagreements. Although ethical arguments exist both for and against accommodating objections to BD, most clinicians (and medical scientific societies) advocate against continuing organ support after BD diagnosis [33]. A brief period of accommodation may be supported.

A few states' laws accommodate objections to BD, such as Illinois considering religious beliefs in determining time of death. In New Jersey, death can be declared only by circulatory-respiratory criteria if a patient has a religious objection to BD.

Organ Donation Process

Counseling Families in Collaboration with Organ Procurement Organizations

After declaring BD, maintaining organ preservation through medication and physiological monitoring is crucial. Counseling families about organ donation following a brain death diagnosis is sensitive and challenging. Conversations about donation opportunities should occur separately after the declaration of death, ideally by knowledgeable personnel separate from the primary care team. The request for organ donation should ideally be performed by trained personnel belonging to the local Organ Procurement Organization. Family consent is essential for organ donation to proceed, in cases that the deceased had not previously declared their intent for donation. Coordinating with the healthcare team and donor coordinator before approaching families is recommended to ensure proper timing, location, and consideration of potential conflicts. Communicating with families may encounter challenges like decision-making issues, attention span, and concentration. Healthcare professionals must use a sensitive and compassionate approach to support families in making optimal decisions for psychological well-being, respecting both religious beliefs and legal requirements.

Case Studies and Practical Insights

Real-life Neurotrauma Example

On a certain day of 2018, a father arrives home to find his son bloodied and dazed. The kitchen floor was covered in blood, Dog paw prints were also found next to the imprint of where a human body had lain. The patient had suffered an apparent gunshot wound to his head. He was first taken to a local community hospital where his right temple was noted to have a 3 × 5 cm wound with exposed brain matter. The patient's mother was summoned emergently. She extensively researched the University of Chicago and its Level 1 Adult Trauma Center, which had recently reopened after a 30-year hiatus in response to community advocacy. Recognizing its specialized neurotrauma care, 24/7 staffing, and dedicated transportation network, she believed that transferring her son to this facility held the potential for lifesaving interventions, especially considering its success in treating numerous patients with penetrating trauma, including gunshot wounds. Before being flown over to the University of Chicago, the patient's mental status deteriorated, and required endotracheal intubation. A head CT (Fig. 1) scan at the University of Chicago demonstrated his penetrating injury along with multiple areas of bleeding in his brain: small right frontal and interhemispheric subdural hematomas, right parietal subarachnoid hemorrhage, and multifocal small hemorrhagic contusions. As a result of these injuries, his brain was becoming overwhelmed with edema—every ridge and groove was swollen, and one hemisphere was starting to shift over and compress the other. As the swelling continued to increase over the subsequent 24 hours, the buildup of pressure was threatening to cause further brain damage, and his medical team decided that it was imperative to place invasive monitors. Initially resistant, his parents were hesitant about invasive procedures, such as placing a bolt into his head, but the doctor's insistence on monitoring intracranial pressure and addressing swelling ultimately proved crucial, contributing vital hours to his life during the critical period. Considering persistently elevated intracranial pressures, the neurocritical care team elected to put him in a medically induced coma for about 2 weeks, and his body temperature was also slightly cooled to slow his metabolism. Then, once his high intracranial pressures had subsided, he underwent a series of reconstructive surgeries to repair his complex craniofacial injuries, performed as a collaborative effort between multiple surgical teams. Twenty-four days after he first arrived in the Neuro ICU, he was noted to have followed his first command. Every day thereafter he started doing more of what was asked of him, and he was able to be transferred to a rehabilitation facility a little over a month after he was first admitted to the hospital. He has since then made a remarkable recovery and continues to make steady progress receiving outpatient rehabilitation at a specialized institution. Amidst emotional upheaval, his family found solace in the unwavering support of a compassionate chaplain, appreciating the crucial role played by the neurocritical care team's effective communication, understanding, and patience. Her mother, spiritually grounded, saw divine intervention in her son's survival, and the efforts of

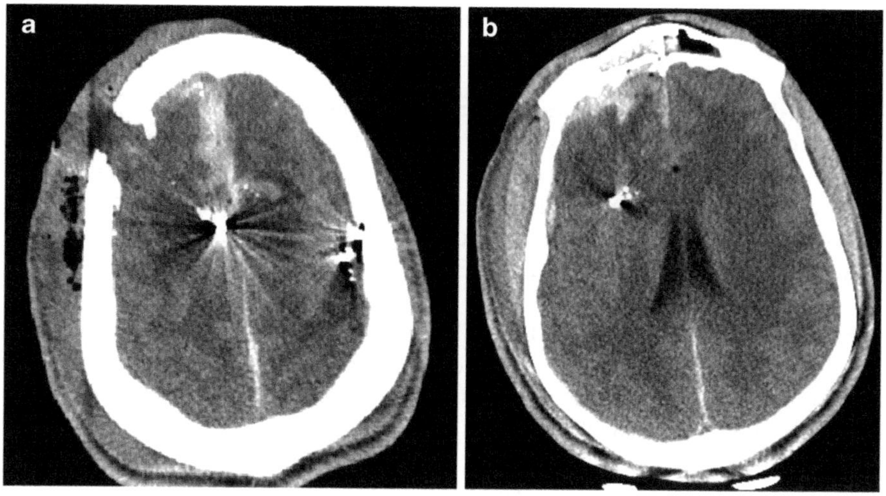

Fig. 1 (**a** and **b**) show intracranial metallic fragments corresponding to penetrating gunshot wound to the head, skull fractue, subarachnoid hemorrhage and subdural hematoma as well as diffuse brain swelling

the nursing and medical staff, who tirelessly encouraged her son during his coma, played a pivotal role in his courageous recovery, reinforcing the importance of love, support, and positive engagement in challenging medical situations.

Future Directions in Neurotrauma Care

Advancements and Emerging Technologies

Precision Medicine The advent of precision medicine will likely revolutionize neurotrauma care by tailoring treatments to individual patient profiles. Genetic profiling and molecular diagnostics will enable a deeper understanding of the underlying mechanisms of injury and patient-specific responses to interventions. Targeted therapies, including drugs designed to modulate specific pathways implicated in neurotrauma, are emerging as promising options for personalized treatment plans. One recent example in the field of neurotrauma is the use of Glial Fibrillary Acidic Protein (GFAP), now cleared by the Food and Drug Administration (FDA) to determine need for head computed tomography (CT) within 12 h after mild TBI [34].

Neuroprotection Strategies Neuroprotection remains a key focus area of research in advancing neurotrauma care. Pharmacological agents targeting excitotoxicity, oxidative stress, and inflammation show promise in minimizing secondary damage. While promising in multiple animal models of traumatic cerebral lesions, the use of these potential interventions in humans has remained limited [35], but remains the topic of aggressive research.

Advanced Imaging Modalities Advanced imaging modalities play a pivotal role in refining the diagnosis and treatment planning for neurotrauma. Functional MRI (fMRI) provides insights into brain function and connectivity, aiding in understanding the impact of trauma. Diffusion Tensor Imaging (DTI) maps of white matter tracts offer valuable information on axonal injuries, while PET scans detect metabolic changes and neuroinflammation [36, 37].

Telemedicine in Neurocritical Care Telemedicine has emerged as a transformative force in neurocritical care. Remote monitoring enables real-time tracking of vital signs, neurological status, and treatment responses, providing a comprehensive approach to acute and post-acute care even in resource limited locations. Virtual consultations bridge geographical gaps, ensuring that patients, particularly those in rural or underserved areas, receive expert guidance.

Artificial Intelligence (AI) and Machine Learning AI and machine learning algorithms have ushered in a new era of data analysis in neurotrauma care. These technologies can process complex neuroimaging data, automating tasks such as lesion detection, segmentation, and quantitative assessments. Predictive models leverage AI to forecast patient outcomes, optimizing treatment strategies and enabling early identification of potential complications [38–40].

Monitoring and Sensing Technologies Wearable sensors and implantable devices are emerging as integral components of continuous monitoring in neurotrauma care [41]. Wearable sensors track physiological parameters, such as heart rate and oxygen saturation, offering real-time insights into patient status. Implantable neurosensors can provide continuous monitoring of brain activity, eventually facilitating personalized and adaptive neurocritical care interventions.

Neuroinformatics and Big Data Analytics Neuroinformatics platforms and big data analytics aggregate diverse datasets, including clinical, genomic, and imaging data. This wealth of information enables researchers to uncover patterns, correlations, and novel insights, contributing to evidence-based decision-making in neurotrauma care. The collaborative nature of neuroinformatics platforms facilitates multi-institutional research, pooling resources, and data to accelerate the pace of discoveries in neurotrauma care [42, 43].

Conclusion

In summary, our journey through neurotrauma care has uncovered a profound impact on our community of patients, care providers, policy makers and researcher. From the imperative of early neurocritical care engagement to the challenges of prognostication, our understanding has evolved, emphasizing the need for personalized interventions, collaborative research, and holistic support systems.

Moving forward, the evolution of neurotrauma care hinges on recognizing the collaborative efforts of dedicated and trained neurocritical care professionals. Embracing precision medicine, incorporating emerging technologies, avoiding nihilism, and nurturing a compassionate approach are integral aspects. The call to action echoes a commitment to ongoing learning, promoting resilient paradigms that not only cater to immediate clinical requirements but also acknowledge the emotional and social aspects affecting patients and their families. Through collective endeavors, the aim is to propel neurotrauma care forward, ensuring its adaptability, evidence-based nature, and alignment with the ever-evolving intersection of medical science and empathetic patient care.

References

1. Prevention CfDCa. National center for health statistics: mortality data on CDC WONDER. 2023.
2. Finkelstein ECP, Miller T, et al. The incidence and economic burden of injuries in the United States. New York: Oxford University Press; 2006.
3. Badhiwala JH, Wilson JR, Fehlings MG. Global burden of traumatic brain and spinal cord injury. Lancet Neurol. 2019;18:24–5.
4. Pham X, Ray J, Neto AS, et al. Association of neurocritical care services with mortality and functional outcomes for adults with brain injury: a systematic review and meta-analysis. JAMA Neurol. 2022;79:1049–58.
5. Chesnut RM, Marshall LF, Klauber MR, et al. The role of secondary brain injury in determining outcome from severe head injury. J Trauma. 1993;34:216–22.
6. Hinson HE, Rowell S, Schreiber M. Clinical evidence of inflammation driving secondary brain injury: a systematic review. J Trauma Acute Care Surg. 2015;78:184–91.
7. Fuller G, Hasler RM, Mealing N, et al. The association between admission systolic blood pressure and mortality in significant traumatic brain injury: a multi-centre cohort study. Injury. 2014;45:612–7.
8. Roberts CJ, Barber J, Temkin NR, et al. Clinical outcomes after traumatic brain injury and exposure to extracranial surgery: a TRACK-TBI study. JAMA Surg. 2023;
9. Kuchler J, Tronnier F, Smith E, Gliemroth J, Tronnier VM, Ditz C. The impact of intrahospital transports on brain tissue metabolism in patients with acute brain injury. Neurocrit Care. 2019;30:216–23.
10. Martin M, Cook F, Lobo D, et al. Secondary insults and adverse events during intrahospital transport of severe traumatic brain-injured patients. Neurocrit Care. 2017;26:87–95.
11. Trofimov AO, Agarkova DI, Trofimova KA, Atochin DN, Nemoto EM, Bragin DE. Dynamics of intracranial pressure and cerebrovascular reactivity during intrahospital transportation of traumatic brain injury patients in coma. Neurocrit Care. 2023;
12. Cronberg T, Greer DM, Lilja G, Moulaert V, Swindell P, Rossetti AO. Brain injury after cardiac arrest: from prognostication of comatose patients to rehabilitation. Lancet Neurol. 2020;19:611–22.
13. Pratt AK, Chang JJ, Sederstrom NO. A fate worse than death: prognostication of devastating brain injury. Crit Care Med. 2019;47:591–8.
14. Steyerberg EW, Mushkudiani N, Perel P, et al. Predicting outcome after traumatic brain injury: development and international validation of prognostic scores based on admission characteristics. PLoS Med. 2008;5:e165. discussion e

15. Izzy S, Compton R, Carandang R, Hall W, Muehlschlegel S. Self-fulfilling prophecies through withdrawal of care: do they exist in traumatic brain injury, too? Neurocrit Care. 2013;19:347–63.
16. McCrea MA, Giacino JT, Barber J, et al. Functional outcomes over the first year after moderate to severe traumatic brain injury in the prospective, longitudinal TRACK-TBI study. JAMA Neurol. 2021;78:982–92.
17. Barbiellini Amidei C, Salmaso L, Bellio S, Saia M. Epidemiology of traumatic spinal cord injury: a large population-based study. Spinal Cord. 2022;60:812–9.
18. Moller F, Rupp R, Weidner N, Gutenbrunner C, Kalke YB, Abel RF. Long term outcome of functional independence and quality of life after traumatic SCI in Germany. Spinal Cord. 2021;59:902–9.
19. Stensman R. Adjustment to traumatic spinal cord injury. A longitudinal study of self-reported quality of life. Paraplegia. 1994;32:416–22.
20. Carney N, Totten AM, O'Reilly C, et al. Guidelines for the management of severe traumatic brain injury, fourth edition. Neurosurgery. 2017;80:6–15.
21. 2021 data brief the state of health for blacks in Chicago 2021.
22. Aarabi B, Tofighi B, Kufera JA, et al. Predictors of outcome in civilian gunshot wounds to the head. J Neurosurg. 2014;120:1138–46.
23. Joseph B, Aziz H, Pandit V, et al. Improving survival rates after civilian gunshot wounds to the brain. J Am Coll Surg. 2014;218:58–65.
24. Cernak I, Noble-Haeusslein LJ. Traumatic brain injury: an overview of pathobiology with emphasis on military populations. J Cereb Blood Flow Metab. 2010;30:255–66.
25. Stone JL, Lichtor T, Fitzgerald LF. Gunshot wounds to the head in civilian practice. Neurosurgery. 1995;37:1104–10. discussion 10-2
26. Mansour A, Powla PP, Fakhri F, et al. Comparative effectiveness of early neurosurgical intervention in civilian penetrating brain injury management. Neurosurgery. 2023;
27. Mansour A, Rowell S, Powla PP, Horowitz P, Goldenberg FD, Lazaridis C. Comparative effectiveness of intracranial pressure monitoring vs no monitoring in severe penetrating brain injury management. JAMA Netw Open. 2023;6:e231077.
28. Zakrison TL, Essig R, Polcari A, et al. Review paper on penetrating brain injury: ethical quandaries in the trauma bay and beyond. Ann Surg. 2023;277:66–72.
29. Verhaeghe S, Defloor T, Grypdonck M. Stress and coping among families of patients with traumatic brain injury: a review of the literature. J Clin Nurs. 2005;14:1004–12.
30. Trowbridge A, Walter JK, McConathey E, Morrison W, Feudtner C. Modes of death within a children's hospital. Pediatrics. 2018;142
31. Practice parameters for determining brain death in adults (summary statement). The Quality Standards Subcommittee of the American Academy of Neurology. Neurology. 1995;45:1012–4.
32. Greer DM, Shemie SD, Lewis A, et al. Determination of Brain Death/Death by Neurologic Criteria: The World Brain Death Project. JAMA. 2020;324:1078–97.
33. Lewis A, Adams N, Varelas P, Greer D, Caplan A. Organ support after death by neurologic criteria: results of a survey of US neurologists. Neurology. 2016;87:827–34.
34. Okonkwo DO, Puffer RC, Puccio AM, et al. Point-of-care platform blood biomarker testing of glial fibrillary acidic protein versus S100 calcium-binding protein B for prediction of traumatic brain injuries: a transforming research and clinical knowledge in traumatic brain injury study. J Neurotrauma. 2020;37:2460–7.
35. Stocchetti N, Taccone FS, Citerio G, et al. Neuroprotection in acute brain injury: an up-to-date review. Crit Care. 2015;19:186.
36. Lee AL. Advanced imaging of traumatic brain injury. Korean J Neurotrauma. 2020;16:3–17.
37. Smith LGF, Milliron E, Ho ML, et al. Advanced neuroimaging in traumatic brain injury: an overview. Neurosurg Focus. 2019;47:E17.
38. Courville E, Kazim SF, Vellek J, et al. Machine learning algorithms for predicting outcomes of traumatic brain injury: a systematic review and meta-analysis. Surg Neurol Int. 2023;14:262.

39. Moyer JD, Lee P, Bernard C, et al. Machine learning-based prediction of emergency neurosurgery within 24 h after moderate to severe traumatic brain injury. World J Emerg Surg. 2022;17:42.
40. Wang J, Yin MJ, Wen HC. Prediction performance of the machine learning model in predicting mortality risk in patients with traumatic brain injuries: a systematic review and meta-analysis. BMC Med Inform Decis Mak. 2023;23:142.
41. Schmid W, Fan Y, Chi T, et al. Review of wearable technologies and machine learning methodologies for systematic detection of mild traumatic brain injuries. J Neural Eng. 2021;18
42. Flechet M, Grandas FG, Meyfroidt G. Informatics in neurocritical care: new ideas for Big Data. Curr Opin Crit Care. 2016;22:87–93.
43. Foreman B. Neurocritical care: bench to bedside (Eds. Claude Hemphill, Michael James) integrating and using Big Data in neurocritical care. Neurotherapeutics. 2020;17:593–605.

Orthopaedic Trauma

Jason Strelzow

The orthopaedic traumatologist plays a critical role in trauma care. Fundamentally, musculosketetal injuries are present in over 50% of all Level 1 trauma patients with trauma databases reporting nearly 80% of trauma related surgeries are orthopaedic in nature [1–3]. The successful integration of orthopaedic surgery into modern trauma care is paramount to provide timely, effective care and optimize outcomes. Modern urban trauma care and the creation of successful orthopaedic trauma program requires a number of steps for success including:

- Assessing the need
- Developing a business plan
- Establishing partnerships
- Recruiting Skilled staff
- Set up infrastructure and facilities
- Develop protocols and guidelines
- Implement quality improvement initiatives
- Promote the program
- Monitoring progress and adapting to changes

Many of these factors are self-evident however, a number require exploration as critical and orthopaedic specific aspects of these factors can ensure success.

J. Strelzow (✉)
Department of Orthopaedic Surgery, The University of Chicago, Chicago, IL, USA
e-mail: jstrelzow@uchicagomedicine.org

S. O. Rogers, Jr (ed.), *Creating a Modern Trauma Center*,
https://doi.org/10.1007/978-3-031-66524-0_8

Assessing the Need

Successfully building a trauma center and orthopaedic trauma program requires the careful, thoughtful planning which often begins with understanding the local health-care market, the expected trauma volumes and the role that a new trauma center may play in environment. Understanding the patient demographics, expected trauma epidemiology, and the established local trauma networks is critical. Furthermore, gauging the potential trauma volume helps determine the remainder of the required steps for trauma program success.

Globally, orthopaedic trauma care needs are tied closely to the overall trauma volume at a specific level 1 trauma center [1, 3, 4]. The demands of modern trauma suggest that injury severity, complexity, and the proportion of peri-articular, pelvis and acetabular injuries is rising with a proportional fall in long bone and less complex fractures as these are managed in community level or non-Level 1 trauma centers [3, 4]. Furthermore, true poly-trauma patients with multiple musculoskeletal injuries is common [1, 2, 5]. Effective, established high acuity trauma centers can provide efficient, high-quality care that improved mortality while not being associated with high commensurate increases in resources and cost [6]. While trauma patterns differ based on location, environment, and time most typically road accidents, pedestrian struck and fall mechanisms make up the majority of injuries seen in trauma centers, with a smaller proportion made up of penetrating causes [5, 7, 8]. Therefore, understanding and adapting the needs of the trauma center to the community is critical. Fundamentally this establishes and hones the central question that must be asked before moving forward, 'what our goals' as a trauma center are, and orthopaedic trauma center.

In establishing our recent modern urban trauma center these questions were simple. In an urban trauma care desert, with a high rate of gun-violence, and surrounded by highways and a socioeconomically disadvantaged population we had immediate and clear establishment of priorities and focus. There was an understanding that trauma care would challenge conventional notions of patient trauma pathology—expectations of somewhere on the order of 30–50% of trauma would result from penetrating injuries with the remainder from high energy motor vehicle accidents. High acuity, high severity injuries that required prompt attention and likely consideration of damage control surgery. Additionally, given the location of our center we would be providing much needed care to an underserviced, and vulnerable population that would necessitate navigating social and financial challenges to optimize access to care.

Developing a Business Plan

Logically establishing a business plan in medicine feels counterintuitive to the ethos of medicine and the delivery of just healthcare however, to provide such care is both expensive and financially fraught with challenges. Orthopaedics is a high cost, financially expensive service line and the addition of level 1 trauma care in the setting complex orthopaedic cases can be expensive. The challenges of trauma system fiscal solvency can be exacerbated by well publicized impacts of type of trauma, payer mix and complex case loads [9, 10]. Despite these challenges several publications have demonstrated the financial viability and effect of orthopaedic trauma programs on hospital systems [9, 11–15]. Thus, a sounds business plan is critical to allow for the delivery of high-quality, efficient, and comprehensive care to, while ensuring financial sustainability and growth for the center such that it can continue to provide care long-term. Consider the following:

- Services to offer –
  - Fracture management
  - Joint Reconstruction
  - Limb Salvage & Infection
- Facilities & Equipment requirements –
  - Surgical suites
  - Equipment & Tools
  - Rehabilitation partnerships
- Referral network –
  - Primary care physicians
  - Physical medicine and rehabilitation (PMR)
  - Occupational & Physical Therapy
- Staffing –
  - Number of surgeons
  - Associated support (nursing, physician extenders, social workers)
- Financial projections –

Within the business plan establishing the overall desire and breadth of services to offer is important. Orthopaedic Trauma focuses primarily on the delivery of fracture care however, adjunctive interests and skills allows for trauma surgeons to also provide associated care. Associated programs can be offered in reconstructive joints, as well as robust programs focused on limb salvage and infection in partnerships with plastic surgery, vascular injury and PMR can help provide more robust trauma aftercare. Additionally, these programs can be financially positive to the institution [15, 16].

This business plan provides a comprehensive roadmap for establishing and operating an orthopaedic trauma center. By focusing on delivering exceptional care, building strong referral networks, and implementing effective marketing strategies, the center can achieve long-term success while positively impacting the lives of patients with orthopaedic trauma injuries.

Set Up Infrastructure and Facilities

Orthopaedics remains a specialty that requires large quantities of equipment, tools and supplies which represent a significant cost expenditure of the institution. These costs include the purchase and maintenance of surgical instruments, implants, and other devices necessary for orthopedic procedures. Additionally, there is a need for specialized equipment such as X-ray machines, MRI scanners, and fluoroscopy machines to aid in diagnosis and treatment. The cost of orthopedic supplies can be high as a result of materials, largely titanium or cobalt-chromium alloys, and production expenses. In order to manage these costs, institutions must carefully plan their budget and procurement processes. Hospitals may negotiate with suppliers to secure favorable pricing or explore alternative options for purchasing equipment and supplies. Furthermore, orthopedic departments can implement strategies to optimize resource utilization. The implementation of evidence-based practices and standardized protocols can help streamline processes and reduce unnecessary expenditures. Additionally, involvement in stewardship programs and surgeon price containment strategies have demonstrated success in optimizing cost (up to 20% decrease in equipment costs in some studies) without effects on patient safety and outcomes [17–21]. Overall, managing the costs associated with orthopedic equipment, tools, and supplies is essential for healthcare institutions. By implementing efficient procurement processes, optimizing resource utilization, and exploring cost-saving alternatives, institutions can ensure the provision of high-quality orthopedic care while minimizing financial burdens.

At our facility we established a single vendor contract model for implants and equipment to drive down overall costs. We established exceptions for injury specific injuries and circumstances and negotiated improved pricing for equipment not otherwise covered under the single vendor contract. Additionally, trauma equipment trays were specially built to optimize critical need equipment to minimize tray numbers, reduce equipment purchases and standardize trays. Once such tray was the spanning external fixator tray which incorporated the basic equipment required for the common injuries needing stabilizing fixators (pelvic ring, femur, knee dislocations and periarticular lower extremity injuries). This tray was light weight, simple and reduced the standard external fixator tray from 4 trays to 1 (Fig. 1).

While specific discussion of the aggregate payer mix and the role of mechanism on the effects of institutional financial analysis are beyond the scope of this chapter little is established in the literature to help guide these discussions. Overall, it is

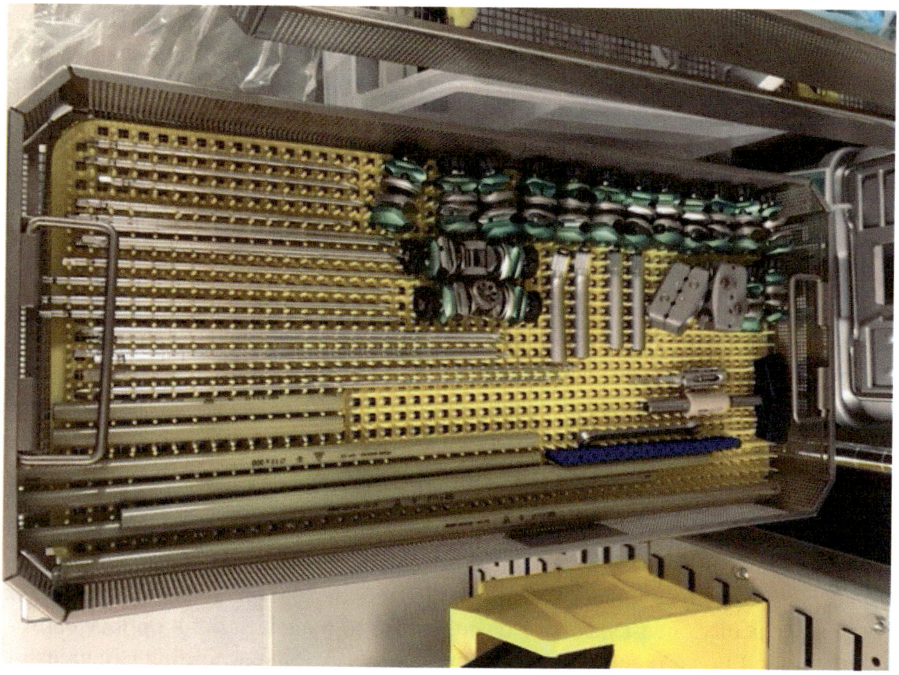

Fig. 1 A customized standard external fixator tray developed with an optimized set of equipment to allow for reduced tray weight, and the most configurations of potential Ex-fix constructs

important to understand the financial impact orthopaedic trauma can provide to an institution and recent analysis has demonstrated positive contribution margins, and direct financial effects of an orthopaedic trauma program.

Hiring Staff

Determine the required staffing levels, including orthopaedic surgeons, nurses and physician extenders is important to establish the required staffing levels to ensure efficient and effective operations. Factors such as patient volume, complexity of cases, and the desired level of patient care should be considered. It is important to have enough surgeons to handle the workload and provide timely care to patients. Appreciating the expected patient and operative volume to mitigate burnout is important [22]. This can be particularly challenging when first building a trauma center as many of these issues are unknown, however, if planned appropriately the expected volume and targeting operative workload can be generally estimated. As the program matures understanding the next 'growth' phase is critical to ensure a steady and sustainable staffing level. Using wRVU or case load volumes can be helpful to ensure onboarding physicians feel fulfilled and appropriately valued is critical [23]. Although benchmarks exist each facility must appreciate the specifics of their program, institution, and patient population. The Medical Group Management Association and the Association of American Medical Colleges provide productivity benchmarks however significant limitations exist in their applicability [23]. Fundamentally, building a team of similarly focused, diverse and talented individuals is paramount for success of the programmatic mission. In trauma this continues to be a challenge as the number of trauma fellows training compared to available jobs is one of the lowest across the specialities [24]. Critically, finding the right person includes establishing common goals, expectations, and aligning skill sets to complement the group. In academic centers this may requiring understanding the institution needs, expectations and requirements for success, such as research requirements, educational involvement, and administrative roles while in the private or employed models this may be a simpler calculus.

Nursing support and physician extenders also play a crucial role in the orthopaedic department, providing direct patient care, assisting in surgeries, and coordinating patient education and follow-up care. Their value cannot be overstated from both an efficiency and patient care perspective with established indirect economic impacts for the hospital [25]. The number of nurses needed will depend on factors such as patient volume, the acuity of cases, and the desired nurse-to-patient ratio for optimal care.

At our facility we successful transitioned our work force according to increasing trauma volumes, complexity demands and a growing program. The program has expanded to 4 full time faculty with 2 advanced practice providers, 3 nurses and an administrator who oversees our trauma group. Additionally, we have plans to add a fifth surgeon and additional trauma nursing coordinator to help patient flow and transitions of care (Fig. 2).

One critical aspect of hiring to understanding trauma call coverage as this can be a source of burnout, exhaustion, and provider unhappiness. Trauma call coverage can be facilitated several ways without any specific superiority of one over another. Initially, given our limited number of adult traumatologists we established a paradigm of all adult orthopaedic surgeons cover call with a clear adult traumatologist backup schedule (Table 1). This allows surgeons who were not comfortable with adult level 1 call to have an established line of communication and help if required while providing autonomy for them to cover cases they felt were appropriate. The management of long bones injuries (tibias, femurs), irrigation and debridement of open wounds and septic joints, and application of external fixators were cases established as within the realm of all orthopaedic surgeons and thus expected to be managed by the on-call attending barring any unforeseen issues. This allowed the trauma surgeons flexibility to avoid a 1 in 2 call schedule and established a culture of trust and support within the department. Fracture cases were placed in the dedicated orthopaedic trauma room for the next day in priority sequence based on need ensuring timely access for patients and avoiding the need for non-trauma surgeons to bump their elective cases or wait for add-ons to complete their call cases. As the adult non-trauma attendings grew more confident the backup schedule evolved to be weekends only which further balanced the call burden for the traumatologists (Table 2).

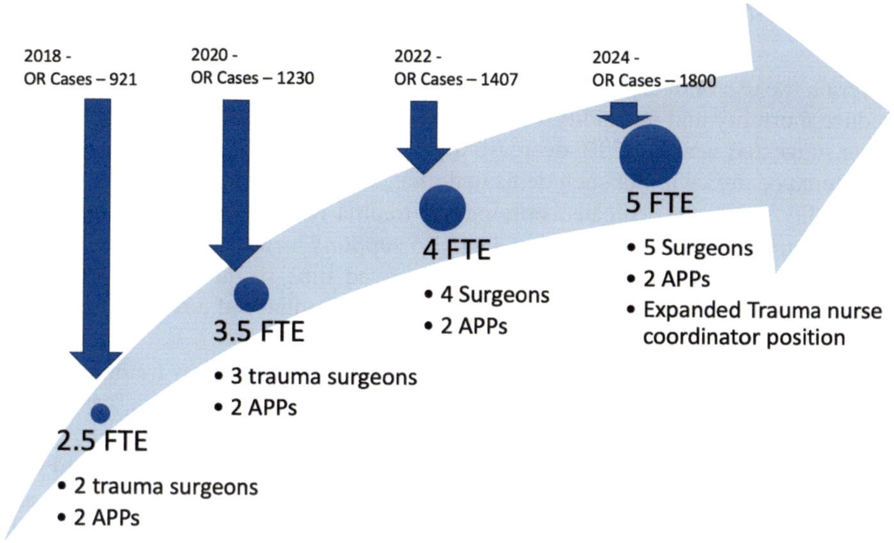

Fig. 2 Case volumes and the expansion of FTE (Full Time Equivalent) Trauma surgeons in our department. 2024–2025 is a prediction based on current trajectory of volumes and case mix

Table 1 Call schedule during the first 2 years as a trauma center. The Primary call pool included all adult faculty at our facility. A Trauma back up call pool included the 2 traumatologists who would be available as required

	Monday	Tuesday	Wednesday	Thursday	Friday	Sat	Sun
Primary	Surgeon 1	Surgeon 2	Surgeon 3	Surgeon 4	Surgeon 5	Surgeon 5	Surgeon 5
Trauma Back-up	Trauma 1	Trauma 2	Trauma 1	Trauma 2	Trauma 1	Trauma 1	Trauma 1

Table 2 Call schedule after the second year. Primary call covered by all adult faculty at our facility. A Trauma back up call pool included the 3 traumatologists who were available on weekend as required

	Monday	Tuesday	Wednesday	Thursday	Friday	Sat	Sun
Primary	Surgeon 1	Surgeon 2	Surgeon 3	Surgeon 4	Surgeon 5	Surgeon 5	Surgeon 5
Trauma Back-up					Trauma 2	Trauma 2	Trauma 2

Overall, it is important to assess the current staffing levels and compare them to the determined requirements. If there is a shortfall, steps should be taken to recruit and hire the necessary staff. On the other hand, if there is an excess of staff, it may be necessary to reassign or redistribute responsibilities to ensure optimal utilization of resources. Regular monitoring and evaluation of staffing levels should be conducted to ensure that the department is adequately staffed to meet the needs of patients and provide high-quality care.

Resources/Facilities

Overall, the use of dedicated fracture/orthopaedic trauma rooms has been shown to reduce mortality and morbidity while being cost effective [26, 27]. Several studies have suggested nearly a 50% decrease in morbidity and operative delay compared to trauma centers without such dedicated time. These and other studies have led to the reality that such dedicated orthopaedic trauma room time has become a best practice guideline [28–30]. Further data also supports weekend orthopaedic access demonstrating reduced lengths of stay, improved time to the OR and enhanced access for patients during work week hours all with enhanced cost savings for the hospital [31, 32].

At our center, a dedicated orthopaedic trauma room is staffed by traumatologists 5 days a week. This room remains available for orthopaedic trauma cases until 630 am in the morning and then becomes open time for add-on and emergency cases across all specialties. This room is dedicated to orthopaedic trauma, supported with an orthopaedic scrub and circulator who are familiar with the requirements and urgency of trauma cases. This room is excluded from our Operative room bump policies and protected where possible to facilitate prompt and timely trauma care to our trauma patients. In additional to this room the hospital has opened additional overflow OR time to help decompress trauma backlog. Thoughtful, data-based discussion has demonstrated the continued need and growth of orthopaedic trauma at our facility making the case for additional dedicated and protected time. We expect to expand our current dedicated orthopaedic trauma room time to include 3 additional days per week and protected time over the weekend days allowing for 7 days a week of trauma room coverage.

One key aspect to this process has been the establishment and adherence to our Urgent emergent list of procedures. In contrast to General Surgery trauma few injuries in orthopaedic trauma care are truly emergent. In the early stages of our discussions about trauma care we established a hierarchy for trauma cases at the perioperative level. Each specialty developed and was responsible for the adhering to the case classification schema that they developed. We established our list based while not exhaustive it was illustrative of case urgency based on established good standards, evidence and best practices as outlined below:

Case Classification

Class A Procedure—30 Minutes

- Traumatic fractures causing hemorrhage of life-threatening extent
- Open pelvic fractures (motorcycle/pedestrian versus vehicle accidents)—massive hemorrhage, major vessel injury and sepsis

Class B Procedure—2 Hours

- Replantation of digit or extremity
- Fasciotomy for compartment syndrome

- Vascular injury requiring repair
- Unstable pelvic ring injury in patient with hemodynamic instability
- Herniated disc or cauda equina syndrome (leg weakness and numbness, loss of bowel or bladder control)
- Spine injury with skeletal instability and neurologic compromise or the possibility of impending neurologic deterioration (i.e. Occipito-atlanto dissociation)

Class C Procedure—4 Hours

- Mangled hand injuries
- Open reduction and internal fixation (ORIF) with neurological deficit
- Markedly displaced fracture or dislocation with soft tissue or nerves at risk (e.g., supracondylar fracture of the humerus in child's elbow or irreducible knee dislocation)
- Grossly contaminated (Grade III) open fracture requiring spanning external fixation

Class D Procedure—24 Hours

- Any high energy periarticular fracture requiring spanning external fixation
- Incision and drainage of septic joint (excluding septic patient)
- Open fractures
- Suspected abscess or wound infection
- Incision and drainage of spine
- Irreducible joint
- Intramedullary (IM) fixation of the femur or tibia
- Spine injuries with skeletal instability requiring stabilization

Within 24–48 Hours

- Fractured hip per protocol (goal within 24 hours and must be performed within 48 hours of admission)

Add-On Procedure—24 Hours

- Fractures with no immediate threat to life or limb
- Ruptured or lacerated tendons
- Pelvic fractures, patient stable
- Removal of foreign bodies—wood, metal, nail

Develop Protocols and Guidelines

Trauma care is particularly suited to the application and development of evidence-based protocols and guidelines for the evaluation, treatment, and management of patients given the high stress, multiple services and concomitant pathologies common in the trauma scenario. Protocols help to ensure standardized care and improved outcomes. Highlighting the areas of clinical overlap between services helps to ensure a streamlined, commonality of care between services in these high stress environments [33]. This focus also helps bring trauma services together as they focus on the common goals of patient care, despite often disparate medical backgrounds and training. In orthopaedics the focus of these multi-service guidelines are typically:

- Open fractures
- Pelvic and acetabular fractures
- Mangled limbs
- Dysvascular extremities
- Compartment syndrome
- Anticoagulation
- Hip Fractures

Additionally, within the orthopaedic trauma group additional protocols focused on isolated MSK related trauma are also necessary to help standardize workflows, improve efficiencies and enhance patient care pathways. These typically include:

- Hip Fractures
- Bone Healthy/Fragility pathways
- Rehab protocols

Establishing establish evidence-based protocols and guidelines requires that several steps be taken. First, a comprehensive review of the existing literature and research is conducted. This identifies the most up-to-date and reliable evidence regarding the evaluation, treatment, and management of these patients. Once gathered, a multidisciplinary team, typically including the invested parties who then analyze the evidence and develop protocols and guidelines based on the best available research. While disagreements and discussions are expected and encouraged to formalize and ensure adoption of such protocols and treatment guidelines these sessions should not be rushed. Across the orthopaedic and trauma literature data demonstrates the utility of adopting evidence-based practice including improved clinical outcomes, reduced patient and system health expenditure and reduced morbidity and mortality [34–37]. Critical to this process is the adoption and monitoring of protocol adherence as this may suggest protocol or personal concerns that need addressed [37–39]. Regular updates and revisions of the protocols and guidelines should also be conducted to incorporate new evidence and advancements in orthopaedic trauma care. This will help ensure that the protocols and guidelines remain evidence-based and reflect the best practices in the field.

To ensure standardized care, the protocols and guidelines should be disseminated to all healthcare providers involved in trauma care and easily available on hospital intranet or online locations. Educational programs, training sessions, and the development of easily accessible resources, such as online platforms or mobile applications also ensure adoption.

At our facility protocol generation was of paramount importance as we developed novel institutional protocols applicable to our facility. During the creation of a novel trauma center the programs are afforded the luxury of a blank slate—starting from scratch without preconceived institutional memory or guidelines that challenge or conflict with modern or up-to-date protocol. On the other hand, developing novel evidence-based strategies from scratch is a labour intensive, challenging experience requiring multiple rounds of revisions, discussion and give and take to develop protocols that a multi-disciplinary team feels reflects best-practice, available evidence, and institutional constraints. One such protocol that our institution was particularly proud of was the open fracture protocol (Fig. 3). This protocol includes a shift to modern antibiotic inclusion way from historical aminoglycosides and is based on bacterial nomograms at our local facility.

By establishing evidence-based protocols and guidelines for the evaluation, treatment, and management of orthopaedic trauma patients, healthcare providers can deliver standardized care that is based on the most current and reliable evidence. This will ultimately lead to improved outcomes for orthopaedic trauma patients, including faster recovery times, reduced complications, and enhanced overall patient satisfaction.

Implementation of Quality Improvement Initiatives

Quality improvement (QI) initiatives are critical for any and all programs investigated in achieving at the highest level [40–42]. These are fundamentally critical to ensure that programs are delivering the best possible care to patients. QI initiatives involve the systematic evaluation of current practices, identification of areas for improvement, and implementation of evidence-based interventions to enhance the quality of care and optimize health care value. One key aspect of QI initiatives is the focus on patient safety. Identifying and addressing potential risks, errors, and adverse events, empowers all involved to create a safer environment for patients. This includes implementing and monitoring adherence to protocols and guidelines, improving communication and teamwork among healthcare providers, and promoting a culture of safety. Concurrently QI initiatives improve the value of healthcare. This is critical to orthopaedic health care delivery given the high equipment and supply costs. By pursuing health care value, we can reduce unnecessary costs, eliminating waste, and optimizing resource utilization. Often this is as straightforward as streamlining processes and implementing efficient practices, while minimizing expenses [43].

Finally, QI initiatives can enhance the overall quality of care provided to patients. The measurement and monitoring of health outcomes and patient satisfaction allows for objective evaluations of interventions and practices, allowing for the adjustment of interventions to ensure effectiveness [44]. By regularly assessing performance and outcomes, healthcare organizations can identify areas for improvement and make necessary changes to enhance patient care [45].

At our facility we find multi-disciplinary approaches to quality improvement is critical to facilitate a team atmosphere, enhance adoption, adherence and optimize care. Our orthopaedic department engages in multiple levels of QI including department wide, subspecialty specific and globally at the institutional level. Each of these levels includes multidisciplinary opportunities. Currently, our departmental QI process includes nursing, administration, physician extenders and physicians

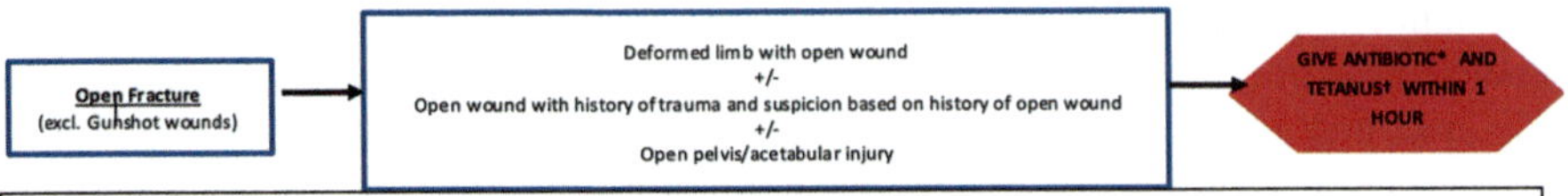

TETANUS PROPHYLAXIS†

Tetanus prone wound (*=>6hrs from injury, irregular margin, >1cm deep, projectile injury, crush, burn, frostbite, devitalized tissue, gross contamination*):

- Immunized, but >10 years since booster: Give Td Booster (0.5mg IM), then full series later
- Not immunized or status unknown: Give Td Booster (0.5mg IM) PLUS Tetanus Immunoglobulin (TIG) (250mL IM)
  - Give Td and TIG in separate sites

NON-Tetanus prone wound:

- Immunized, but >10 years since booster: Give Td Booster (0.5mg IM)
- Not immunized or status unknown: Give Td (0.5mg IM), then full series later

ANTIBIOTIC PROPHYLAXIS*

Gustilo-Anderson Classification System

Type I fracture	Open fracture with clean wound <1 cm long
Type II fracture	Open fracture with laceration >1 cm long without extensive soft tissue damage
Type III fracture	Open segmental fracture, open fracture with extensive soft tissue damage, or traumatic amputation, GSW Tibia

Injury	Preferred Regimen	Severe Beta-Lactam Allergy	High-Risk for MRSA (*See notes section below for patient stratification*)		Antibiotic Prophylaxis Duration	Infusion Duration
			Without Severe Beta-Lactam Allergy	Severe Beta-Lactam Allergy		
Type I/II Fractures	**Cefazolin*** 2G IV Q8H	**Clindamycin** 600mg IV Q8H	**Cefazolin*** 2G IV Q8H (3G if TBW >120kg) AND **Vancomycin*** (1gm if 40-70kg, 1.5gm if 71-90kg, 2gm if 91->120kg)	**Vancomycin*** (1gm if 40-70kg, 1.5gm if 71-90kg, 2gm if 91->120kg)	Maximum 24 hours Cefazolin 3 doses (based on renal function) Clindamycin 3 doses Vancomycin 1-2 doses (based on renal function)	**Cefazolin:** 3-5 min IV push OR 30min IVPB **Ceftriaxone:** 1-4 min IV push OR 30min IVPB **Ciprofloxacin:** 60 min IVPB only **Clindamycin:** 30min IVPB only **Vancomycin:** 1000mg: 60 min 1500mg: 90 min 2000mg: 120 min
Type III Fractures / Open Acetabulum† / Pelvis or delayed presentation						
No gross contamination Contamination with soil or fecal material	**Ceftriaxone** 2G Q24H	**Ciprofloxacin*** 400mg IV Q12H AND **Clindamycin** 600mg IV Q8H	**Ceftriaxone** 2G Q24H AND **Vancomycin*** (1gm if 40-70kg, 1.5gm if 71-90kg, 2gm if 91->120kg)	**Ciprofloxacin*** 400mg IV Q12H AND **Vancomycin*** (1gm if 40-70kg, 1.5gm if 71-90kg, 2gm if 91->120kg)	24 hours after wound closure	
Contamination with standing/ fresh water	**Cefepime** 1G Q6H (2G Q8H if TBW >80kg)	**Ciprofloxacin** 400MG Q8H AND **Clindamycin** 600mg IV Q8H	Cefepime 1G Q6H (2G Q8H if TBW >80kg) AND **Vancomycin*** (1gm if 40-70kg, 1.5gm if 71-90kg, 2gm if 91->120kg)	Ciprofloxacin* 400MG Q8H AND **Vancomycin*** (1gm if 40-70kg, 1.5gm if 71-90kg, 2gm if 91->120kg)	24 hours after wound closure	

NOTES

Severe beta-lactam allergy includes anaphylaxis, hives, angioedema, Stevens-Johnson syndrome (SJS), toxic epidermal necrosis (TEN).

- Patients with a reported rash to penicillin can still safely receive cephalosporins (cefazolin, cefoxitin)

High-risk for MRSA

- *History of MRSA infection or colonization*
- *Hemodialysis*
- *Recent hospitalization (within 90 days)*

The recommendations provided in this document are meant to be used as general guide to antimicrobial prophylaxis based on available evidence, there may be additional situations for which prophylaxis is needed based on the potential risk of infectious complications (which should be considered on case-by-case basis and should be discussed with Infectious Diseases).

Fig. 3 Example protocol for open fractures developed for a new urban trauma center focused on current evidence-based practices and local nomogram data

themselves. Submissions for QI review are actively encouraged from all members of the department regardless of the size or significance of the potential topic and trends or repetitive concerns are flagged for specific review and potential intervention and protocol/guideline creation. An early success in this program was our Hip fracture pathway which developed from the hardwork of our surgeon champion, nurse champion, and counterparts in the Emergency room, Anesthesia, and Medicine. This program has led to substantial decreases in length of time to the OR and improved patient care during their inpatient stay.

In summary, QI initiatives play a vital role in ensuring that programs deliver high-quality care, improve healthcare value, and enhance patient safety. By focusing on these key areas, healthcare organizations can continuously strive for excellence and provide the best possible care to their patients.

Clinical Pearls

- Establishing early goals and purpose during the establishment of an orthopaedic trauma team will lead to a sound foundational base to build a successful program. Such goal setting will act as a compass for future decision making and ensure practical, goal oriented development.
- Active understanding and appreciation for the financial implications of orthopaedic trauma care are critical during the development, establishment, and ongoing growth of a nascent trauma center. A solid grasp of these principles will ensure physicians can 'play ball' with administrators who may not fully appreciate the value-add that orthopaedic trauma has both on the community it serves as well as on the financial backbone of the institution.
- Establishing daily dedicated orthopaedic trauma operative space is critical to successful delivery of trauma care. Such protected access is well supported in the literature with clear benefits on patient morbidity, mortality and patient flow elements.
- Multidisciplinary support and teamwork is critical to success of a trauma center and is particularly important for the orthopaedic trauma surgeon. They will be required to interact with multiple members of the trauma team.
- Constant program monitoring and evaluation is critical to allow for adaptations that are necessary through programmatic growth and changing health care landscapes.

Fundamentally, remember, starting an orthopaedic trauma program requires a multidisciplinary approach, collaboration with other healthcare providers, and a commitment to providing high-quality, evidence-based care to trauma patients.

References

1. Holtenius J, Berg HE, Enocson A. Musculoskeletal injuries in trauma patients: a Swedish nationwide register study including 37,266 patients. Acta Orthop. 2023;94:171–7. https://doi.org/10.2340/17453674.2023.11960.
2. Banerjee M, Bouillon B, Shafizadeh S, et al. Epidemiology of extremity injuries in multiple trauma patients. Injury. 2013;44(8):1015–21. https://doi.org/10.1016/j.injury.2012.12.007.
3. Lunevicius R, Mesri M. A profile of a major trauma Centre of north West England between 2011 and 2018. Sci Rep. 2021;11(1):5393. https://doi.org/10.1038/s41598-021-84266-x.

4. Tarabadkar N, Alton T, Gorbaty J, Nork S, Taitman L, Kleweno C. Trends in orthopedic fracture and injury severity: a level I trauma center experience. Orthopedics. 2018;41(2):e211–6. https://doi.org/10.3928/01477447-20180103-01.
5. Heim C, Bosisio F, Roth A, et al. Is trauma in Switzerland any different? Epidemiology and patterns of injury in major trauma—a 5-year review from a Swiss trauma Centre. Swiss Méd Wkly. 2014;144(1314):w13958. https://doi.org/10.4414/smw.2014.13958.
6. Schwartz AM, Staley CA, Wilson JM, Reisman WM, Schenker ML. High acuity polytrauma centers in orthopaedic trauma: decreasing patient mortality with effective resource utilization. Injury. 2020;51(10):2235–40. https://doi.org/10.1016/j.injury.2020.06.043.
7. Agarwal-Harding KJ, von Keudell A, Zirkle LG, Meara JG, Dyer GSM. Understanding and addressing the global need for Orthopaedic trauma care. J Bone Joint Surg. 2016;98(21):1844–53. https://doi.org/10.2106/jbjs.16.00323.
8. Mock C, Cherian MN. The global burden of musculoskeletal injuries: challenges and solutions. Clin Orthop Relat Res. 2008;466(10):2306–16. https://doi.org/10.1007/s11999-008-0416-z.
9. Ziran BH, Barrette-Grischow MK, Marucci K. Economic value of orthopaedic trauma: the (second to) bottom line. J Orthop Trauma. 2008;22(4):227–33. https://doi.org/10.1097/bot.0b013e31816bae67.
10. Medicine I of IOM report: the future of emergency care in the United States Health System. Acad Emerg Med. 2006;13(10):1081–5. https://doi.org/10.1197/j.aem.2006.07.011.
11. Althausen PL, Hill AD, Mead L. Hospital fundamentals. J Orthop Trauma. 2014;28:S18–24. https://doi.org/10.1097/bot.0000000000000139.
12. Anderson TJ, Althausen PL. The role of dedicated musculoskeletal urgent care centers in reducing cost and improving access to orthopaedic care. J Orthop Trauma. 2016;30:S3–6. https://doi.org/10.1097/bot.0000000000000712.
13. Moody AE, Gurnea TP, Shul CP, Althausen PL. True cost of operating room time: implications for an orthopaedic trauma service. J Orthop Trauma. 2020;34(5):271–5. https://doi.org/10.1097/bot.0000000000001688.
14. Vallier HA, Patterson BM, Meehan CJ, Lombardo T. Orthopaedic traumatology: the hospital side of the ledger, defining the financial relationship between physicians and hospitals. J Orthop Trauma. 2008;22(4):221–6. https://doi.org/10.1097/bot.0b013e31815e92e5.
15. Flanagan CD, Rascoe AS, Wang DM, Vallier HA. The trauma service line: revenue from subsequent injury- and noninjury-related care. J Orthop Trauma. 2019;33(9):e345–51. https://doi.org/10.1097/bot.0000000000001501.
16. Rascoe AS, Flanagan CD, Kim CY, Vallier HA. Variations in revenue generation for the care of orthopaedic trauma patients. J Am Acad Orthop Surg. 2020;28(4):e151–7. https://doi.org/10.5435/jaaos-d-17-00871.
17. Morellato J, Baker M, Isaac M, et al. Does an implant usage report card impact orthopaedic trauma implant stewardship? J Orthop Trauma. 2019;33(11):e427–32. https://doi.org/10.1097/bot.0000000000001557.
18. Morellato J, O'Hara NN, Baker M, O'Toole RV, Pollak AN. What is the long-term impact of an implant stewardship program on orthopaedic trauma implant pricing? J Orthop Trauma. 2021;35(5):e153–7. https://doi.org/10.1097/bot.0000000000001967.
19. Okike K, Pollak R, O'Toole RV, Pollak AN. Red-yellow-green. J Bone Joint Surg. 2017;99(7):e33. https://doi.org/10.2106/jbjs.16.00271.
20. Wasterlain AS, Melamed E, Bello R, et al. The effect of price on surgeons' choice of implants: a randomized controlled survey. J Hand Surg. 2017;42(8):593–601.e6. https://doi.org/10.1016/j.jhsa.2017.05.005.
21. Ayoub M, Bassett WP, Seuffert P, Matijakovich D, O'Hara DA, Butler MS. Perception versus reality in the cost of orthopedic trauma implants. J Surg Educ. 2018;75(5):1333–41. https://doi.org/10.1016/j.jsurg.2018.02.015.
22. Waldron J, Denisiuk M, Sharma R, Boura J, Afsari A, Best B. Does seasonal variation in orthopaedic trauma volume correlate with adverse hospital events and burnout? Injury. 2022;53(6):2053–9. https://doi.org/10.1016/j.injury.2022.02.042.

23. Blasier RD, Gagnon MR, Iannotti JP, Jarvis-Selinger S. Hiring your next partner. J Bone Joint Surg. 2014;96(17):e150. https://doi.org/10.2106/jbjs.m.00725.
24. Chan JY, Charlton TP, Thordarson DB. Analysis of orthopaedic job availability in the United States based on subspecialty. JAAOS: Glob Res Rev. 2020;4(11):e20.00195. https://doi.org/10.5435/jaaosglobal-d-20-00195.
25. Althausen PL, Shannon S, Owens B, et al. Impact of hospital-employed physician assistants on a level II community-based orthopaedic trauma system. J Orthop Trauma. 2016;30:S40–4. https://doi.org/10.1097/01.bot.0000510721.23126.48.
26. Lemos D, Nilssen E, Khatiwada B, et al. Dedicated orthopedic trauma theatres: effect on morbidity and mortality in a single trauma centre. Can J Surg J Can Chir. 2009;52(2):87–91.
27. Elder GM, Harvey EJ, Vaidya R, Guy P, Meek RN, Aebi M. The effectiveness of orthopaedic trauma theatres in decreasing morbidity and mortality: a study of 701 displaced subcapital hip fractures in two trauma centres. Injury. 2005;36(9):1060–6. https://doi.org/10.1016/j.injury.2005.05.001.
28. Featherall J, Bhattacharyya T. The dedicated orthopaedic trauma room model: adopting a new standard of care. J Bone Joint Surg. 2019;101(22):e120-1-4. https://doi.org/10.2106/jbjs.19.00352.
29. Althausen PL, Kauk JR, Shannon S, Lu M, O'Mara TJ, Bray TJ. Operating room efficiency. J Orthop Trauma. 2016;30:S15–20. https://doi.org/10.1097/01.bot.0000510720.85008.87.
30. Bhattacharyya T, Vrahas MS, Morrison SM, et al. The value of the dedicated orthopaedic trauma operating room. J Trauma Inj Infect Crit Care. 2006;60(6):1336–41. https://doi.org/10.1097/01.ta.0000220428.91423.78.
31. Runner R, Moore T, Reisman W. Value of a dedicated saturday orthopaedic trauma operating room. J Orthop Trauma. 2016;30(1):e24–9. https://doi.org/10.1097/bot.0000000000000441.
32. Wixted JJ, Reed M, Eskander MS, et al. The effect of an orthopedic trauma room on after-hours surgery at a level one trauma center. J Orthop Trauma. 2008;22(4):234–6. https://doi.org/10.1097/bot.0b013e31816c748b.
33. Baker H, Erdman MK, Christiano A, Strelzow JA. Team approach: the unstable trauma patient. JBJS Rev. 2023;11(6):e22.00226. https://doi.org/10.2106/jbjs.rvw.22.00226.
34. Ahmed I, Khan MA, Nayak V, Mohsen A. An evidence-based warfarin management protocol reduces surgical delay in hip fracture patients. J Orthop Traumatol. 2013;15(1):21–7. https://doi.org/10.1007/s10195-013-0274-7.
35. Khan MH, Rihn J, Steele G, et al. Postoperative management protocol for incidental dural tears during degenerative lumbar spine surgery: a review of 3,183 consecutive degenerative lumbar cases. Spine. 2006;31(22):2609–13. https://doi.org/10.1097/01.brs.0000241066.55849.41.
36. Khan H, Hussain N, Bhandari M. The influence of large clinical trials in orthopedic trauma. J Orthop Trauma. 2013;27(12):e268–74. https://doi.org/10.1097/bot.0b013e31829642f9.
37. Nicolay RW, Tawari AA, Kempegowda H, Suk M, Mullis B. How often are protocols followed at level I trauma centers? J Surg Orthop Adv. 2018;27(2):109–12.
38. Vallier HA, Moore TA, Como JJ, et al. Teamwork in trauma. J Orthop Trauma. 2015;29(11):e446–50. https://doi.org/10.1097/bot.0000000000000383.
39. Vallier HA, Wang X, Moore TA, Wilber JH, Como JJ. Timing of orthopaedic surgery in multiple trauma patients. J Orthop Trauma. 2013;27(10):543–51. https://doi.org/10.1097/bot.0b013e31829efda1.
40. Azar FM. Quality, value, and patient safety in orthopedic surgery. Orthop Clin North Am. 2018;49(4):xvii. https://doi.org/10.1016/j.ocl.2018.07.001.
41. Jevsevar DS, Shea KG, Styhl A, Koenig K. Practical quality improvement implementation in orthopaedic clinical practice. Instr Course Lect. 2016;65:601–8.
42. Jevsevar DS, Karl JW, Bhandari M, Bozic KJ, Piasio MA, Weinstein SL. Evidence, quality, costs, and reimbursement: connecting the dots. Instr Course Lect. 2016;65:567–75.
43. Saleh KJ, Bozic KJ, Graham DB, et al. Quality in orthopaedic surgery—an international perspective. J Bone Joint Surg. 2013;95(1):e3. https://doi.org/10.2106/jbjs.l.00093.

44. Bosco JA, Sachdev R, Shapiro LA, Stein SM, Zuckerman JD. Measuring quality in orthopaedic surgery: the use of metrics in quality management. Instr Course Lect. 2014;63:473–85.
45. Beaulé PE, Roffey DM, Poitras S. Continuous quality improvement in orthopedic surgery: changes and implications with health system funding reform. Can J Surg. 2016;59(3):149–50. https://doi.org/10.1503/cjs.005416.

Vascular Trauma

Kenneth L. Wilson

History

The city of Chicago is dubbed "Chiraq," infamously associating the West and Southside Chicago neighborhoods to being akin to the former war zone in Iraq. The University of Chicago (UChicago) re-opened the trauma bay doors in 2018, after a 28-year absence of providing trauma care on the Southside, specifically to young black men in Chiraq. The trauma patients from Southside neighborhoods are currently experiencing penetrating trauma rates of 30–40%, well above the national rate of 12%. Like Iraq during the height of the war campaign, the most common vascular injury was an injury to the superficial femoral artery. An entire damage control triage system was set in motion to address salvaging limbs conjoining temporary vascular shunts (TVS), fasciotomies and a balanced blood resuscitation or whole blood administration with the intent of counteracting an extremity injury. There were no traumatic vascular cases that penetrated the outer hull of UChicago in 28 years, but the city nicknamed Chiraq indubitably has the femoral artery as its most common vascular injury after the 2018 opening of the trauma center.

Our initial query about trauma management at UChicago produced zero examples of a vascular injury being handled at UChicago within the last 20 years. There was no institutional memory of how the hospital system would react in the evaluation of vascular injuries. Therefore, the system we elected to put into place was damage control limb salvage mimicking combat medic early tourniquet application and wartime tenants in the name of limb salvage.

K. L. Wilson (✉)
University of Chicago Medicine & Biologic Sciences, Chicago, IL, USA
e-mail: kwilson9@bsd.uchicago.edu

S. O. Rogers, Jr (ed.), *Creating a Modern Trauma Center*,
https://doi.org/10.1007/978-3-031-66524-0_9

The System We Built

Hemorrhage from injured limbs was a leading source of battlefield death [1, 2] and in the past conflict in Iraq and Afghanistan emergency tourniquet use improved survival rates in patients with major limb trauma [3]. The experience with tourniquets placed in austere environments crossed into civilian practice leading to liberal tourniquet application by EMS, Police and civilians. The pre-hospital tourniquet does not solve the problem from a blast injury, but only controls the obvious bleeding from a limb. UChicago has evaluated several trauma activations presenting concomitantly with penetrating limb injuries initially controlled with a tourniquet with still other bleeding sources needing to be elucidated from the torso. The system we built is predicated upon the default being "damage control" approach. The unstable injury patterns from multiple gunshot wounds and the simultaneous trauma activations with multiple patients with unstable injuries is what led to damage control as the default. The management from trauma bay to OR is a 4-minute time clock with a run across a bridge into operating room six floors above the emergency room. The tourniquet eventually has to be released and a temporary vascular shunt needs to be deployed or definitive repair completed depending on patient stability. This is the charge of every trauma surgeon taking call at UChicago, shunt placement for definitive fixation in the daylight hours. The other intent was to improve a trauma vascular skillset without a phone call to a vascular surgeon sleeping at home. This was a bold statement to make in a system uninitiated in all aspects of vascular trauma care.

The unreciprocated increase in penetrating vascular injuries from gun violence has not been counterbalanced by the number of trauma surgeons comfortable nationwide with completing vascular trauma cases from skin to skin. Seven trauma surgeons launched the Uchicago trauma center. Four of the surgeons were fresh graduates without any unsupervised vascular experience beyond fellowship training. The new recruits would also face the training deficit currently gripping all general surgery residents which is a paucity of open vascular procedures. Major vascular cases completed by general surgery residents over the past 20 years has decreased despite an increase in the national cohort of chief general surgery resident graduates increasing per year [4]. UChicago general surgery residents would rely upon outside rotations prior to 2018 to participate in the treatment of penetrating vascular trauma. The gleaned experience from outside rotations would be further obfuscated by only observing as junior residents during the outside trauma rotations. The general surgery residents' significant inexperience in an open operative vascular trauma, and the shift to learning endovascular skills, would further challenge proficiency. Potentially, Southside Chicago residents were being denied surgeons with the necessary surgical technique and muscle memory not inherent in surgical training to complete the exsanguinating cases that would soon await them at their neighborhood institution.

This mismatch of vascular complexity and poorly prepared surgeons is the paradigm that plagued active-duty surgeons during deployment. I strongly believe that being in an austere environment where definitive vascular repairs have proven to be unwarranted during all armed US conflicts, serendipitously helped UChicago, the newest level one academic center, quickly convert to an austere treatment plan adding the placement of a temporary vascular shunts. A low budget insertion of a piece of plastic in a vessel became an innovative concept for training novices to become experts. The lowering of the threshold to remove the tourniquet, clear clot and place a shunt allayed anxiety. We soon discovered that shunt placement became the most expeditious way to rotate repeatedly from emergency room to operating room if the revenge shooting trailed only minutes to hours behind the vascular injury requiring shunting. However, bullets find vessels beyond the extremities.

The first week of the May 2018 launch was a harrowing start. A brand-new trauma attending was unenviably greeted with two abdominal trauma cases with exsanguinating vascular injuries from the inferior vena cava. Both patients did not survive and the blood bank was depleted for both cases. The shunt is not the answer to all vascular injuries. Speed, accuracy and precise decision making had to overtake anxiety and hesitancy. It has been a delight to watch the conversion from unease and indecision become converted into confidence.

The planning stages of vascular coverage obviously mandated a conversation and an agreement with the vascular service. As previously mentioned, there was not a recent recollection of taking a vascular trauma case to operating room. The UChicago vascular service covered both adult and pediatric cases with the additional expertise of endovascular procedures. The perceivable future advent of a trauma service could become exhaustive at night and interfere with a busy elective caseload the following morning. While many institutions will get vascular control and call the vascular team for definitive repair, this is not the model we intended to champion. We were seeking to match the match the passion and fervor that it took to build this trauma center with complete care. Every trauma surgeon will become an "old school" trauma surgeon where vascular surgery is woven into the DNA of trauma surgeons. This would not dismiss the need for occasional vascular surgery help or intraoperative consultations.

A study conducted at Harborview promoted vascular surgeons as being essential members of the trauma team. The importance of having vascular surgeons on the team was predicated upon the number of intraoperative vascular consultations steadily increasing and the call for consults could not be attributed solely to an increase in endovascular hemorrhage control. Instead the increase number of consults reflected the declining experience of trauma surgeons with vascular trauma. When consulted, Harborview vascular surgeons were effective in quickly gaining control of "the situation" to provide exposure, hemorrhage control, or revascularization [5]. The model of vascular coverage at Harborview highlights the differences in the identities of trauma centers. Harborview's immense geographical coverage extending across multiple state lines, including Alaska. In addition trauma in Seattle does not rival Chiraq with less penetrating trauma rates. Although, this would not become our vascular model, we are in agreement with Harboview's assement about the deteriorating experience of trauma surgeons nationally who may not be comfortable with vascular repairs. We feel strongly about the reverse being true, where the trauma surgeons take the lead with the vascular surgeons on standby.

The opportunity to become incrementally better and steeped in confidence for repairing injured vessels exists in Chicago. What one could not shunt, sew, ligate or balloon tamponade one week is more than likely to show up again the following next week in the Southside of Chicago. Our trauma surgeons have repaired every named vessel from the base of the skull to below the knee and out to the wrists. Vascular control is always the responsibility of the on-call trauma surgeon with an immediate call to another trauma surgeon. While in the operating room, the UChicago trauma surgeon's primary consideration is if the placement of a temporary vascular shunt is warranted. This process preserves the experience for another team member (trauma surgeon) to repair during daylight hours, but the surgeon who placed the shunt has the right to complete the case when the resuscitation has become optimal.

The Early Compromise Leading to a Complete Vascular Coverage

The introduction of vascular trauma to the hospital system created a unique opportunity to not only restore the proper role of trauma surgeons as vascular surgeons, but it also created a training paradigm allowing for the development of young trauma surgeons and vascular fellows. The University of Chicago, with newly minted trauma surgeons and new vascular fellows, both having experienced reduced numbers of open operative procedures inherent in training, would simultaneously share decision-making and combined efforts in the management of peripheral vascular trauma.

The preferred call as mentioned is to an experienced trauma surgeon, which could not be mandated but only be strongly suggested. The vascular surgery consult would initially bring the vascular fellow to the operating room for assistance. The graduate medical education (GME) stipulations protected this arrangement. The requirement to have an attending present, which was the role occupied by the junior trauma surgeon, while allowing both the fellow and the trauma surgeon the opportunity to jointly share in decision-making about repairing an injured vessel. If the case was deemed too difficult, the vascular fellow could opt to call in a vascular attending for further guidance and assistance. This relationship between the trauma service and vascular service in my opinion was a 2-year compromise that greatly favored the maturation of the young trauma attending. The vascular fellows also gained valuable open vascular experience, with one of the vascular fellows becoming permanent staff at the end of the two-year fellowship. It was unlikely and inevitable that a trauma attending with three or more years of operative vascular trauma experience would no longer allow themselves to be bumped down the table by a more junior vascular fellow. As predicted, the muscle memory and technical skills grew alongside confidence. The call to the vascular service is never for immediate hemorrhage control but for vascular consultation that pulls a vascular attending into the decision making process. The need for endovascular expertise is not championed by the trauma service at this moment.

Why We Shunt

Temporary vascular shunts quickly restore perfusion until definitive repair can be accomplished, and this is a lesson learned from Afghanistan and Iraq [6]. Temporary Vascular shunts as damage control adjuncts were utilized up to 25% of extremity vascular injuries in Iraq and were subsequently mandated by military practice guidelines (CPGs) to be utilized in both theaters of operations in Iraq and Afghanistan [7]. In the civilian practice temporary vascular shunting has not been fully embraced because most vascular trauma develops from a blunt mechanism. Our most common presenting mechanism of injury is penetrating, with gunshot wounds leading the way. Similar to the military experience, the femoral artery is the most targeted vessel. The obvious comparison of Iraq to Chiraq leant support for a similar approach of mimicking what worked well for deployed active-duty surgeons for our new surgeons. The massive transfusion protocol of 1:1:1 with the later addition of whole blood became adjuncts further imitating a Role-2 austere forward resuscitative team (FRST). The trauma nurses and techs also "drank the Kool-Aid" and perceived themselves as resuscitating and evacuating expeditiously to a higher echelon of care, a Role-3, the operating room. We truly became an FRST-minded team. The vigilance to salvage lives cloaked our Southside patient population from treatment biases, as the focus became about team efficiency toward saving a limb and a life.

The maximum duration of the shunt has never been explicitly defined for our team. Placement of a shunt for a range of 6 until the daylight for femoral and brachial artery injuries is a simple guess. Shunt placement could extend beyond 3 days if the injured vessel was associated noncompressible hemorraghe such as an iliac artery or concomitant intraabdominal injuries. The learning curve of placing the shunts was done without morbidity and no bleeding concerns after departing the operating room. Only a few went down without an associated amputation.

The day definitive repair after shunt placement lends to a pace as close to as a trauma surgeon can get toward being an elective vascular surgeon. There is no need to even make a skin incision in that once the temporary closure is removed, the anatomy is beautifully displayed with the temporary vascular shunt highlighting the two ends of the vessel that need to be joined. The controlled viewing allows understanding of the associated anatomy, deconstruction of the trauma injury pattern and allowing conceptualization of how to achieve a successful salvage for one's self. The insight into how the emergency exposure was obtained especially for infrequently encountered exposures, such as the subclavian vessels is invaluable. We believe that the injury notion rarely encountered vascular injuries not seen by other trauma centers will never be our fate. A keen knowledge concerning exposure, hemorrhage control and repair is invaluable. We vehemently reject the argument of this space belongs to anyone else than the trauma surgeon and repetition as in all things proves performance.

Did You Call an Expert?

There is an exasperating academic discussion pitting supporters of vascular surgeons against trauma surgeons as to who is best suited to manage patients presenting with injured peripheral vascular injuries. The conversations highlight that there is no difference detected in vascular-related complications between the two groups [8]. The service most likely to consult a vascular surgeon will remain the trauma service for extremity malperfusion [9] but not for hemorrhage control. Preceding the trauma surgeons arrival to UChicago, vascular trauma triage meant shipping an injured patient to Northwestern Hospital. No one in a 28 year span could rightfully claim expertise in vascular-related hemorrhage control beyond tourniquet placement and triage away from UChicago. The introduction of the trauma service has had the residual effect of better trained residents able to initiate the resuscitation and vascular repair especially when the attending is already in the operating room. The appearance of another trauma surgeon or the back-up trauma surgeon at night is expected to make the drive to assist in the operating room. We will still occasionally allow a vascular fellow assist when malperfusion is suspected, but never for assistance with the stoppage of bleeding.

Despite being incessantly greeted with Monday morning quarterbacking (which takes place Wednesdays) of "did you call an expert," our trauma surgeons do not falter and maintain steely fighter pilot confidence. I believe the trauma services internal quality review allows for greater detailed dissection of our vascular outcomes. However, the most grueling account is our internal quality meeting when deviations occur as minimal as not exiting the emergency room fast enough to a delayed amputation.

We are thankful for our partnership with the vascular team but the honing of confidence for vascular trauma is clear thinking when the bombardment of decision waypoints is channeled into a single resuscitative action while hypotension is taking place. Trauma surgeons arrive quicker to the operating and have no difference in short-term clinical outcomes of brachial and femoral artery repairs compared with patients treated by vascular surgeons [10].

Ongoing Challenges

The original trauma seven consider it an eminence honor to be reestablish a trauma center in the Southside of Chicago. We consider ourselves summoned to be guests by the disenfranchised young community advocates that rallied and protested to support the opening of the trauma center. These young advocates represent the demographic of individuals experiencing the brunt of intentional gun violence. We recognize the tremendous reluctance of the University of Chicago to engage in conversations that were essentially thrust upon them by a community activism. The risk of financial ruin and to absorb an entirely new service line that admits patients counter distinctive to the reputation of a renowned academic research institution. The University of Chicago distinguished themselves as a truly eminent institution to create an immediately impactful trauma service. UChicago has been able to gave access to the hospital but to the vexation of others who never wanted to lower the draw bridge to this particular patient population. Despite positive momentum not all encounters have been positive and ongoing challenges remain.

Pediatrics

The only component of the UChicago hospital system that participated in trauma care was Comer Children's Hospital. The pediatric age of 15 years +364 days was under the auspices of pediatric surgery. The heavy life would be opening the adult trauma center with relative little adjustments required. The pediatric trauma system is unfortunately receiving injury patterns that no child should have such as gunshot wounds and stabbings. In the pediatric realm, kids may not be viewed as "little adults" but the injury patterns sustained in the zip codes surrounding the University of Chicago mimic the adult population. Our initial introduction to pediatric vascular trauma occurred well ahead of the May 2018 inauguration of the adult trauma service. The very first day of the school year 2017, an eighth grader died from a gunshot wound to the abdomen. This is a vascular injury pattern that immediately caught the attention of the trauma surgeons awaiting an opportunity to help.

There are two portals of entry for adult and pediatric trauma patients at night. The pediatric trauma patient is under the auspices of pediatric surgery, with call taken outside of the hospital and the adult trauma patient is under the auspices of trauma surgery, with call taken inside the hospital. The femoral artery represents the primary vascular injury for our pediatric population as well. To date our most serious noncompressible vascular cases include retrohepatic inferior vena cava injuries to the iliac arteries and veins. Penetrating heart injuries have been salvaged on and off cardiopulmonary bypass. ECMO support combined with temporary vascular shunt placement followed subsequent revascularization has taken place. The temporary vascular shunt in our pediatric population has not led to a single immediate or delayed amputation. The delayed repair, allowed by temporary vascular shunting, allow daylight hour conversation assuring that a growing child is receiving the appropriate vascular repair. All children are eventually repatriated to the Children's hospital if less than 16 years of age.

Hand Coverage

Upper extremity management is anatomic splitting between the vascular service and our two hand services, plastic surgery, and orthopedic surgery. The agreed upon division was at the elbow prior to the arrival of the trauma service. Operative coverage distal to the elbow belonged to the realm of the hand services, and operative coverage above the elbow belonged to the vascular surgeons. The coverage model for south of the elbow had one glaring problem. Even with the participation of two services participating in nighttime coverage, we were not assured that the attending backing the resident was trained to repair the main two arteries to perfuse the hand. For example, the attending covering hand call may be an expert in gender reassignment and may have only seen hand surgery as a resident. This highlights just one example of subspecialty participation encountered by a trauma surgeon in our institution. We have perfected shunting and repairing in a delayed fashion for allowing daytime "expert" evaluation. However, we may elect to repair the artery ourselves. The subclavian vessels seem to not have a home with either service and the trauma service receives little to no interference from either service.

Summary

The penetrating rate presenting to UChicago is 38–42%, and during the summer season with more human targets outside, the penetrating rate has reached 50%. This unfortunate redundancy in injury patterns allows the entire team a chance to perfect vascular repairs. A significant portion of the vascular injuries occur during "trauma alley" in the middle of the night with multiple patients presenting simultaneously or with shootings occurring in rapid succession in short intervals of rest throughout a long summer night. In order to mitigate activating an additional team in the middle of the night, we have adopted a "damage control" philosophy surrounding vascular repairs which translates into the placement of temporary vascular shunt delaying definitive repair. The definitive revascularization can then be deferred until the critical phase with overwhelming influx of wounded patients has passed. In Iraq, this vascular adjunct represents a safe and effective damage control technique and is preferable to attempted reconstruction in severe conditions [11, 12]. The same approach is safe and effective in Chicago.

There are several physiologic advantages to delays that we have found to be beneficial as well. In addition to having a revived patient with better physiologic parameters, there is an additional opportunity to observe the operation or complete the vascular repair in a more controlled setting. This in our system has become a way to overcome a lack of exposures to open vascular repairs endemic in the modern residency training paradigm.

The philosophy is to have redundancy in our system, where each and every trauma attending has the responsibility and the same opportunity to maximize their confidence with vascular pairs. Temporary vascular shunts at night with definitive daytime repairs allows for a viewing of the anatomy with unhurried exposures. Senior residents who once observed vascular operations when the trauma service launched, now have an opportunity to be ahead of the vascular deficit curve. Confidence at achieving our minimum expectation of shunt and fix later is evident. The anxiety has subsided and the swagger more profound each time a repair goes well. Instead of being apprehensive about the next exsanguinating vascular repair, the chance to prove mettle is what has occurred when the trauma pager blares a vascular injury is inbound.

Our most common penetrating vascular injury after 5-years still remains the injury to the superficial femoral artery. We have grown the trauma service to 13 trauma surgeons with the expectation that all members of the trauma service participate in vascular surgery. For the novices, the expectation for halting exsanguination follows the same understanding to get a little better and further in the understanding of the vascular operation. The minimum anticipation for a win is placing a temporary vascular shunt in an alive patient for an anticipated return to the operating room.

References

1. Bellamy RF. The causes of death in conventional land warfare: implications for combat casualty care research. Mil Med. 1984;149(2):55–62.
2. Holcomb JB, McMullin NR, Pearse L, et al. Causes of death in U.S. special operations forces in the global war on terrorism. Ann Surg. 2007;254:986–91.
3. Kragh JF Jr, Baer DG, Walters TJ. Extended (16-hour) tourniquet application after combat wounds: a case report and review of the current literature. J Orthop Trauma. 2007;21:274–8.
4. Kim Y, Cui CL, Williams ZF, Long CA. Impact of integrated vascular surgery residency on general surgery resident and vascular fellow operative volume: a national analysis. Vasc Endovasc Surg. 2023;
5. Hemingway JF, Desikan S, Dasari M, Tran C, Hoffman R, Gobble A, Spurlock A, Singh N, Quiroga E, Tran N, Starnes BW. Intraoperative consultation of vascular surgeons is increasing at a major American trauma center. J Vasc Surg. 2021;
6. Woodward EB, Clouse WD, Eliason JL, Peck MA, Bowser AN, Cox MW, Jones WT, Rasmussen TE. Penetrating femoropopliteal injury during modern warfare: experience of the Balad vascular registry. J Vasc Surg. 2008;47(6):1259–64.
7. Goredon W, Balsamo L, et al. Joint trauma system clinical practice guideline: amputation: evaluation and treatment. Joint Trauma Syst. 2016;
8. Gallagher S, Sozzi M, Gallegos H, Ugarte C, Park S, Schellenberg M, Matsushima K, Magee GA, Inaba K, Martin M. Epidemiology and outcomes of traumatic vascular injury repair by trauma surgeons and vascular surgeons in a collaborative model. J Trauma Acute Care Surg. 2023;95(5):628–34.
9. Hemmingway JF, Desikan S, Dasari M, et al. Intraopeartive consultation of vascular surgeons is increasing at a major academic trauma center. Vasc Surg. 2021;74(5):–1587.
10. Karam BS, Haberman K, Nguyen P, Eddine SBZ, Boyle K, Baskaran A, Figueroa J, Milia D, Carver T, Somberg L, Webb T, Davis CS, Dodgion C, Elegbede A, de Moya MA. Trauma surgeon–performed peripheral arterial repairs are associated with equivalent outcomes when compared with vascular surgeons. J Trauma Acute Care Surg. 2022;92(4):754–9.

11. Rasmussen TE, Clouse WD, Jenkins DH, Peck MA, Eliason JL, Smith DL. The use of temporary vascular shunts as a damage control adjunct in the management of wartime vascular injury. J Trauma Inj Infect Crit Care. 2006;61(1):8–15.
12. Hornez E, Boddaert G, Ngabou UD, Aguir S, Baudoin Y, Mocellin N, Bonnet S. Temporary vascular shunt for damage control of extremity vascular injury: a toolbox for trauma surgeons. J Visc Surg. 2015;6:363–8.

Integration of PM&R Consultation Services at a Level 1 Trauma Center

Dana Branch and Stephen Leb

Physical Medicine & Rehabilitation

Physiatrists and Physical Medicine & Rehabilitation (PM&R)

Physiatrists are physicians who have completed residency training in Physical Medicine & Rehabilitation (PM&R). Physiatrists specialize in caring for patients with disabilities, including loss of function due to injury or illness. Physiatrists prescribe physical medicine (e.g. thermotherapy, hydrotherapy, electrotherapy, manual therapy and therapeutic exercise), medications, injections, and prosthetics/orthotics in addition to overseeing a multi-disciplinary team (e.g. physical/occupational therapists, speech-language pathologists, nurses, dieticians) to help restore a person's function.

Physiatrists can be found throughout the healthcare system.

Outpatient

In the outpatient setting, PM&R physician care is broad. Physiatrists may practice spasticity management (e.g. botulinum toxin injection, intrathecal baclofen pump refills and dose adjustment), post-amputee care (e.g. prosthesis prescription, wound management), or specialized care following spinal cord injury (SCI), traumatic brain injury (TBI), or stroke. Physiatrists may also evaluate and care for patients with neuromuscular disorders (e.g. Amyotrophic lateral sclerosis, Guillain-Barré syndrome, peripheral neuropathy), gait disorders, debility, or any person who has

D. Branch (✉) · S. Leb
Department of Physical Medicine & Rehabilitation, Shirley Ryan AbilityLab, Chicago, IL, USA
e-mail: Dbranch@sralab.org; sleb@metrohealth.org

S. O. Rogers, Jr (ed.), *Creating a Modern Trauma Center*,
https://doi.org/10.1007/978-3-031-66524-0_10

experienced a functional loss. Some physiatrists may specialize further by completing fellowship training in areas such as sports medicine or pain management.

Post-Acute Rehabilitation Facilities

Physiatrists are also found in post-acute rehabilitation facilities, including Long Term Acute Care Hospitals (LTACH), Skilled Nursing Facilities (SNF), or Inpatient Rehabilitation Facilities (IRF). This chapter will focus on the role of physiatrists in the IRF setting as it is most relevant to the changes made to promote the integration of PM&R physician expertise at UChicago Medicine (UCM).

IRFs can be:

- **Free-standing rehabilitation hospitals**. Some examples in the Chicago area include:
  - Shirley Ryan AbilityLab
  - Schwab Rehabilitation Hospital
  - Marianjoy Rehabilitation Center
- **Rehabilitation units in acute care hospitals**. Some examples in the Chicago area include:
  - Shirley Ryan AbilityLab Inpatient Rehabilitation at Uchicago Medicine Ingalls Memorial Hospital
  - Advocate Illinois Masonic Medical Center Rehabilitation
  - Jesse Brown VA Rehabilitation

IRF care includes:

- **Intensive therapies** (3 hours therapy/day over 5 days or 15 hours therapy/week over 7 days in certain situations)
- **Physician oversight** via face-to-face visit at least 3 days/week
- **Multiple therapy disciplines**, including physical therapy (PT), occupational therapy (OT) and speech-language pathology (SLP)
- **Multi-disciplinary team conference** at least once/week

In an IRF, physiatrists act as the primary physician overseeing the medical and rehabilitation needs for patients receiving intensive rehabilitation. Physiatrists manage a patient's medical problems, including work-up and treatment of acute medical problems, ongoing treatment of chronic medical problems, and medication management to optimize a patient's capacity to benefit from the rehabilitation process. Physiatrists also lead an interdisciplinary team including nursing, PT/OT/SLP, prosthetist/orthotist, psychologist, dietitian, wound care specialist, and social worker/case manager to tailor the rehabilitation program to a patient's needs and remove barriers to a safe discharge.

Acute Care

In the acute care setting, PM&R physicians primarily lend their expertise as consultants. Physiatrists may be asked to see patients who require specialized management, such as patients with **major multiple trauma** (e.g. optimization of weight bearing and range of motion precautions, pain management), **acute spinal cord injury** (e.g. American Spinal Injury Association (ASIA) Impairment Scale to identify neurologic level of injury, neurogenic bowel/bladder management, autonomic dysreflexia management, patient/family education), **acute traumatic brain injury** (e.g. agitation management, addition of neurostimulants, paroxysmal sympathetic hyperactivity management, spasticity management, patient/family education), impending or new **amputation** (e.g. advise optimal level of amputation, prognosticated functional outcomes, phantom limb pain management, contracture prevention, prosthesis counseling, patient/family education), and **burn injury** (e.g. contracture prevention, compression garment and orthotic recommendations).

Physiatrists may also be consulted in the acute care setting to assist with **transition of patients to the appropriate post-acute care setting**. In this role, physiatrists utilize their expertise to assist with comprehensive evaluation and care of a patient including:

- **Medical** history and ongoing medical needs
- **Functional** history, current functional status including review of PT/OT/SLP evaluations, and prognosis for functional recovery
- **Social** history and barriers to discharge home, including home setup and support
- **Physical examination** including in-depth musculoskeletal and neurological examination
- **Coordination of care** including discussion with medical teams, RN, PT/OT/SLP, registered dietitian, social work/case management, post-acute rehabilitation facilities, insurance providers, family members
- **Disposition** including determination of appropriate discharge destination and level of post-acute rehabilitation
- **Recommendations** to optimize patient for transition to home or post-acute rehabilitation facility

Physiatrists' Role in Trauma

PM&R and Trauma

Physiatrists have a long history of caring for patients with traumatic injuries [1]. Part of the establishment of the Physical Medicine & Rehabilitation specialty (first recognized by the American Board of Specialities in 1946 [2]) stems from the comprehensive rehabilitation services developed for wounded soldiers returning from World War II. Today, the scope of the PM&R specialty has expanded, but continues to encompass the care of trauma patients with the aim "**to enhance and restore functional ability and quality of life** to those with physical impairments or disabilities affecting the brain, spinal cord, nerves, bones, joints, ligaments, muscles, and tendons" [3].

In regards to patients with traumatic injuries, physiatrists are involved in the care of these patients from initial injury through recovery (e.g. acute care, rehabilitation facilities, outpatient care). This section will focus on how physiatrists contribute to the comprehensive care of trauma patients in the acute care setting.

Impact of Physiatrist Involvement in Specialized Patient Populations

Involving physiatrists in the care of hospitalized patients has multiple benefits for both patients and hospital systems.

- Acute care PM&R consultation for **trauma patients** 8 days or less after admission is associated with [4]:
  - Shorter length of stay (12 vs. 30 days, $p < 0.001$).
  - Fewer complications.
  - Less use of benzodiazepines and antipsychotics.
- Early physiatry involvement for **trauma patients** is associated with [5]:
  - Increased rates of return to work.
- Physiatry involvement in cases of **acute traumatic SCI** results in [6]:
  - Significant survival benefit at 30 days (92.6% vs. 78.6%, $p = .004$).
  - Reduced risk of mortality.
  - Increased discharge to an IRF (52.9% vs. 19.6%, $p < .01$).
- Brain injury medicine (BIM)-certified physiatrist consultation on hospitalized **TBI** patients results in [7]:
  - Shorter acute care length of stay.
  - Decreased unplanned transfers to acute care from rehabilitation.
  - Increased likelihood of emerging from a minimally conscious state during inpatient rehabilitation.
- Addition of a dedicated BIM-specialized physiatrist to a trauma team results in the following regarding care of hospitalized **TBI** patients [8]:
  - Significant improvement in Functional Independence Measure (FIM) motor and cognitive scores ($p < 0.05$).
  - Significantly more neurostimulants ($p < 0.001$) and sleep medications ($p = 0.02$) received.
- Early PM&R consultation less than 48 hours after admission on hospitalized **TBI** patients results in [9]:
  - Significantly better Functional Independence Measure (FIM) scores with transfers and locomotion.

  - Significantly shorter length of stay (p = .001).
  - Reduced health care costs.
  - Increased discharge to community.
- Receiving acute post-operative specialized rehabilitation following transtibial or transfemoral **amputation** results in [10]:
  - Improved physical functioning at rehabilitation discharge.
  - Increased likelihood of receiving a prescription for a prosthetic limb within 1 year post amputation.
  - Increased likelihood of home discharge.
- Addition of PM&R consultation service to an acute **burn** program and subsequent inpatient rehabilitation results in [11]:
  - Significant reduction in inpatient rehabilitation length of stay.
- PM&R consultation for **stroke** patients in acute care results in [12]:
  - Increased likelihood of discharge home after inpatient rehabilitation (p = 0.042).

Physiatrist Involvement in Level 1 Trauma Centers

A level I trauma center is defined as "capable of providing total care for every aspect of injury – from prevention through rehabilitation" [13]. Physiatrist involvement in level 1 trauma centers is widespread and growing due to the value that physiatrists can add to comprehensive trauma care and due to updated guidelines on best practice care of trauma patients.

The **Committee on Trauma, American College of Surgeons (ACS)** released new guidelines in 2022 regarding "Resources for Optimal Care of the Injured Patient".

Standard 4.26 of the guidelines state that **level I trauma centers must have specialists in physiatry** [14].

Excerpts from Standard 5.27 of the guidelines [14] state all trauma centers must meet the rehabilitation needs of trauma patients, including:

- "Developing protocols that **identify which patients will require rehabilitation services** during their acute inpatient stay"
- "Establishing processes that **determine the rehabilitation care, needs, and services required** during the acute inpatient stay"
- "**Early multidisciplinary assessment of patients to determine their rehabilitation needs** and provide the relevant services during the acute phase of care is critical to ensuring optimal functional recovery. Multidisciplinary assessment might include input from physicians (including **physiatry**, where applicable)."

Standard 5.28 of the guidelines [14] recommend:

- "All trauma centers must have a process to determine the **level of care patients require after trauma center discharge**, as well as the **specific rehabilitation**

care services required at the next level of care. The level of care and services required must be **documented in the medical record**."

- "The specific services required might include **rehabilitation expertise** that focuses on spinal cord injury, TBI, musculoskeletal rehabilitation, or others relevant to the needs of the patient."

In a survey of 164 PM&R departments [15], the following was reported:

- Physiatrists **consult in 91%** of the responding level 1 trauma centers.
- Of PM&R departments at level 1 trauma centers, **67% participated in multidisciplinary rounds** with the trauma service and **89% reported a good or excellent relationship** with the trauma service.

Early physiatry consultation at level 1 trauma centers can ensure that guidelines regarding rehabilitation and discharge planning are met in a timely fashion and documented in the medical record for the highest quality care of the trauma patient.

Demographics of UCM Trauma Population

Unique Characteristics at UChicago Medicine

The UChicago Medicine adult trauma population has many unique characteristics that make successful discharge to home or post-acute rehabilitation a challenge. Many of these patients experience a significant functional decline after sustaining traumatic injuries and can benefit from the expertise of physiatrists to help restore function and quality of life.

Injury Characteristics

The Uchicago Medicine Level 1 adult trauma center opened on May 1, 2018. Prior to 2018, South Chicago was without an adult trauma center for 27 years [16].

As of May 2023 [16], the Uchicago Medicine adult trauma population demographics included:

- 58% from **falls**, **vehicle accidents**, other **blunt trauma**
- 40% from **penetrating injuries** (gunshots and stabbings)

Population Characteristics

Uchicago Medicine mainly services 12 different zip codes in South Chicago (Figs. 1 and 2) with the following characteristics [17]:

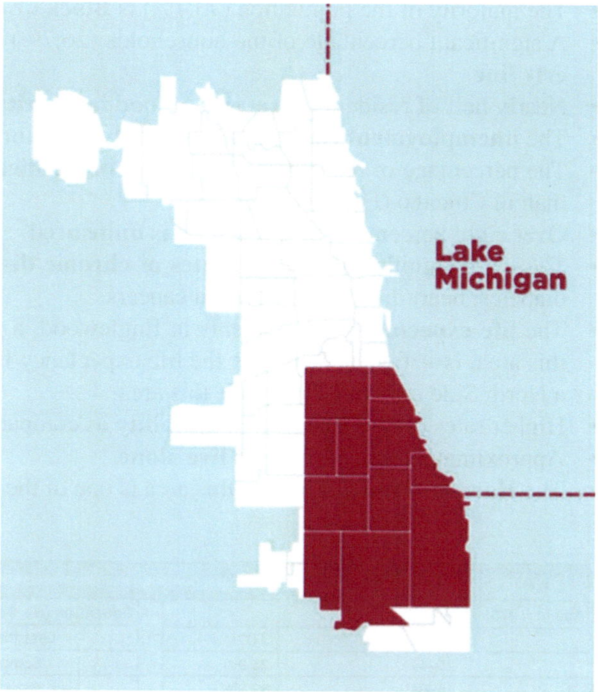

Fig. 1 University of Chicago Medical Center (UCMC) Service Area in South Chicago [17]

Zip Codes					
60609	60615	60617	60619	60620	60621
60628	60636	60637	60643	60649	60653

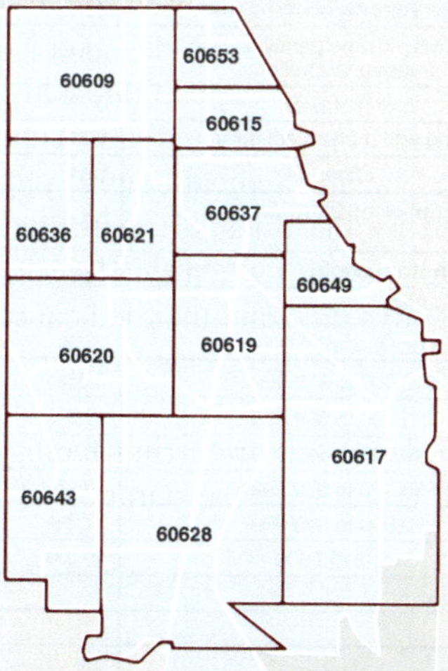

UCHICAGO MEDICINE SERVICE AREA
Zip Codes and Community Areas*

60609
Armour Square
Bridgeport
Douglas
Fuller Park
Gage Park
Grand Boulevard
McKinley Park
New City
Washington Park

60615
Grand Boulevard
Hyde Park
Kenwood
Washington Park

60617
Avalon Park
Calumet Heights
East Side
Hegewisch
South Chicago
South Deering

60619
Avalon Park
Burnside
Calumet Heights
Chatham
Greater Grand Crossing
Roseland
South Shore

60620
Ashburn
Auburn Gresham
Beverly
Chatham
Englewood
Greater Grand Crossing
Roseland
Washington Heights

60621
Englewood
Greater Grand Crossing
Washington Park

60628
Pullman
Riverdale
Roseland
Washington Heights
West Pullman

60636
Chicago Lawn
Gage Park
West Englewood

60637
Greater Grand Crossing
Hyde Park
South Shore
Washington Park
Woodlawn

60643
Beverly
Morgan Park
Washington Heights
West Pullman

60649
South Shore
Woodlawn

60653
Douglas
Grand Boulevard
Kenwood
Oakland

* Some community areas stretch across multiple zip codes. Out community benefit service area extends only to those parts of a community area within the 12 zip codes identified.

Fig. 2 University of Chicago Medical Center (UCMC) Service Area by zip code [17]

- The majority of the population (73.7%) is **Black or African American** (Fig. 3).
- A significant percentage of the households (26.7%) are **below the federal poverty line**.
- Nearly half of residents are at risk of **food insecurity**.
- The **unemployment rate** (15.8%) is nearly three times the national rate (5.4%).
- The percentage of residents in this area with **Medicaid coverage** is 45% higher than in Chicago (Fig. 4).
- Over eight percent of the population is **uninsured**.
- There are significantly **higher rates of chronic disease** in this area, including diabetes, heart disease, and certain cancers.
- The **life expectancy** for residents in Englewood, a Chicago community within this area, is ~30 years less than the life expectancy for residents in Streeterville, a North Side community outside this area.
- Higher rates of residents with a **disability** as compared to Chicago.
- Approximately 4 in 10 **seniors live alone**.
- The **Hardship Index score** of this area is one of the highest in Chicago (Fig. 5).

Table 1. Demographics of Community Input Survey Respondents in UCMC Communities

Age (n = 975)	
18–24	3.0%
25–44	25.9%
45–64	39.9%
65 and older	31.2%
Gender Identity (n = 974)	
Male	16.3%
Female	82.0%
Transgender man, FTM	0.0%
Transgender woman, MTF	0.0%
Genderqueer/gender-nonconforming	0.4%
Other	0.22%
Decline to answer	1.0%
Orientation (n = 964)	
Straight or heterosexual	87.6%
Lesbian or gay	2.3%
Bisexual	4.4%
Queer, pansexual, and/or questioning	0.9%
Other	0.5%
Don't know	0.5%
Decline to answer	3.8%
Race (n = 972 with multiple answers allowed)	
American Indian or Alaska Native	1.5%
Asian or Mideast Asian	1.5%
Black or African-American	70.7%
Choose to not disclose	3.1%
Hispanic/Latino(a)	5.3%
More than one race	5.2%
Unknown	0.7%
White	15.2%

Education (n = 963)	
Less than high school	0.7%
Some high school	1.9%
High school graduate or GED	6.7%
Vocational or technical school	1.5%
Some college	20.5%
College graduate	30.1%
Advanced degree	38.6%
Current Living Arrangements (n = 963)	
Own my home	58.9%
Rent my home	33.7%
Living in emergency or transitional shelter	0.3%
Living outside	0.2%
Living with a friend or family	5.3%
Other	1.6%
Average Number of Children in Home	0.54
Disability in Household	151
Income (n = 885)	
Less than $10,000	7.7%
$10,000 to $19,999	5.6%
$20,000 to $39,999	12.3%
$40,000 to $59,999	16.8%
$60,000 to $79,999	16.9%
$80,000 to $99,999	11.3%
Over $100,000	29.3%

Fig. 3 Overview of demographics in UCMC Communities [17]

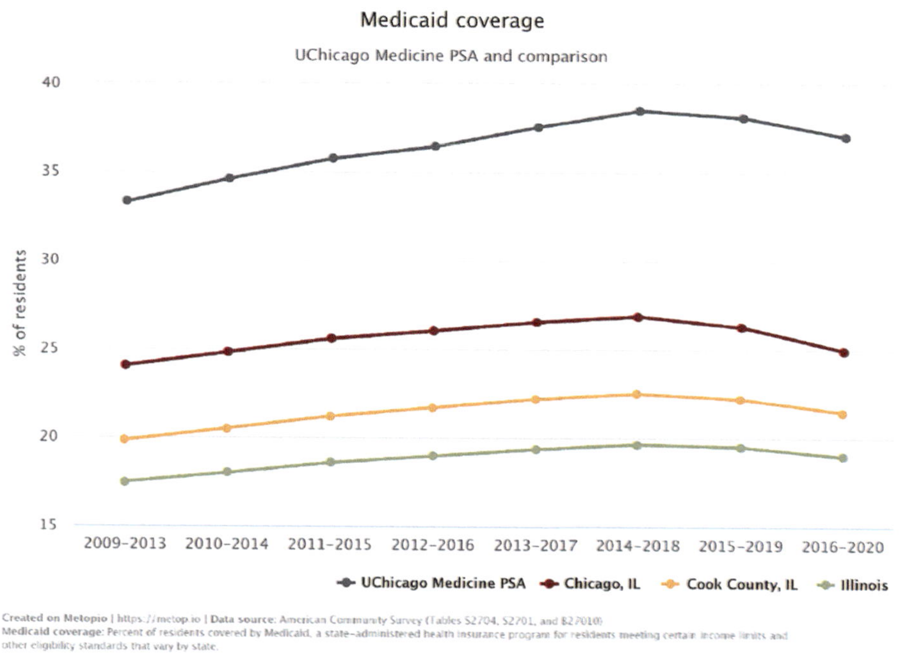

Fig. 4 Comparison of percentage of residents with Medicaid coverage in UCMC service area as compared to citywide, county, and state [17]

- The percentage of **Disconnected Youth** (ages 16–19 neither working nor enrolled in school) is higher in this area (11.6%) compared to Chicago (8.3%).
- The **crime rate** (per 100,000 residents) in this area is higher than the citywide average (Fig. 6).
- The hospitalization rate for **assault by firearms** in this area ranks in the 95th percentile for IL.

These characteristics introduce major challenges into this population's daily life. With an increased rate of crime and hospitalization for assault by firearms, this population is more susceptible to trauma and the resultant injuries and functional loss that often follow. Adding a serious injury or disability to the challenges this population already faces (e.g. uninsured status, reduced support at home, food insecurity, unemployment, poverty, chronic disease, increased Hardship Index) results in significant barriers to safe post-hospitalization discharge planning and access to necessary resources.

The unique demographics of the Uchicago Medicine trauma population and the challenges they face are the driving force behind many of the initiatives led by physiatrists at UChicago Medicine to care for this distinctive population.

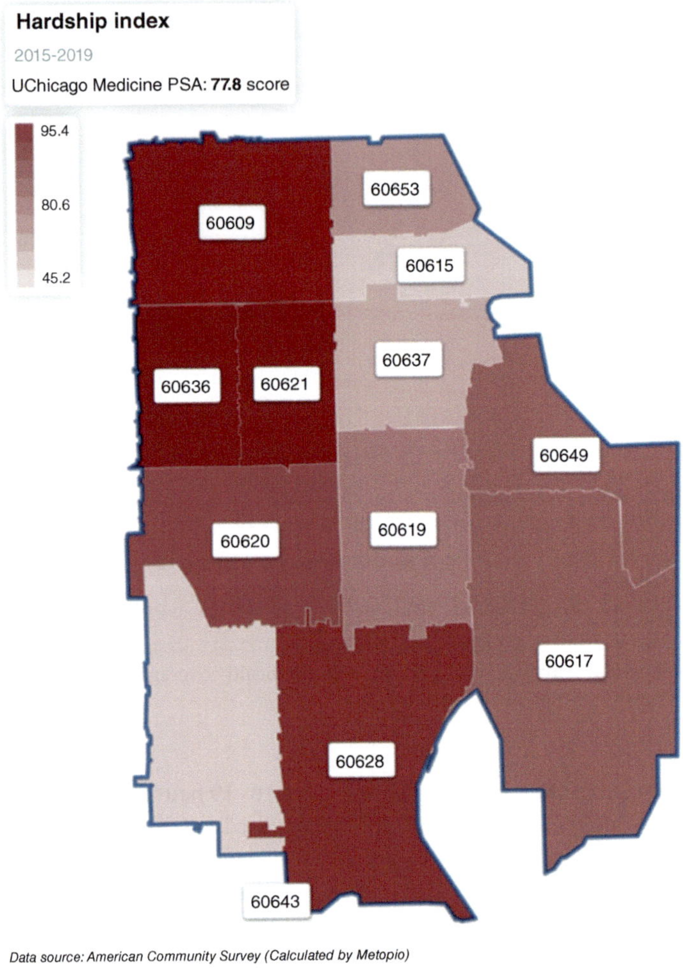

Fig. 5 Hardship Index Scores in the 12 zip codes of the UCMC service area [17]

Topic	UChicago Service Area	Chicago, IL	Illinois
Violent crime *crimes per 100,000 residents, 2020*	1,616.8 ± 0.0	1,125.6 ± 0.0	425.9 ± 0.0
Aggravated assault/battery *crimes per 100,000 residents, 2020*	1,054.1 ± 0.0	695.2 ± 0.0	278.9 ± 0.0
Burglary *crimes per 100,000 residents, 2020*	527.7 ± 0.0	351.0 ± 0.0	246.4 ± 0.0
Homicide *crimes per 100,000 residents, 2020*	55.7 ± 0.0	36.6 ± 0.0	9.1 ± 0.0
Larceny (theft) *crimes per 100,000 residents, 2020*	1,786.6 ± 0.0	1,686.3 ± 0.0	1,143.5 ± 0.0
Arson *crimes per 100,000 residents, 2020*	35.0 ± 0.0	24.9 ± 0.0	12.2 ± 0.0
Property crime *crimes per 100,000 residents, 2020*	2,919.4 ± 0.0	2,510.0 ± 0.0	1,559.4 ± 0.0
Robbery *crimes per 100,000 residents, 2020*	432.5 ± 0.0	339.0 ± 0.0	97.4 ± 0.0
Criminal sexual assault *crimes per 100,000 residents, 2020*	74.5 ± 0.0	49.7 ± 0.0	40.4 ± 0.0
Motor vehicle theft *crimes per 100,000 residents, 2020*	570.1 ± 0.0	447.8 ± 0.0	169.5 ± 0.0

Fig. 6 Crime rate per 100,000 residents in UCMC service area as compared to city and state [17]

Integration of PM&R Consultation Services into the UCM Trauma Center

Trauma Center: Pre-Opening

Before the opening of the trauma center, there were two physiatrist consultants at UCM in the Department of Orthopaedic Surgery and Rehabilitation Medicine. These physiatrists were involved in multidisciplinary planning meetings that included the two physiatrists, members from the Therapy Services Department, various surgical services, and the Director of the trauma center.

With the goal of presenting tested strategies to the Director of the trauma center, the physiatrists gathered information from colleagues at other major trauma centers around the country with a specific interest in learning ways to integrate PM&R consultants into a trauma center as well as other tips for the development of a successful trauma program from a PM&R perspective.

Proposed Strategies: Physiatrist Integration into a Major Trauma Center

- **PM&R physician dedicated to trauma**
  - Rounding with the trauma team (e.g. ICU patients, floor patients).
  - Consults for management and disposition recommendations.
  - Patient/family education.

- **Required evaluations by a physiatrist** for certain diagnoses (e.g. SCI, TBI, traumatic amputation, major multi-trauma with weight bearing precautions)
- **PM&R Service under the Department of Trauma**

Proposed Strategies: Physiatrist Perspectives for a Successful Trauma Center

- **Geographic organization** of trauma patients (e.g. patients, trauma RNs, trauma PT/OT located in one area of hospital).
- **Specialty population care** (e.g. social work with trauma experience, specialty psychiatric/psychological care, specialty PT/OT/SLP).
- **Rehabilitation throughput** (e.g. discussion with nearby rehabilitation centers to prepare for the influx of trauma patients with unique social circumstances).
- **Multidisciplinary rounds** formalization.
- **PM&R outpatient** follow-up care.

The major takeaway from the informal survey of other major trauma centers was that a dedicated PM&R physician was often embedded in the trauma team with time specifically allotted for the care of trauma patients. Additionally, this trauma PM&R physician was often employed as part of a PM&R department at the trauma center. At the time of this writing, the physiatrists at UCM remain in the Department of Orthopaedic Surgery and Rehabilitation Medicine and do not have dedicated time alotted for the trauma team.

Therapy Interventions

Multiple preparatory initiatives were also undertaken by the management team of therapy services. There were informal discussions with members of the PM&R faculty in the planning stages as well as conversations with the trauma center leadership. A number of the therapists were members of the American Congress of Rehabilitation Medicine (ACRM) trauma working group and shared information about best practices from that organization. Therapists were also sent to established trauma centers to learn best practices, including at UChicago Medicine Comer Children's Hospital, which was already a level I trauma center at that time. These interventions led to the creation of TBI and SCI treatment guidelines. Additionally, therapists received Crisis Prevention Institute training to learn de-escalation techniques.

Environmental modifications to aid in rehabilitation were also instituted. The unit which was planned to receive the majority of trauma patients was made into a locked unit. This was part of patient and staff security measures, but also for protection of patients with TBI who can be prone to elopement. Additionally, overhead slings were installed in each of the patient rooms in this unit to facilitate transferring patients with significant functional impairments in and out of bed.

Trauma Center: Early Days

There was variable involvement of PM&R physicians in the early days following the trauma center opening.

PM&R Consult Timing

PM&R consults were requested on some trauma patients, but inconsistently. Consults were requested via phone call from the trauma service or social worker, usually for management recommendations in patients with SCI or TBI. Furthermore, the timing of the consult requests for disposition planning was variable. Frequently, PM&R services were requested late in a patient's hospital course, usually when the primary team had cleared the patient for discharge. This late involvement made it challenging to optimize the patient for the rehabilitation setting in a timely manner and made coordination of discharge to the appropriate rehabilitation setting more difficult.

Length of Stay

Trauma patients with the need for rehabilitation interventions, but with particularly challenging barriers for discharge– such as legal issues, uninsured status, or complex medical problems—had particularly long hospitalizations. To the knowledge of the PM&R physicians, there were limited protocols in place to solve for these barriers to discharge.

Multidisciplinary Rounds

Physiatrists attended in-person multidisciplinary rounds twice weekly led by a trauma APN or resident. Also in attendance at these rounds were social work, RN, and PT/OT. Physiatrists found these rounds to be both valuable and productive. The primary team efficiently entered orders during rounds based on multidisciplinary team recommendations. RN input was up to date and reliable regarding a patient's bowel, bladder, suctioning needs, nutritional intake, and family dynamics, all of which play a role in rehabilitation recommendations and discharge planning.

Activity Precautions

Patients with polytrauma frequently have injuries that require complex activity precautions. This may include limitations on weight bearing or range of motion (ROM) of multiple limbs at specific joints. Determining these activity precautions is essential prior to engagement in therapeutic activity in order to clarify the direction of therapy, including how to safely mobilize a patient without inducing further injury or harm.

At UCM, there were occasions of differing recommendations from surgical teams or discordance in documentation of activity precautions in the chart. Often, this presented a barrier to therapeutic activity for these complex patients as therapists would rightfully abstain from mobilizing a patient prior to clarification of the patient's activity precautions.

There were additional challenges when a patient transitioned from the acute care hospital to the rehabilitation setting. It was sometimes unclear what was required to de-escalate activity precautions (e.g. specific duration of time of precautions, timing of follow-up imaging) in order to optimize a patient's functional progress. At times, the activity precautions used in acute care were not clearly communicated to the accepting rehabilitation unit.

Trauma Center: Current/Ongoing

Despite the longstanding and continuously growing relationship between physiatrists and the trauma department, usage of the PM&R consultation service remained initially inconsistent. This was in part due to the lack of a formalized hospital-wide consult process. An opportunity for improvement came when the hospital system as a whole transitioned to a new Epic Consult Process. The new process required a provider to place a consult order in Epic that triggered an automatic page to the consulting service and added the patient to the consult service's system list. The PM&R consultation service was enrolled in the new process in December 2022.

Following this shift in UChicago Medicine consult order culture, the PM&R consult service was able to reinforce multiple initiatives to integrate further into the care of the trauma population.

Initiatives for Integration of PM&R Consultation Services

1. **Compulsory Consults**

One of the first initiatives implemented was the development of the compulsory consult process. This process called for providers to automatically place a consult to PM&R for patients with any of the following diagnoses:

- Traumatic **spinal cord injury**
- Traumatic **brain injury** (moderate to severe)
- Traumatic **amputation**

This initiative ensured early involvement of physiatrists who could provide invaluable recommendations in the management of neurogenic bowel/bladder, disorders of consciousness, agitation, and appropriate level of amputation. Physiatrists were also involved in early education to patients and families about these specialized diagnoses and rehabilitation expectations.

2. **Participation in ICU Rounds**
With the compulsory consult model in place, the trauma team was more consistently consulting PM&R than ever before. However, the PM&R consultants still noted a delay in the timing of the consult order in comparison to the patient's length of stay. It was concluded that the delayed consults were often on patients who were admitted to the Surgical ICU (SICU) or the Neurological ICU (NICU). Thus, the physiatrists began attending **weekly rounds in the SICU and the NICU** to promote early physiatrist involvement for trauma patients in the ICU's. During rounds, physiatrists would provide education, offer management recommendations, and, if appropriate, recommend a PM&R consult for formalized involvement. This initiative was successful in promoting a culture of earlier PM&R consults in the ICU's and in solidifying the relationship between physiatrists, trauma surgeons, and neurointensivists.

3. **PT/OT Enter Consult Orders**
With the above initiatives in place, physiatrists were seeing increased involvement in the trauma population. There were, however, many instances of patients with traumatic injuries and/or functional decline that were brought to the attention of the physiatrists only by informal discussion with the physical and occupational therapists. In these instances, there was a delay in physiatry care for these patients as the therapist would then have to contact the patient's primary team to recommend a PM&R consult. Due to the frequency of these occurrences, and following discussion with administrators, a process was implemented where **physical and occupational therapists could enter orders to consult PM&R**. This initiative empowered the therapists to involve physiatrists in the care of patients with a functional decline and resulted in more widespread and earlier involvement of physiatrists in the trauma population.

4. **Educating key players**
It was recognized early on that many members of a patient's care team participate in optimizing the patient's rehabilitation outcomes. To that end, education sessions, both formal and informal, were created to broadcast important principles regarding rehabilitation and to build team camaraderie.

Members of the physiatry team met with the **physical, occupational, and speech-language therapists** to review appropriate times to consider consulting PM&R. In light of the evolving insurance environment with increasing numbers of denials for rehabilitation services, education was also provided to therapists regarding optimal documentation to support their rehabilitation recommendations. Discussion with PM&R consultants also became part of the onboarding process for newly hired physical and occupational therapists starting at UCM, ensuring that these fundamentals were ingrained early on.

It was also recognized that, from the perspective of many other medical disciplines, the inpatient rehabilitation setting can be a "black box"—a mysterious place where patients go after hospitalization. Thus, meetings were held with **internal medicine and neurology residents** to provide education on the different rehabilitation settings and the patients that they treat, as well as how to optimize a patient for the inpatient rehabilitation setting. This included the creation of a **"Med Ready Guide"**, or a handout that outlines common criteria for transferring a patient to the acute rehabilitation setting.

ACUTE REHAB DISCHARGES

The below guidelines can decrease **length of stay** and facilitate discharge to acute rehab facilities sooner

Delays can occur when the **estimated date of discharge** provided to facilities is incorrect.

MEDICAL READINESS GUIDELINES

In addition to patient medical clearance, it is important that the following are in place:

- Patient is able to **tolerate & participate in 3 hours** of daily therapy
- Accepting facility can manage patient's **medical needs**
- Follow up **appointments** and upcoming **diagnostic testing** should be scheduled after discharge from rehabilitation (unless approved by accepting facility). Average length of stay is 21 days.

NOTE: These are guidelines. **Contact admission liaisons** and/or **PM&R consulting physicians** for additional information.

Remember: Patients must be able to participate in therapy 3 hours per day in acute inpatient rehabilitation and the following are guidelines to help meet this requirement.

MEDICAL STATUS

- **Work-up** completed and treatment plan agreed upon by primary and consulting services
- **Agreement** of discharge readiness among consulting services
- No active **psychiatric** issues that would prevent participation in rehabilitation program.

TREATMENT and LAB DATA

- No continuous/overly frequent **suction** or **irrigation**
- Documented orthopedic or spinal **precautions**
- **Dialysis** stable 3 days/week (or less) & OP community chair established.
- No **telemetry** monitoring
- Blood product **transfusions** no more than 3 times per week

MEDICATIONS/ THERAPEUTICS

- Enteral/SubQ only, except IV antibiotics with PICC line
- No IV push meds
- No continuous IV drips or IV heparin.
- Established anticoagulation/DVT ppx
- No IV chemo/immunotherapy (PO meds only without need for tele. Patient may need to bring own supply).
- No radiation therapy

RESPIRATORY

- **Suctioning** needed at a maximum frequency of every 4 hours
- **Respiratory treatments** maximum frequency of every 6 hours
- O2 per **nasal cannula** < 4 lpm
- O2 per **trach collar** FiO2 < 40%
- If trach in place, change to **cuffless tracheostomy tube**

DIET

- **Oral diet** or able to tolerate tube feeding to provide caloric and fluid requirements
- **Gastrostomy tubes** recommended.
- **DHT** cannot be primary nutrition source
- **TPN** patients need to be on a stable solution, cycled at night with a plan for discharge to home on TPN. Some facilities don't accept any TPN.

INFECTION CONTROL

- No **active TB**
- No **airborne/droplet precautions** (except in unique situations for COVID19 patients)
- **COVID isolation** protocols vary among facilities

PM&R consultants also met with the **social work/case management department**. As central members of multidisciplinary rounds, social workers and case managers are uniquely situated to identify patients who may benefit from the involvement of physiatrists. The physiatrists reviewed with the social workers and case managers strategies for working with insurance companies to reduce length of stay including education about when to submit for insurance authorization as well as unique or challenging features of certain insurance plans. The physiatrists also reviewed the nuances of different rehabilitation units that have specialized programs for TBI or SCI patients. This effort helped reduce referrals to inappropriate levels of care.

5. **Therapy Services Initiatives**
A number of changes were instituted to meet the challenges that came with providing rehabilitation treatments to a level I trauma center patient population. These changes were driven by the therapy services leadership team.

- *Staff Knowledge*
  - Education sessions to work through challenges of working with a new patient population.
  - Education sessions for working with patients in custody.
  - Developed trauma therapy core competencies.
- *Environmental*
  - Additional overhead slings added in other units.
  - All units became locked units.
  - Obtained High-back reclining wheelchairs.
  - Identified community resources for equipment for patients with significant financial barriers.

Initiatives to Streamline Discharge & Improve Access to an Inpatient Rehabilitation Facility

1. **Partnership with Ingalls Inpatient Rehabilitation Facility (IRF)**
In 2016, UCM completed a merger with Ingalls Memorial Hospital, a general medical and surgical community hospital located in Harvey, IL, a south suburb of Chicago. This merger also included the acquisition of the Ingalls inpatient rehabilitation facility with 43 licensed beds, which allowed rehabilitation referrals within the network of care. This partnership provided numerous benefits to the UCM trauma population because the care of these complex patients became easily coordinated across the continuum of care.

- Therapy expertise and training was shared between the acute care hospital and the Ingalls IRF.
- Physiatrists who performed consultations at UCM trauma center also provided inpatient rehabilitation care at Ingalls IRF, allowing for continuity of care.
- In August 2022, after the integration of Epic electronic health records system at Ingalls, the medical record system for these two entities was also effectively merged.

The increased level of professional trust and electronic health record transparency between the acute care hospital and Ingalls IRF allowed for more clinically tenuous patients to transition to post-acute care at Ingalls IRF when other rehabilitation facilities may otherwise have been more hesitant.

2. **Single Case Agreement**
The UCM population encompasses a large percentage of uninsured and underinsured patients [17]. These financial factors can be a significant barrier to timely discharge and medically appropriate post-acute care resources. In instances where patients are appropriate for IRF, but are otherwise unable to be discharged to IRF due to uninsured or underinsured status, a single case agreement is utilized. A single case agreement is a contract between UCM and an accepting IRF (most often Ingalls IRF) whereby UCM agrees to financially cover the cost of a patient's post-acute care rehabilitation, just as an insurance company may do under typical circumstances. The single case agreement facilitates transition of patients with financial barriers to the appropriate level of post-acute care in a timely manner and thus reduces the patient's acute care length of stay.

Additionally, the single case agreement and the partnership with Ingalls IRF are used to counteract delays in discharge due to pending insurance authorization. Oftentimes, patients are medically ready for discharge to IRF, but discharge is delayed solely due to pending insurance authorization. At UCM, an operating procedure was put in place for these situations where patients were given the opportunity to transfer to Ingalls IRF as soon as medically appropriate by utilizing a single case agreement. In this single case agreement between UCM and Ingalls IRF, UCM agrees to financially cover the cost of the patient's rehabilitation course, allowing the patient to discharge to IRF despite lack of insurance authorization. If insurance authorization for IRF is ultimately denied, UCM incurs the cost of the patient's rehabilitation. If insurance authorization is obtained retroactively, rehabilitation costs are instead covered by the patient's insurance company. At the time of this writing, every patient transferred from UCM to Ingalls IRF via insurance pending single case agreement has had insurance authorization obtained retroactively. This usage of the single case agreement to facilitate transfers prior to obtaining insurance authorization has led to **117 hospital days saved** for 61 patients as of November 2023.

3. **Activity Precaution Form**
Patients with major multiple trauma present a unique challenge when it comes to weight bearing and ROM precautions. A careful balance must be struck between the detriments of immobility and the necessity to protect surgical sites and avoid exacerbating injuries. When treating a patient following a traumatic injury involving multiple limbs (often multiple joints of the same limb) and/or the spine, comprehensive management frequently requires the involvement of multiple surgical teams (e.g. orthopedic surgery, neurosurgery, plastic surgery). The challenge in this situation is the risk for miscommunication and confusion surrounding the appropriate precautions for each limb. Thus, an "**Activity Precaution Form**" was created to **consolidate precautions from multiple surgical teams into one document**. The form outlines the weight bearing and range of motion precautions for each limb, the recommendations for surgical wound care, and the contact information for each surgeon should questions arise. The PM&R consultants discussed the form with the trauma team, the orthopedic surgery team, the trauma social workers, and the

therapy department. After consensus agreement to use the form, PM&R consultants recommended that the form be used for **any patient with a traumatic injury involving more than one limb** and recommended the form be completed once the patient was considered operatively complete for the hospital admission.

ACTIVITY PRECAUTION FORM

RIGHT UPPER EXTREMITY:
Injuries: Right distal radius fracture
Procedures: s/p ORIF
Primary surgeon contact: Dr. Bones. Please call 312-1234 if needed.
- **Weight bearing, ROM restrictions**:
  - NWB.
  - ROM as tolerated.
  - Duration: follow-up
  - Limitations: None
- **Orthosis/splint**: Type short arm splint. Duration Until follow up. may be removed for hygiene.
- **Dressings**: can be changed at rehab as needed. Type foam. Frequency daily and prn.
- **Sutures/Staples**: can be removed at rehab. Removal date on 11/22. Imaging not required prior to removal.
- **Follow-up**: Appointment scheduled -.

Right upper extremity comments:

LEFT UPPER EXTREMITY:
Injuries: Left elbow dislocation
Procedures: s/p closed reduction
Primary surgeon contact: Dr. Bones. Please call main orthopedic office if needed.
- **Weight bearing, ROM restrictions**:
  - WBAT
  - ROM as tolerated. Avoid ROM through NA
  - Duration: follow-up
  - Limitations: No lifting more than 15 lbs
- **Orthosis/splint**: Type NA.
- **Dressings**: NA
- **Sutures/Staples**: NA
- **Follow-up**: Appointment scheduled 11/26.

Left upper extremity comments: No aggressive stretching in to extension. Pronation/Supination as tolerated

---

RIGHT LOWER EXTREMITY:
Injuries: Right femoral neck fracture; Right ankle bimalleolar fracture
Procedures: s/p right hip IMN and right ankle ORIF
Primary surgeon contact: Dr. Oucsh. Please message via pager if needed
- **Weight bearing, ROM restrictions**:
  - WBAT and CAM boot
  - ROM as tolerated. posterior hip precautions.
  - Duration: follow-up
  - Limitations: ambulation distance 200 feet
- **Orthosis/splint**: Type CAM boot. Duration until follow up. When out of bed
- **Dressings**: can be changed at rehab as needed.
- **Sutures/Staples**: cannot be removed at rehab. Follow up with surgeon
- **Follow-up**: Please call office to arrange appointment in 2 weeks after rehab.

Right lower extremity comments:

LEFT LOWER EXTREMITY:
Injuries: Left tibial plateau fracture; lower leg degloving injury
Procedures: s/p skin grafts with plastic surgery
Primary surgeon contact: Dr. Barby. Please call hotline if needed.
- **Weight bearing, ROM restrictions**:
  - hinged knee brace
  - no knee extension past 30 degrees.
  - Duration: follow-up
  - Limitations: avoid shear to the skin grafts
- **Orthosis/splint**: Type hinged knee brace. When out of bed. may be removed for hygiene
- **Dressings**: can be changed at rehab as needed. Type acquacel. Frequency daily or as needed.
- **Sutures/Staples**: cannot be removed at rehab unless images of wound reviewed by surgeon
- **Follow-up**: Appointment scheduled 12/23.

Left lower extremity comments:n/a

SPINE
Injuries: C4 burst fracture
Procedures: s/p Occiput to C6 PSF
Primary surgeon contact: Dr. Geraff. Please call office if needed.
- **Dressings**: can be left open to air
  - Spine stability: Spine only stable WITH orthosis to be worn AT ALL TIMES. Orthosis type: Aspen Collar.
  - Brace may be removed for hygiene while maintaining spinal precautions.
  - Patient may not be placed in prone position with brace.
  - Duration: Brace to be worn until follow-up.
- **Sutures/Staples**: can be removed at rehab. Removal date on/after 11/24.

VTE prophylaxis:
- **VTE ppx**: Type Aspirin 81 mg BID. Duration 35 days

The Activity Precaution Form has helped to streamline communication in the acute care setting between the trauma team, surgical teams, physiatrists, and physical/occupational therapy. With the weight bearing and ROM precautions clarified and easily accessible in one document, patients' ability to participate safely in therapies was optimized, which oftentimes led to updates or changes in recommendations for post-acute rehabilitation.

Results of PM&R Consultation Service Integration

At the time of this writing, there are four physiatrists at UCM, an increase from the two physiatrists present prior to the opening of the UCM trauma center. The integration initiatives reviewed in this chaper, have resulted in earlier and more frequent involvement of physiatrists in the care of the UCM trauma patient population, which has streamlined delivery of rehabilitation services, fostered improved interdisciplinary relationships, and improved patient access to IRF care despite financial and medical barriers.

Trauma Center: Future Directions

1. Optimizing care for patients with traumatic brain injury
   - Introducing more objective scales for measuring agitation (e.g. Agitation Behavior Scale).
   - Nursing education on caring for agitated patients (e.g. de-escalation techniques).
   - Initiating use of enclosure beds for patients at risk of fall due to impulsivity.
2. Optimizing care for patients with traumatic spinal cord injury
   - Nursing education on management of neurogenic bowel/bladder and autonomic dysreflexia.
   - Peer support during acute care hospitalization.
3. Optimizing care for patients with traumatic amputation
   - Fabrication of rigid removable dressing for limb protection and shaping during acute care hospitalization.
   - Peer support during acute care hospitalization
4. Equipment
   - Installment of overhead gait tracks to allow for earlier patient gait training after traumatic injury while secured in a body harness.
   - Increased number of overhead slings to improve ability to transfer patients out of bed.
   - Increased access to specialized wheelchairs to optimize patient positioning when out of bed.

5. Outpatient PM&R clinics
    - Post-IRF follow-up visits.
    - Ongoing care for sequelae of TBI (e.g. mood changes, agitation management, spasticity management).
    - Ongoing care for sequelae of SCI (e.g. neurogenic bowel/bladder management, spasticity management, durable medical equipment, wound care).
    - Expansion of post-amputation care (e.g. prosthetics, wound care, pain management).
6. Research
    - Leverage integrated electronic medical record systems to investigate relationships between acute care clinical factors and subsequent rehabilitation outcomes.
    - Identify factors present in acute care to better predict unplanned readmissions from IRF.

Conclusion

Trauma patient care requires numerous medical, surgical, nursing and allied health disciplines to achieve quality outcomes. Once the life of the patient is out of danger, there is often a long path to the ideal functional outcome and associated quality of life. With their interdisciplinary and holistic approach, the physiatrist can be a valuable resource for helping patients navigate the path of recovery. An integrated PM&R consult service at a level I trauma center that stretches across the healthcare system and continuum of care can improve the efficient delivery of high-quality care and improve patient outcomes.

Clinical Pearls
- An integrated PM&R consultation service at a level 1 trauma center helps to transition patients to the appropriate level of care.
- Having a partnership with an IRF can facilitate earlier transfer to IRF despite socioeconomic barriers.
- Physiatry involvement reduces length of stay and complications in patients with specific trauma diagnoses.
- Physiatry interventions help to prepare patients for future rehabilitation interventions.
- Initiatives to consider for successful PM&R integration into a trauma center include:
    - Physiatry involvement in all cases of traumatic spinal cord injury, moderate-severe traumatic brain injury, and traumatic amputation.
    - In-person multidisciplinary and ICU rounds.
    - Regular education to key groups.

References

1. Sandel E. 2012. The early history of physical medicine and rehabilitation in the United States. PM&R Knowledge Now. https://now.aapmr.org/the-history-of-the-specialty-of-physical-medicine-and-rehabilitation/
2. ABPMR. 2023. ABPMR's history. https://www.abpmr.org/About
3. AAPM&R. 2023. What is physical medicine and rehabilitation? https://www.aapmr.org/about-physiatry/about-physical-medicine-rehabilitation
4. Robinson LR, Tam AKH, MacDonald SL, Hanada EY, Berbrayer D, Abdullahi A, Camilotti BG, Tien H. The impact of introducing a physical medicine and rehabilitation trauma consultation service to an academic level 1 trauma center. Am J Phys Med Rehabil. 2019;98(1):20–5. https://doi.org/10.1097/PHM.0000000000001007. PMID: 30063526.
5. Tam AK, Berbrayer D, Robinson LR. What should be the role of physiatrists in early acute care rehabilitation? Current literature, models of care, and thoughts for the future. Am J Phys Med Rehabil. 2016;95(3):225–9. https://doi.org/10.1097/PHM.0000000000000406. PMID: 26495815.
6. Tracy BM, Hoover E, Jones N, Hinrichs MJ, Gelbard RB. The effect of physiatry involvement for patients with acute traumatic spinal cord injury at a level 1 trauma center. Top Spinal Cord Inj Rehabil. 2022;28(4):76–83. https://doi.org/10.46292/sci21-00050.
7. Weppner JL, Linsenmeyer MA, Wagner AK. Effects of an acute care brain injury medicine continuity consultation service on health care utilization and rehabilitation outcomes. PM&R. 2021;13(11):1227–36. https://doi.org/10.1002/pmrj.12563. PMID: 33527710.
8. Greiss C, Yonclas PP, Jasey N, Lequerica A, Ward I, Chiaravalloti N, Felix G, Dabaghian L, Livingston D. Presence of a dedicated trauma center physiatrist improves functional outcomes following traumatic brain injury. J Trauma Acute Care Surg. 2016;80(1):70–5. https://doi.org/10.1097/TA.0000000000000890.
9. Wagner AK, Fabio T, Zafonte RD, Goldberg G, Marion D, Peitzman A. Relationships with acute functional outcome, length of stay, and discharge planning after traumatic brain injury. Am J Phys Med Rehabil. 2003;82:526–36. https://doi.org/10.1097/01.PHM.0000073825.09942.8F.
10. Kurichi JE, Small DS, Bates BE, Prvu-Bettger JA, Kwong PL, Vogel WB, Bidelspach DE, Stineman MG. Possible incremental benefits of specialized rehabilitation bed units among veterans after lower extremity amputation. Med Care. 2009;47(4):457–65. https://doi.org/10.1097/MLR.0b013e31818b08c6.
11. Robinson LR, Godleski M, Rehou S, Jeschke M. The impact of introducing a physical medicine and rehabilitation consultation service to an academic burn center. J Burn Care Res. 2019;40(5):648–51. https://doi.org/10.1093/jbcr/irz079.
12. Ikramuddin FS, Guarino AJ, Seidel E, Vonderhor K, Larson E, Battaglino R, Morse L. Physical medicine and rehabilitation consultation for stroke patients in acute care setting may be associated with an increased rate of discharge to the community from the inpatient rehabilitation facility. Am J Phys Med Rehabil. 2022;101(5):429–32. https://doi.org/10.1097/PHM.0000000000001842.
13. Soto JM, Zhang Y, Huang JH, Feng DX. An overview of the American trauma system. Chin J Traumatol. 2018;21(2):77–9. https://doi.org/10.1016/j.cjtee.2018.01.003. Epub 2018 Feb 21. PMID: 29605432; PMCID: PMC5911730.
14. ACS/American College of Surgeons. Resources for optimal care of the injured patient. 2022. https://www.facs.org/quality-programs/trauma/quality/verification-review-and-consultation-program/standards/
15. Melchiorre PJ. Status of physiatry and physical medicine and rehabilitation departments in adult level I trauma centers. Arch PM&R. 1998;79(1):62–6. https://doi.org/10.1016/S0003-9993(98)90210-6.
16. Wang J. Five years after launching level 1 adult trauma center, UChicago Medicine set to exceed 18,800 adult trauma patients. 2023. https://www.uchicagomedicine.org/forefront/trauma-articles/adult-trauma-center
17. UCMC CHNA. Community health needs assessment & strategic implementation plan: University of Chicago Medical Center. 2021–2022. uchicagomedicine.org/ucmc-chna

Penetrating Pediatric Trauma

Kenneth L. Wilson

The Tale of Two Cities

Highland Park, Illinois is an idyllic small town located adjacent to the northern shore of Lake Michigan. It is a patriotic town with the streets lined with American flags and regalia in anticipation of the annual Fourth of July parade. However, on July 4, 2022 the parade turned deadly in a way community members could not have imagined [1]. What was initially mistaken for fireworks were bullets reigning down from an elevated position killing seven and wounding numerous unsuspecting victims. The wounded were evacuated to the nearest hospital, NorthShore Highland Park Hospital, where the staff rose to the occasion and performed valiantly triaging injured patients and performing lifesaving operations. One of the youngest victims, an 8-year-old boy, suffered a thoracoabdominal gunshot wound that required operative intervention by several surgeons. The abdomen was temporarily closed for the possibility of re-exploration, and the University of Chicago Aeromedical Network (UCAN) helicopter launched to fly the young boy thirty-four miles to the University of Chicago's Children's Hospital for further evaluation and treatment. UCAN provides rapid helicopter transport to critically injured pediatric and adult patients is entrusted to call for a hot offload from the roof for immediate transport directly to the operating room. The clinical situation did decline in route to UChicago, and UCAN requested to be met on the helipad for direct operating room evaluation.

K. L. Wilson (✉)
Department of Surgery, Section of Trauma and Acute Care Surgery, University of Chicago, Chicago, IL, USA
e-mail: kwilson9@bsd.uchicago.edu

S. O. Rogers, Jr (ed.), *Creating a Modern Trauma Center*,
https://doi.org/10.1007/978-3-031-66524-0_11

This heartbreaking event would was highlighted by this young child becoming the first pediatric patient with a penetrating injury trauma flown down the north Lake Michigan shoreline to the south shoreline, skipping the closer pediatric hospital, Lurie Children's Hospital. The UCAN flight crew followed the rehearsed playbook and radioed for the adult trauma team to meet the young man on the roof out of concern for continued bleeding. In the operating room, an additional intra-abdominal injury was discovered. The operation was led by the adult trauma service with participation by the pediatric surgery attending and pediatric surgery fellow. The case concluded without complication, and the patient transferred to the pediatric intensive care unit (PICU) where the remainder of his care was concluded with the pediatric surgery service directing his care while recovering in Comer Children's Hospital at the University of Chicago.

Aspects of this young man's life are searchable in the media, and it is well-known that he left Comer Children's hospital with an additional surgeries, but without the use of his legs do to a thoracic spinal cord injury from the shooting. He is a remarkable young man with a supportive family and community that happily continues to support him. He has received public crowdfunding and was invited to throw out the ceremonial first pitch at a Milwaukee Brewer's game. Recently, he and the Comer PICU team appeared at the Society of Critical Care Medicine, praising the pediatric team for the clinical care rendered in support of this remarkable 9-year-old boy in achieving a clinical outcome that would not have been possible without their dedication. Unceremoniously, UCAN and adult trauma team modestly returned to work. The care for this young man has been heralded, but for the Southside of Chicago it was business as usual.

The eyes of the nation were on Highland Park with little outcry over the bloodshed adjacent to the south shore of Lake Michigan that took place the same 4th of July. Chicago's bloody 4th of July weekend eclipsed the Highland Park toll. The same weekend of the Highland Park Shooting, the city of Chicago's death toll surpassed the Highland Park shooting. According to Chicago police department data, 68 people were shot in 51 separate shootings over the Fourth of July weekend. Paradoxically, the Fourth of July weekend in 2022 compared to 2021, shootings were down 14%. The total number of shooting victims in 2022 decreased 21%, and the number of homicides dropped by 53% [2]. There is no reported data about shootings during the same period in the affluent town of Highland Park (presumably not shared because there was no appreciable increase or decline in the homicide rate as violence in the lakeside suburb is an anomaly). There were no crowdsourced charity drives raising millions for victims and families in South Chicago, where the holiday weekend death count seemed ordinary.

It is the tale of two cities only separated by 34-miles. The same Fourth of July weekend, the University of Chicago pediatric and adult trauma surgeons continued to dole out the same measure of pediatric trauma care whether an injured child over flew the downtown skyline or scooped up by ground ambulance in an adjacent neighborhood. It highlighted that our system is coveted for what we bring to the realm of pediatric trauma.

Pediatric Penetrating Trauma

The University of Chicago, almost exclusively services South Chicago and Northern Indiana for level I trauma care. Gunshot wound injuries are the leading mechanism of injury in the adult trauma population static at 38% and peaking to nearly 50% during the summer months. Violence in Chicago's Southside communities and Northern Indiana does not spare children. Forty-five percent of the pediatric penetrating cases involve children who are less than fourteen years of age, and 60% of pediatric trauma happens at night when the operating room in the Children's Hospital is ratcheting down to perform low level traumas and the operating room reduces capability for on call general pediatric cases (no trauma). The University of Chicago's rate of pediatric penetrating trauma in 2022 was a horrifying one out five pediatric traumas arriving with an gunshot wound injury, and the rate 20% has not decreased despite the increase in the pediatric trauma volume. In 2019, the total number of children killed in Chicago was 39. The city saw 49 youth killings the following year. In all of 2022, 66 juveniles were shot and killed in Chicago. Fifty-five kids aged 17 and younger were shot to death in Chicago at the start of 2023. At the tail end of 2023, twelve children between the ages of 10 and 17 were shot in Chicago between the dates Oct. 30th and Nov. 10th alone. Police records show the South Chicago District is one of two CPD patrol districts to see an increase in the number of shooting incidents from 2022 to 2023, and 73 people were shot July 4th weekend 2023 that began and ended with mass shootings [3, 4].

Barriers to Success

Prior to the reemergence of adult trauma services at the University of Chicago, Comer Children's Hospital participated solely in pediatric trauma care under the auspices of the general pediatric trauma service. The adult trauma service was provided a shocking glimpse into the trauma burden facing children living in Southside shortly after arriving to the hospital campus ahead of the opening of the adult trauma center in August of 2017. The very first day of the academic school year, September 2017, an eighth grader presented with a devastating vascular injury with reverberating repercussions that drew the adult trauma service into the contested management strategy surrounding the future state of pediatric trauma care. The death of this young boy led to the realization that significant retooling needed to take place for the anticipated onslaught of pediatric penetrating trauma that would take place when the adult trauma system became a fully functioning. The real likelihood of responding to both adults and children gunshot injuries arriving simultaneously by drop-off or ambulance with two separate locations available requiring lifesaving resuscitations with a closed operating suit requiring transport across the street to the awaiting adult trauma center created consternation.

A new algorithm needed formulation. The stipulation for management by the Illinois Department of Health (IDPH) is that children should present to Comer Children's Hospital. The 16-year and above by IDPH designation should be treated as an adult. Physiologically, the 16-year and above rarely requires adjustment in trauma management, but emotionally they are better suited for a children's hospital versus an adult hospital. The injury patterns sustained in the zip codes surrounding the University of Chicago mimic that of the adult population. An immediate problem to solve became does a pediatric weight-based approach or a physiology-based system matter more. In the pediatric realm, kids may not be viewed as "little adults" but when penetrating injuries across multiple body cavities requiring resections for multiple bleeding points this is a trauma presentation seldom encountered or written about in resuscitation manuals outside of cities like Chicago. Another critical decision to be discussed was who would lead resuscitations for children when penetrating trauma presented. In Comer, the resuscitating team was expanded to included a pediatric intensivist, pediatric resident and a child life specialist none of which are trained to perform and emergency room thoracotomy. The resuscitation focuses presented a serious barrier to success in the critical first five minutes.

As astonishing consequence of a pediatric shooting death elucidated two different mobilization practices for the mobilization of the massive transfusion protocol (MTP). The pediatric system relied upon blood products arriving via a tubing system from the blood bank. This system allows for the patient and the blood to miss each other while the patient is moving from the location of the emergency department to the operating room. In one particular instance, the blood did not arrive to the emergency room because it was stuck in the tubing system. The adult trauma service is an amalgamation of best practices from the most relevant trauma systems in the United States in that the newly arriving trauma attendings trained as residents and fellows in notable trauma hospitals. The MTP is stored in all critical locations. MTPs can be provided to patients in Indiana by UCAN as they begin the race back to the University of Chicago with bleeding patients. Patients can receive whole blood in flight as well. MTP blood refrigerators (stocked) are available in the adult trauma bay, adult operating room and interventional radiology. Beyond the initial MTP, multiple MTPs are brought to the patient's location by a runner going back and forth to receive a cooler of blood, fresh frozen plasma and platelets packaged in a 1:1:1 ratio. What constitutes a runner is "anybody" with legs that knows how to find the blood bank!

The alums of these premier trauma programs debated best practice guidelines and were asked to minimize their training biases about superiority, and decide upon treatment algorithms and best practices that we know dub the "UChicago Way." The philosophy of the UChicago Way places emphasis on speed the speed of decision-making, hemorrhage control from the emergency room setting to the operating room with emphasis on immediate hemorrhage control. This includes championing vascular trauma. This is a forward military team approach—a limited number of people focused on accuracy and speed to maximize the saving of multiple lives. The expanded team in the Children hospital where multiple bodies appear focused on feelings and cannot perform an emergency room thoracotomy or run to retrieve a MTP was initially an unwelcomed paradigms shift at higher headquarters. The coverage model lingered and stayed stagnant for several more years in our pediatric level I trauma center.

The coverage model at a level I pediatric trauma system, where the whole trauma system is devoted to around the clock pediatric trauma coverage is rarity without the coverage of adult trauma surgeons. The larger urban areas prevailing model is a hybrid model where children are shuttled into the care of the adult trauma service and the pediatric surgeons are consulted after stabilization has occurred. The hybrid model of trauma surgeons with pediatric consultation is at mostly at a central location since freestanding pediatric hospital are limited, and both adult and pediatric surgeons work collaboratively.

There are two portals of entry into the University of Chicago trauma system. The pediatric trauma patient is under the auspices of pediatric surgeons when entering the children's hospital and the adult trauma patient is under the auspices of trauma surgeons when entering the adult hospital. I believe the journey toward our own fusion model after the Highland Park shooting is occurring. The hospital roof capable to support the UCAN helicopter is the adult hospital with the drop into the operating room. The alert to meet on the roof sends security to freeze the elevators for a rapid ascent up to the roof by the trauma service and a quick descent into the operating room. A yellow phone hangs at the entrance of the doors exiting the helipad. This phone rings directly to the operating room desk and allows the trauma surgeon to communicate physiologic parameters, a call for the appropriate instruments and trays. If a decision is made to bypass the operating room and divert into the emergency department it can all be communicated from the rooftop as well. This is the expectation when UCAN flew with whole blood and blood products to Highland Park that when the trauma service would meet them on the roof. The pediatric surgeons were consulted to assist in the operation and to be made aware of what needed to happen next when the patient would be admitted to the PICU under their care. This approach, although not policy highlights the one portal of entry for the sickest pediatric trauma patients needing to occur where the adult team and the operating room is available.

The best-case scenario for the current dual entry points is to insure that the adult trauma service should be alerted when pediatric penetrating trauma is inbound. We have discovered that our experience is invaluable. The general surgery residents have also expressed a greater comfort when am adult trauma attending is at the helm for the resuscitation. For example, a 4-year-old girl shot in the chest was brought to Comer and a consultation was made to the in-house trauma surgeon who responded immediately. A decision was made to split the sternum in the children's hospital for the suspicion of a penetrating cardiac injury. The trauma surgeon opened the chest and discovered a hole in the left ventricle. A finger was held over the hole in the heart temporizing the situation until the arrival of pediatric cardiothoracic surgeon arrived placing the child on cardiopulmonary bypass to repair the hole in the backside of the left ventricle. The coordination between adult trauma and the phonecall made by the pediatric surgeon was invaluable.

As another example, a 12-year-old girl received a thoracoabdominal gunshot wound that injured her left lung, liver, duodenum and the most difficult portion of her inferior vena cava to access, obstructed from view as it passes behind the liver, the retrohepatic inferior vena cava. This unfortunate young recipient of this injury was sleeping at home when gunfire was directed at her grandmother's home. She was brought by EMS to the Children's Hospital early Saturday morning, the nadir of operating room availability in the children's hospital. Her injury to the retrohepatic inferior vena cava presents a major challenge is are associated with a high rate of mortality [5]. The patient was transferred to the adult hospital at the request of the pediatric surgeon for the procedure.

Based upon her thoracic injuries and other concomitant intra-abdominal injuries, she received a damage control operation. The trauma surgeon and the pediatric surgeon mutually agreed upon her overnight recovery in the adult ICU to avoid traveling underneath both hospitals to the PICU as she was requiring active MTPs and would need a return to the operating room within the next 48 hours. She received an operation within 48 hours, and with all operations completed, she was returned to the PICU not requiring any more operative procedures. She recently celebrated her fifteenth birthday.

A final example of combined involvement included a case initially managed by the pediatric service with late but minimal involvement of the adult trauma service. The case is a 16-year-old male shot in the right chest while driving with his parents taken to an outside facility before being transferred to the University of Chicago. A CT scan was obtained in the emergency department at Comer Children's Hospital revealing a major intrathoracic vascular injury, the innominate artery. The responding trauma team was a fourth year general surgery resident and a covering endocrine surgery fellow meeting the minimal IDPH standard for coverage. Together, they elected to consult the vascular service instead of the trauma. The vascular surgery service recommended that the pediatric cardiothoracic surgery service should be contacted because the vascular injury would require opening the chest with a median sternotomy incision. The pediatric cardiothoracic service felt that the age of the patient matched the physiology of an adult, and that the adult cardiac service should come to evaluate the patient. The patient was ultimately transferred from the pediatric hospital emergency room to the adult operating room, monitored by the on-call trauma surgeon until the perfusionist and the full cardiac team and the perfusionist arrived to the hospital. Ultimately, a sternotomy and synthetic graft was sewn in place to repair the injured vessel. The patient went to the PICU for recovery. Although, we can celebrate this procedure as a victory for the patient and his family, the inherent delays are unexceptable when an the presence of an adult trauma surgeon would have moved with forward surgery military efficiency.

Each of the three cases highlights an interplay of how the system can interact collaboratively, but also underpins the potential avoiding catastrophe by assigning a trauma surgeon to the care of the patient. The last case came at the request of the operating room staff, who knew that a trauma surgeon was available with the known capability of opening the chest for emergency vascular control if the hemodynamic status of the child began to falter.

The question of "little adults" living in the Southside needing a trauma surgeon ahead of the pediatric surgeon is not a question of competency, but a statement about muscle memory when it comes to curtailing bleeding. The intricacies of critical care manage for our youngest victims of trauma are better served recovering in the PICU after by the pediatric surgery service able to better coordinate care in their facility with a PICU specialist.

Coverage Models

Then

The pediatric trauma coverage model prior to 2018 did not require the pediatric surgeon to be in house, although preferable. The weekend and the nighttime coverage was frankly porous. IDPH regulations required the immediate availability of a "clinical" fifth year general surgery resident. Prior to the opening of the trauma center, the evaluating surgical resident was reliant upon their trauma rotation at Cook County Hospital and an Advanced Trauma Life Support course completed (ATLS). A stairstep approach to reaching the attending entailed the presence of the pediatric fellow prior to the arrival of the pediatric surgery attending. A CT scan was routinely ordered that prompted a consultation to the general pediatric surgeon covering pediatric trauma remotely. The Southside rate of penetrating trauma may not allow the time benefit of obtaining preoperative CT scan, which will never be the answer for an unstable bleeding patient. If the fifth-year resident or responding pediatric surgery fellow concluded that the patient needed an operating room it occurred in Comer. If this determination was made for an emergency operation after the daytime closing of the Comer operating rooms trays and instruments were hurried into the hospital from the adult side.

"15-minute rule"

The chances of surviving a traumatic injury has been predicated much upon the belief that interventions need to happen within "the golden hour." This is a timestamp that should be markedly truncated when a vessel is hosing uncontrollably, perhaps shaving the time to 10 minutes before entering an operating room. Vascular injuries involving the chest or abdomen represent a unique challenge for the pediatric general surgeon, as penetrating life- or limb-threatening injuries are rarely encountered beyond general surgery residency. The first day of school abdominal vascular injury became a catalyst to attempt to create a new approach to improve the efficiency for pediatric trauma reaching the operating room at the University of Chicago.

Short of calling this a summit, the pediatric surgery assistant and associate professors devised a plan intended to not erase two portals of entry into the trauma system. The adult trauma center created a pit crew efficiency with techs and nurses that took pride in an expeditious 4-minute run into the operating room from the emergency department. The pediatric and adult surgeons recognized that we needed to design a similar glide path into an awaiting operating room for children.

We decided upon the "first 15-minute rule." A certain clinical history adjoined with mechanism of injury and physiologic parameters would alert the pediatric system for movement toward the portal of entry with the most appropriate operating room. The principals of the first 15-minutes rule would require the creation of checklist that would tell the emergency room call nurse (ECRN) where to send a child when receiving a trauma alert from EMS about an injured child. The ECRN based upon the mutually agreed upon criteria would service as the traffic control. There are still two separate ECRN call locations, one located in the children's hospital and the other in the adult hospital. We chose to focus on having one incoming call center instead of two. The ECRNs would no longer be siloed within one of the two trauma centers but would become one team centrally located. A fall from a crib with altered mental status would require a CT scan of the head, exceeding 15 minutes and could be sent to the children's hospital. The 12-year-old unstable patient with the gunshot wound to the abdomen has a great chance of needing an operation, without a CT scan and an immediate operation. The ECRN taking that phone call at night would divert the ambulance to the adult hospital a block away matching the UCAN plan for an immediate run into an operating room on the adult side.

This approach garnered excitement with the younger pediatric general surgeons. The more seasoned surgeons were relieved and had already wanted to jettison all trauma responsibilities to the adult service. This innovative and moderate plan was flatly rejected without consideration by Comer leadership. We missed an immediate opportunity to flow toward a blended coverage model. The only agreement was to allow Comer to stay separate but the adult trauma service continued to always be available when called upon by the covering resident or at the behest of a pediatric surgery attending.

Now

A shortage of pediatric surgeons exists across the nation and the city of Chicago does not present as an exception to this actuality. The coverage range of the University of Chicago pediatric surgeons extends almost as far north as the young man involved in the Highland Park shooting. Their responsibilities at the suburban hospitals away from the mothership in the Southside are more likely than not to be of a blunt mechanism than the penetrating mechanism of injury that presents in the neighborhoods surrounding the University of Chicago. The outside hospitals are more than likely to offer the opportunity to practice the type of pediatric surgery that inspired many of them to pursue a fellowship in pediatric surgery, such as bread and butter general surgery for small children, pediatric cancer or pediatric reconstructive surgery. The pediatric coverage model resembles a private practice model, where the rounding physicians for the nighttime call have multiple responsibilities and are interconnected throughout the night to make sure all consulting facilities are covered. The stretching of the UChicago pediatric on-call surgeons across the city is reportedly exhausting and when covering Comer, the acuity of the trauma can become harrowing even though necessary. The is a dedicated core that does not find shot children a harrowing reality and look forward to covering pediatric trauma. Most will meet the requirement of trauma coverage but do not look forward to the penetrating trauma and the associated resuscitation and sprint into the tunnel under the hospital and having to reemerge in the adult hospital for a thoracotomy of exploratory laparotomy.

Our Future State

Pediatric trauma care where only the trauma service is involved in the immediate management of children is more likely to occur away from an academic trauma center or in a rural environment out of necessity. Some academic centers have simply chosen to divert all pediatric trauma care into the adult hospital by design or after some agreed upon hour in the evening and during the weekends. Pediatric trauma system models where the pediatric surgeons are asked to participate usually involve a hybrid approach involving trauma surgeons.

Pediatric trauma at the University of Chicago does not operate as a combined entity. There is no fusion of one Trauma Director, and both sides have two separate quality improvement forums. Therefore, there is no true UChicago Way when it comes to pediatric trauma care. The same trauma event by design can have to separate interpretations by the two separate quality reviews. One side sees an opportunity for improvement and the other sees a successful outcome that potentially put a child in peril despite a fortunate outcome.

The lack of merging to one standard is problematic. However, at the level of the clinical staff there is recognition that a hybrid model could exist. Southside pediatric trauma has made the pediatric surgeons to become traumatologist instead of focusing on the rare pediatric anomalies that are unfamiliar to trauma surgeons. None of the pediatric surgeons have ever expressed not wanting to be entrusted with the care of children but call coverage for complex trauma even pushes trauma surgeons to capacity in stamina and mental health. The pediatric coverage at our institution needs to formulate a coverage model where the expertise of both adult and pediatric surgeons blend in the proper sequence for resuscitation, operative care and recovery.

Our adult trauma opening is pressing the issue of when a preponderance of pediatric trauma crosses with a dearth of pediatric surgeons. Do systems using adult trauma surgeons exclusively compare favorably with those using pediatric surgeons? A comparative model between where both centers utilized trauma surgeons to fill the gaps for a lack of pediatric trauma coverage by pediatric surgeons examined could trauma surgeons become the answer for a shortage of pediatric surgeons available to participate in trauma care [6]. This type of service model was not associated with an elevated mortality risk. Adult surgeons alleviate shortages in pediatric surgeon coverage. Adult trauma surgeons should be willing to hand-off care when deemed appropriate.

The one out of 5 children shot is alarming and emotionally draining. The strain like a forward military team are those with a dog in the fight and motivated to see the mortality rate decrease despite the increasing total number of pediatric trauma patients. The nurses and technicians have improved dramatically in the care of penetrating pediatric trauma patients unfortunately as the repetitions increase but also as more children are pushed faster into the operating room (adult side) through the catacombs of heating pipes from the children's hospital and re-emerge in the adult-side and up to the elevator and into an awaiting operating room. That sense of achievement has made the boots on ground nursing in the children's hospital clamor for more support and training from the adult surgeons. The well-intended pediatric surgeons, trained to correct congenital anomalies are also contacting upper echelons of their command structure wanting less acute involvement and to receive greater number of calls for consultation.

The most recent outcome from the fusion of fatigue and wanting to improve in the care of pediatric trauma by the nurses, staff and pediatric surgeons has led to the appointment of a Pediatric Trauma Director under the auspices of one of the adult trauma surgeons. In support of this role, the adult trauma surgeons have created a separate in-house call coverage to specifically supplement decimated in-house pediatric service coverage, as their practice model increasingly requires their presence as satellite facilities. It is a brand new start still but a drastically different conversation is being held since that fateful first day of school several years ago.

Conclusion

Recognition of the scarcity of surgeons trained in the care of injured children means that understanding that the pediatric surgeon cannot shoulder the burden of pediatric trauma alone. There are no gaps in coverage in a blended model of covering the pediatric patient population, which we are adopting with anticipation of the number of call shifts being greater skewed toward adult trauma surgeons. Two separate quality improvement programs need to be unified into one trauma standard. The adult trauma surgeons have no other commitments other than to the mothership. It is the trauma service that by the design of bullets whizzing around the Southside have the greatest muscle memory and repetitions for penetrating trauma. We are motivated for the big win in both adult and pediatric trauma. Once the operation is completed, we welcome PICU care, child life support and the necessary intangibles of the Childrens hospital.

Expanding the number of trauma surgeons with expertise in pediatric surgery may be a possible strategy in providing pediatric care in our community. A formally trained pediatric surgeon with an interest in trauma is equally acceptable but the recruitment and retention of these individuals is more difficult. Trauma skill acquisition and maintenance is for the taking in the Southside, but that responsibility requires dedication to the art of trauma care. It will be important to increase the training opportunities in common pediatric conditions beyond the 20 cases presently required by the American Board of Surgery. Training should cover the common conditions, the workup and initial management of important symptoms of hemorrhage and critical care [7]. A pediatric trauma surgery fellowship can certainly be created with the volume available at the University of Chicago. A new training paradigm launched at the University of Chicago could become a vital resource for Chicago and other urban areas impacted by the increased intentional targeting of children with firearms.

The UCAN flight from Highland Park that landed on our roof with an injured child is the obtainable standard for our hospital system. We are poised to for the sudden arrival of injured children in our zip code and across the state. The system is maturing constantly with the new coverage model improving. The system is strengthening and will set a national standard.

References

1. Chicago tribune. Published: July 6, 2023 at 1:51 p.m. | Updated: July 6, 2023 at 6:04 p.m.
2. https://news.wttw.com, page 197 II Chicago News July, 5. 2022.
3. Chicago Tribune. Published: November 11, 2023 at 6:00 a.m. | Updated: November 11, 2023 at 9:55 p.m.
4. Sun-Times Media Wire Updated July 5, 2023 12:13 p.m.
5. Balachandran G, Bharathy KGS, Sikora SS. Penetrating injuries of the inferior vena cava. Injury. 2020;51(11):2379–89.
6. Stiles PJ, Helmer SD, Ward JG, Reyes J, Harrison PB, Haan JM. Pediatric trauma system models: do systems using adult trauma surgeons exclusively compare favorably with those using pediatric surgeons after initial resuscitation with an adult trauma surgeon? Am J Surg. 2015.
7. Nakayama DK, Randall S, Burd B, Newman KD. Pediatric surgery workforce: supply and demand. J Pediatr Surg. 2009.

Opening a Modern Trauma Center at UChicago Medicine: Ob-Gyn and the Pregnant Trauma Patient

Jennifer Cone

Overview and Background

Trauma affects up to 25% of all pregnancies with the need for hospital admission in 0.4% of all pregnancies [1]. Over 50% of pregnant trauma patients are in the third trimester at the time of trauma [1]. The most common mechanism of trauma is motor vehicle crash, followed by fall and assault [2, 3]. Penetrating trauma in pregnancy has been reported at rates of 6–9% of all pregnant trauma patients. Because trauma is the primary cause of non-obstetric related death during pregnancy, an institutional protocol was necessary to optimize the care of the pregnant trauma patient.

A multidisciplinary team of care providers was assembled to create an optimal pathway for pregnant trauma patients [4]. This team included a trauma surgeon and surgical intensivist, a maternal-fetal medicine specialist, an obstetric anesthesiologist, the head obstetrician at our Labor and Delivery unit, an obstetric quality lead physician, and nursing leadership.

Initial Evaluation

The biggest initial obstacle that our team faced was that the emergency department, inpatient adult hospital, birth center, and post-partum care unit were all located in different buildings. This, of course, provided logistical challenges for the teams that

J. Cone (✉)
University of Chicago, Department of Surgery, Chicago, IL, USA
e-mail: jcone2@bsd.uchicago.edu

S. O. Rogers, Jr (ed.), *Creating a Modern Trauma Center*,
https://doi.org/10.1007/978-3-031-66524-0_12

then needed to appropriately care for patients in multiple locations. The trauma surgeons needed to be present in the emergency department for initial evaluation of trauma patients as well as present in the adult inpatient building where the operating rooms and ICU were present. The obstetricians needed to be present in the labor and delivery unit where their active labor patients were housed and where the obstetric operating rooms were located. They also needed to be able to evaluate post-partum patients, who were located in yet a separate building.

From a trauma surgery standpoint, it was vital that patients meeting trauma activation criteria present to the trauma bay in the Emergency Department. With the chaos that invariably comes with trauma, we needed to ensure that there was consistent evaluation of any trauma patient in a manner that met American College of Surgeons Trauma Center standards. Furthermore, we needed to guarantee the right people, teams, and equipment were present to take care of the patient. Since we had standardized trauma activation criteria and already clarified protocols surrounding the initial evaluation, we decided that pregnant patients that were brought to the Emergency Department who met activation criteria would remain there until the completion of the primary and secondary survey and maternal stability was assessed. Pregnant patients that self-presented to the Labor and Delivery (L&D) Unit that met trauma activation criteria would be brought over to the trauma bay for safe and rapid stability assessment.

The vast majority of pregnant patients presenting with trauma do not have serious or life-threatening injuries. Most commonly pregnant women present to the hospital after falls, physical altercations, and minor motor vehicle collisions where the abdomen hits the steering wheel. From an obstetrician standpoint, the major concern is shearing forces on the uterus causing placental abruption. Because the emergency department and trauma bay are not close to the obstetric operating room and because time to management is of utmost importance in cases of placental abruption, the obstetricians felt strongly that the safest place for pregnant patients that have sustained minor trauma was L&D. We thus decided that patients that self-presented to L&D that did not meet trauma activation criteria would stay in L&D and a trauma consult would be placed. The trauma team could then come to L&D to assess the patient while fetal and uterine monitoring were taking place. Pregnant patients that presented to the Emergency Department who did not meet activation criteria would be immediately sent over to L&D, where the trauma team could still evaluate them.

When to Involve OB in Trauma Activations

In our institution, "Dr. Stork" is an overhead code utilized for patients that have impending delivery. It is utilized if a patient presents in the late stages of labor to any area of the Medical Center other than L&D. The code activates a team of medical personnel including obstetricians, neonatal intensivists, nursing staff for both teams, respiratory therapy, and pharmacists. Because of the potential need for a peri-mortem cesarean section and access to the iliac vessels, "Dr. Stork" codes are activated for any unstable trauma patient with a systolic blood pressure less than 90 who is 18 weeks gestation or more.

The majority of the pregnant trauma patients at our institution have stable physiology. It would be onerous for the obstetric team to constantly run over to the trauma bay, only to wait for the trauma team to complete the assessment of the mother. Thus, it was decided that obstetric consult will be obtained as soon as feasible for any trauma patient with a known pregnancy, regardless of gestational age. Consult to the obstetric team was deemed *emergent* when the pregnant trauma patient was over 24 weeks gestational age and there were suspected uterine contractions, placental abruption, traumatic uterine rupture, or the pregnant patient was emergently being taken to the operating room [4].

Admission

The decision of where to admit the pregnant trauma patient is decided by a discussion between the attending trauma surgeon and the attending obstetrician to determine the best location depending on the most pressing medical issue or injury. As our L&D unit is not staffed for ICU capabilities, any patient requiring ICU admission regardless of gestational age is admitted to the Surgical ICU. Pregnant trauma patients in the third trimester that have any adverse factors including uterine tenderness, abdominal pain, vaginal bleeding, sustained contractions, membrane rupture, fetal heart rate abnormalities, high risk mechanism, or low fibrinogen are admitted for 24 hour observation.

Trauma-Specific Considerations

In developing our protocols regarding care of the pregnant trauma patient, it was important to emphasize that the best initial treatment of the fetus is excellent resuscitation of the mother [2, 4]. Thus, our focus as trauma surgeons needed to remain on the mother. Our typical trauma workup and pathway should not be altered if there was clinical suspicion of injury.

We had valuable conversations with our maternal-fetal medicine specialists and our attending radiologists regarding the amount of radiation a pregnant trauma patient could receive and whether consent was necessary prior to CT scans. After extensive conversation and literature review, it was decided that any radiographic study indicated for maternal evaluation including abdominal CT should not be deferred or delayed due to concerns regarding fetal exposure to radiation [4]. Exposure to under 5 rad has not been associated with an increase in fetal anomalies or pregnancy loss and was deemed to be safe at any point during gestation [2]. However, when possible, females of reproductive age are shielded for x-rays.

Blood transfusion is frequently administered in the trauma bay before patient specific blood typing is completed. To avoid rhesus D (Rh) alloimmunization in Rh-negative mothers, O-negative blood should be transfused when needed in women of childbearing age until cross-matched blood becomes available [4]. If the Massive Transfusion Protocol is initiated, 1 unit of cryoprecipitate is transfused with each MTP pack to ensure appropriate fibrinogen level in the even that delivery is indicated.

Because the gravid uterus can shift the abdominal contents cephalad, especially in the third trimester, thoracostomy tubes should be inserted 1 to 2 intercostal spaced higher than usual to avoid diaphragm and intra-abdominal injury on placement [3, 4].

Tetanus is routinely administered in the trauma bay for patients with penetrating injury. The tetanus vaccine is safe in pregnancy and Tdap should be given to pregnant trauma patients when clinically indicated [4].

Pregnancy-Specific Considerations

Because pregnancy may not be known to the trauma patient or the patient may be too unstable to communicate their pregnancy, every female of reproductive age should receive a quantitative beta-HCG pregnancy test during the initial workup [2].

Supine hypotension syndrome occurs when a gravid uterus of 20 weeks gestational age or more compresses the inferior vena cava when lying supine. This leads to reduced venous return to the heart and systemic hypotension. In pregnant trauma patients, supine hypotension can confound a workup and lead to unnecessary interventions. It can also worsen an already unstable physiology. Thus, one should consider keeping the pregnant patient tilded left-side down 15 degrees to keep the gravid uterus off of the inferior vena cava [2, 4] To assist with spine-stabilizing in a tilted patient, rolled blankets or gel supports can be utilized. It is appropriate to leave a pregnant trauma patient in this position while obtaining adjunct imaging and definitive imaging like CT scans.

Pregnant patients have preexisting hypercoagulation secondary to an increase in procoagulants including fibrinogen and a decrease in anticoagulant activity. However, because a low fibrinogen level is a predictor of postpartum hemorrhage, in addition to the routine blood tests ordered in trauma, which in our institution include a CBC, CMP, PT/INR, it is important to order a fibrinogen level in pregnant patients [4]. As previously mentioned, when administering massive transfusion to a pregnant patient, one unit of cryoprecipitate should be administered with each pack.

RhoGam is a relatively low-risk drug and is given to all Rh-negative pregnant trauma patients within 48 hours of admission. Further, a Kleihauer-Betke test is additionally drawn on presentation for all pregnant trauma patients to determine fetal blood contamination into maternal circulation [2, 4].

After stability of the mother is evaluated, fetal assessment can begin. In pregnancies that are pre-viable and less than 24 weeks, fetal heart tones are checked by Doppler. Viable pregnancies of more than 24 weeks require further evaluation.

Cardiotocographic monitoring should be performed for a minimum of 4-6 hours in these patients [2–4]. If the patient has frequent uterine contractions, vaginal bleeding, abdominal or uterine tenderness, abdominal bruising, or concerning fetal tracings, then monitoring should be extended. Uterine ultrasound is performed in all patients with a viable pregnancy [4].

Finally, because of the vulnerability associated with both pregnancy and trauma, every pregnant patient who sustains trauma should be questioned specifically about intimate partner violence.

Peri-mortem C-section

A peri-mortem cesarean section is considered in any moribund pregnant woman over 18 weeks gestation. Standard fetal viability is generally agreed to be 24 weeks gestational age, however there is a great deal of unknown during trauma activations. Moribund patients cannot usually communicate how far along their pregnancies are and they may not be accurate. In our underserved and vulnerable patient population, prenatal care may not have occurred, and fetal growth restriction may be present. Thus, we felt that we could not fully rely on either information received in the midst of chaos or physical exam. In the midst of this uncertainly, we still wanted to facilitate best chances for survival for both mother and baby. As a result, we agreed to perform peri-mortem cesarean sections at a lower than usual gestational age.

The emergency department, operating room, and Surgical ICU needed to be prepared to perform and manage peri-mortem cesarean sections. Neonatal incubators were stocked in all potential delivery areas and we ensured that intubation equipment suitable for a neonate was available at all locations.

References

1. Leshikar, et al. Chapter 37—Trauma in pregnancy. In: Moore F, Mattox D, editors. Trauma. New York: McGraw Hill; 2017. p. 731–9.
2. Barraco, et al. Practice management guidelines for the diagnosis and management of injury in the pregnant patient: the EAST Practice Management Guidelines Work Group. J Trauma. 2010;69(1):212–4.
3. Mendez-Figueroa, et al. Trauma in pregnancy: an updated systematic review. Am J Obstet Gynecol. 2013;209(1):1–10.
4. Jain, et al. Guidelines for the management of a pregnant trauma patient. J Obstet Gynaecol Can. 2015;37(6):553–74.

Interventional Radiology: Here Comes Trauma!

Jeffrey Leef

For many reasons (some quite valid), the mere utterance of the words "Trauma Center" strikes fear and loathing in the hearts of Interventional Radiologists.

When the announcement was made that The University of Chicago would become a Level 1 Trauma Center, the groans of displeasure from radiologists could surely be heard nationwide.

However, the IR group quickly passed through the first four stages of grief (denial, anger, bargaining and depression) to reach the final stage –acceptance.

In this case, there was one more stage—embracement.

This was achieved in the same manner in which both surgeons and IR's approach and succeed at any difficult task; through planning, education, and training.

By following these critical steps, the path to the seamless integration of Interventional Radiology into the complex construction of a trauma center will be made not only painless but also enormously gratifying.

Name the IR Leadership Team

First, prior to launching into this endeavor, a physician and a non-physician administrator (technologist or nurse) must be named to lead the project. This should occur at least 2 years before opening day.

This IR team then must establish their individual and joint work lists and timelines to completion. Within this framework, a list of "musts" and a separate "wish list" should be created.

J. Leef (✉)
Loyola University Medical Center, Maywood, IL, USA
e-mail: jeffrey.leef@lumc.edu

S. O. Rogers, Jr (ed.), *Creating a Modern Trauma Center*,
https://doi.org/10.1007/978-3-031-66524-0_13

These tasks then must be categorized into levels of urgency and those which will entail approval by the highest level of hospital administrators.

Be prepared for those high-level decisions/approvals to occur at glacial speeds.

Establish Relationships

From the standpoint of the physician Director of Interventional Trauma, the most critical step in the entire process is establishing a rapport with the Head of the Trauma Center.

At the University of Chicago, this was Dr. Selwyn Rogers. Dr. Rogers is a visionary who was introducing a completely new level of care to not only the underserved local southside community, but to the entire Chicagoland area.

It was critically important to understand his vision and goals, but also who he was as a person.

This better allowed the IR team to fully support him in his quest to create the most elite trauma center in the country.

Also of critical importance was learning his "must haves" regarding both IR and other radiology services:

- Will in-house IR be a requirement? If not, what is the expected response time when on call?
- Will IR be needed in the OR or ER?
- Will IR be asked to emergently place vascular occluding devices in the ER?
- Will a hybrid OR/IR suite be built? If so, where?
- What are the expectations for dealing with multiple concomitant traumas, or mass trauma casualties?
- Will trauma surgeons be performing procedures typically performed by interventional radiologists?
- Will cross-training of staff be required?
- Will one of the existing IR labs be required to be "OR ready"?
- What are the expected volumes that IR will see? What percentage from ER vs. OR?
- What is the estimated number of secondary procedures ordered, e.g. IVC filters, gastrostomy tubes, abscess drainages, chest tubes, etc.
- Will the Adult Trauma Surgery Team also be treating pediatric trauma victims?
- What ancillary equipment will be necessary to be immediately available in the IR suite, e.g., Rapid Blood Transfusers, surgical instruments?

As many of these questions and requests overlap with the worklists created by the IR leadership team, one must combine, organize and divide them into manageable units.

IR Worklists and Prioritization

Nearly the entire list of tasks will require the input and help of both IR physicians as well as the non-physician leaders. Only a handful require the sole attention of the IR physician leader.

Responsibilities of the IR Physician Leader

1. Establish the relationship with the lead Trauma surgeon and their staff.
2. Train the physicians in the manner in which trauma patients are to be received and treated.
3. Establish treatment protocols if needed.
4. Assure that all deadlines are met
5. Orchestrate and participate in trial runs of various trauma scenarios
6. Assure that all attending physicians as well as residents and fellows have all necessary contact numbers.
7. Initially (the length of time varies), assume the role of primary contact for all problems.
8. Enforce and monitor the IR physician call-in process.
9. Create IR sectional morbidity and mortality.
10. Participate in Trauma Surgery Sectional morbidity and mortality.
11. Adjust the daily workflow to immediately accommodate the trauma emergencies while managing the expectations and requests of all the other services that refer to IR.
12. Determine if current staffing levels are adequate to handle the significant increase in procedures.
13. Determine the feasibility of performing procedures remote from the IR suites.
14. Review existing hospital policies pertaining to the overall care of patients coming to IR and adjust these policies to better suit the special needs of trauma patients.
15. Cope with and respond to unexpected problems... Like a worldwide pandemic!

Responsibilities of the IR Administrator

1. Become the main liaison with the surgical administrators.
2. Lead the training of technologists in the care of the trauma patient and all newly introduced equipment/technologies.
3. Orchestrate all new trauma processes.
4. Assess inventory and work with the hospital's supply chain to accommodate the substantial increase in access to essential trauma-related devices.

5. Work with hospital leaders to secure space for the storage of the increased inventory.
6. Oversee the construction and layout of new procedure rooms.
7. Work with hospital security to ensure physical safety in the IR care of trauma patients.
8. Work with nursing leaders to facilitate the implementation of new patient care policies.
9. Adjust daytime and after-hours staffing.
10. Lead the interview process of all new staff.
11. Work with directors of Blood Bank to create new guidelines, which not only fulfill the needs but also are compatible with the staffing and workflow of IR.
12. Create and implement new daytime and after-hours communication pathways.
13. Ensure the needs of the anesthesia department are compatible with IR staffing and overall workflow.
14. Work with the IR nurse administrator to create, execute and enforce the technologist and nurse after-hours call-in procedure.
15. Cope with and respond to unexpected problems .... Like a worldwide pandemic!

The Future Is Now

With continued advances in angiography and transcatheter techniques and procedures, interventional radiology has played an increasingly larger role in the management of patients suffering acute traumatic injuries. Particularly at level one trauma centers such as The University of Chicago, interventional radiology plays a major role in treating vascular injuries via transcatheter embolization and endovascular repair, specifically in major arterial injuries. In addition to standard angiography and transcatheter techniques, hybrid CT (also known as Angio-CT or 4DCT) represents an alternative imaging modality for the rapid assessment and management of trauma patients. This specialized room is uniquely equipped with a traditional ceiling mounted C-arm fluoroscopic unit that allows for standard interventional procedures, however, there is also a mobile CT scanner within the room that can be interchangeably used. CT, specifically CT-Angiography is one of the most effective ways of diagnosing acute traumatic injury effectively and efficiently. Combining this imaging modality with trained interventional radiologists allows for optimal patient care in trauma by decreasing time from diagnosis to treatment and avoiding surgical morbidity [1].

This integration of two radiographic modalities within one interventional suite allows for an improved course from diagnosis to treatment of complex medical conditions including acute trauma. This technical combination is beneficial in numerous ways, but one of the most important benefits of the Angio-CT suite is that one can do multiple sequential procedures or a longer complex stepwise procedure in the same room without transport between the CT scanner and IR suite [2]. This allows the patient to remain in the same position with almost no interruption in workflow. Many complex embolization procedures require time and expert technique to optimally access the most proximal location of vascular extravasation. By moving the CT scanner to the patient, room and patient set up is preserved, and the risk of losing vascular access is nearly eliminated.

Additionally, Angio-CT allows for rapid sequence targeted CT imaging which can provide superior anatomic visualization of the area of trauma including the surrounding soft tissues, rather than predominantly the vasculature as seen on conventional angiography. These real-time CT images can also be reformatted and reconstructed including rapid production of 3D reconstructions [3]. By increasing knowledge of the regional anatomy specific to the patient, as well as the 3D course of regional vasculature, the interventional radiologist has a superior roadmap when compared to real time fluoroscopy and 2D DSA images used in conventional angiography. This improvement from a technical standpoint can greatly reduce procedure duration, radiation dose to the patient, and efficiency in appropriate treatment. An example of the utility of Angio-CT and rapid generation of 3D reconstructions is seen in Fig. 1. This example highlights the role of hybrid CT angiography in diagnosing and treating a high flow pudendal artery arterial cavernous fistula resulting in high flow priapism.

In addition to improving the roadmap for the procedure itself, intermittent CT scans can be performed at the area of interest throughout the procedure to monitor procedure effectiveness, improve patient safety, minimize complications, and increase procedural efficiency. There are also technical improvements using CT when compared to conventional fluoroscopy. For example, the CT scanner can be run in multiple phases including non-contrast, arterial weighted, and portal venous phase. Having this technical modality available within the angiography suite allows for delineation of exact location, composition, type of bleed, and adjacent injuries. In addition to improved visualization of regional anatomy and extent of injury, CT can help alleviate simple diagnostic dilemmas frequently seen on conventional fluoroscopy, such as impaired/obscured visualization of the region of interest due to overlying bowel gas.

While only scraping the surface of the impact and utilization of 4D CT, initial data at the University of Chicago argue for improved efficiency and quality of care within the department of vascular and interventional radiology. , specifically in the management of acute trauma. 4D CT has innumerable additional applications including but not limited to renal artery aneurysm embolization, endoleak repair, CT guided biopsy, cryoablation, and Yttrium-90 mapping.

Coping with COVID

As was the case for all hospitals around the world, the COVID-19 pandemic strained the basic fundamentals of hospital workflow making even simple tasks seem monumental. The University of Chicago was faced with a new challenge: Adapting

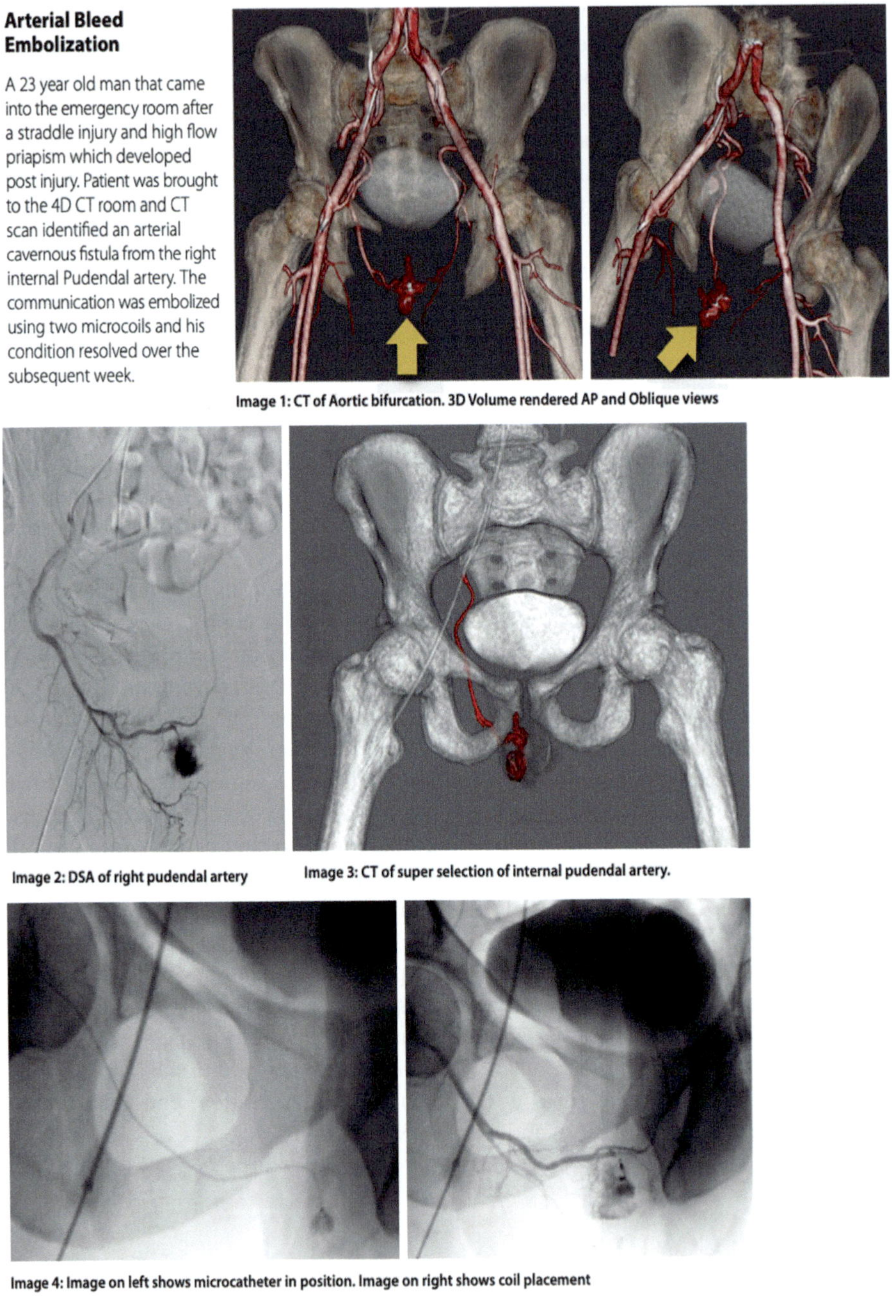

Fig. 1 4D CT in pudendal artery cavernous malformation embolization

practice models during a global pandemic to continue to provide state-of-the-art care while maintaining safe conditions for patients and healthcare workers.

While these changes in practice looked different from department to department, for Interventional Radiology this meant simple modifications to the hybrid angio-CT suite. While case volume may have decreased during the pandemic, trauma never sleeps. This need for acute care in the midst of a worldwide airborne a droplet transmissible disease pandemic required converting the hybrid CT suite into a negative pressure room expeditiously.

A negative pressure room is an isolation technique used in hospitals and medical centers to prevent cross contamination from room to room. A negative pressure room relies on a pressure gradient (lower pressure in the isolation room) which allows air to flow into the isolation room, but not out of the room. This thereby prevents contaminated air from escaping the room. Negative pressure rooms are used to treat patients with airborne diseases such as: tuberculosis, measles, Severe Acute Respiratory Syndrome (SARS-CoV), Middle East Respiratory Syndrome (MERS-CoV), and now Coronavirus disease 2019 (COVID-19).

Due to the rapid onset of the COVID-19 pandemic, a quick but effective solution was paramount. This necessity led to the creation of the negative ante room. This ante room was constructed surrounding the door leading into the angiography suite. Once the temporary walls were put up, an Omniaire 600 Nitro Portable HEPA Air Scrubbers were installed. These devices would draw air in, filter it, and exhaust the clean air into the hallway/control area outside of the ante room. As a matter of quality assurance and patient safety, an Omnigaurd manometer was installed within the ante room to monitor and ensure that negative pressure was maintained at −2.5 Pa (Fig. 2).

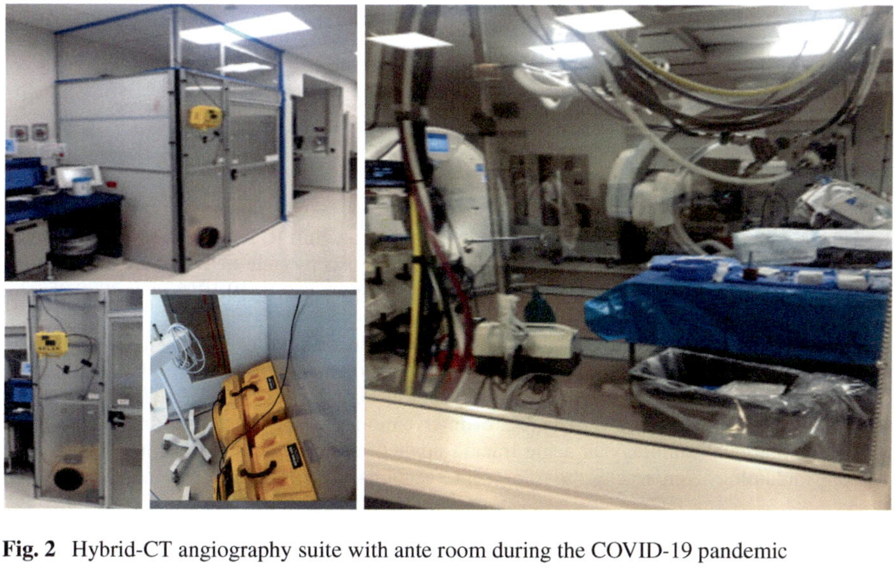

Fig. 2 Hybrid-CT angiography suite with ante room during the COVID-19 pandemic

Successful organizations are able to quickly adapt to change while maintaining their integrity and ability to function. At The University of Chicago we were able to rapidly convert our hybrid-CT room into an airborne precaution OR type environment with little expense. Some achievements of our isolation ante room include but are not limited to:

1. Rapid and cost-effective hybrid-CT room conversion to care for contagious patients in a safe setting.
2. 24/7 availability for trauma and critical care of all patients, especially in light of the fact that all patients were treated as Covid positive in the emergent setting.
3. Maximization of the benefits of the hybrid-CT room regardless of outside conditions and global limitations.

It's Not Over Till It's Over

This general blueprint can be used by any Interventional Radiology Section as a framework for establishing a successful trauma program.

Enormous variability exists, however, between hospitals and institutions.

While financials and available physical space are major factors accounting for these differences, geographic location far and away is the most significant variable.

The needs and requirements of level 1 trauma centers located in all large metropolitan cities in the country are far more complex than those in suburban or rural areas. Further, the percentage of penetrating versus blunt trauma affects many of the categories listed above.

That said, by working in conjunction with the Trauma Surgery leaders, the ultimate goal will be achieved: The Section of Interventional Radiology will become an invaluable tool in the armamentarium of the trauma surgeon, providing state-of-the art-care in the safest and most efficient manner.

References

1. Feinberg N, Funaki B, Hieromnimon M, Guajardo S, Navuluri R, Zangan S, Lorenz J, Ahmed O. Improved utilization following conversion of a fluoroscopy suite to hybrid CT/angiography system. J Vasc Interv Radiol. 2020;31(11):1857–63. https://doi.org/10.1016/j.jvir.2020.05.028. Epub 2020 Oct 9. PMID: 33041175.
2. Kinoshita, et al. The survival benefit of a novel trauma workflow that includes immediate whole-body computed tomography, surgery, and interventional radiology, all in one trauma resuscitation room: a retrospective historical control study. Ann Surg. 2019;269(2):370–6.
3. Martens S, Leef J, Ahmed O. The role of interventional radiology in acute trauma. The role of interventional radiology in acute trauma applied radiology. 2021, December 22. https://appliedradiology.com/articles/the-role-of-interventional-radiology-in-acute-trauma

Emergency Medical Services (EMS)

Katie Tataris and Ameera Haamid

Introduction

Trauma patients enter the Emergency Department from three different access points. There are some that walk into triage through the main entrance, those that are transported by ground EMS (Emergency Medical Services) through the ambulance entrance, or those that are flown by helicopter EMS to the roof helipad. From these three points of entry, the highest percentage of patients coming to the University of Chicago Trauma Center present by ground EMS which is the focus of this chapter. Most patients that present by helicopter EMS are transported by the University of Chicago Aeromedical Network (UCAN) which is further detailed in a dedicated chapter. Emergency Medical Services (EMS) was a critical partner in developing a new trauma center as most patients receive their initial medical care in the field by EMTs and Paramedics and are then transported to the Trauma Center to continue resuscitation. Collaboration with EMS at the state, regional, and local level was part of a successful implementation plan for a new Level 1 Trauma Center at University of Chicago.

K. Tataris (✉) · A. Haamid
Chicago South EMS System, Department of Medicine, Section of Emergency Medicine, University of Chicago Medicine, Chicago, IL, USA
e-mail: ktataris@uchicagomedicine.org; ahaamid@uchicagomedicine.org

S. O. Rogers, Jr (ed.), *Creating a Modern Trauma Center*,
https://doi.org/10.1007/978-3-031-66524-0_14

State EMS Systems

History of EMS and Trauma

The origins of EMS Systems can be traced back to morbidity and mortality from traumatic injuries in the 1960s. At that time, the federal government charged each state to create EMS Systems to address motor vehicle collisions on the newly built highway transportation routes. For Illinois, this new field of Emergency Medical Services (EMS) was placed under the realm of Public Health. In 1971, the Illinois Department of Public Health (IDPH) became the state regulatory body for all pre-hospital care and established the Division of Emergency Medical Services and Highway Safety [1]. Through new this authority, the IDPH was responsible for designating Trauma Centers within EMS Systems for the state of Illinois.

State Designation of Trauma Centers

The regulatory process for opening a new Trauma Center in the state of Illinois is defined by the IDPH Administrative Code. The first step is justification of the need for a new Trauma Center with criteria including the number of expected trauma cases, current EMS transport times for trauma patients in the current system, and recommendation by the local Trauma Regional Advisory Board and EMS Regional Advisory Board. This need was clear on the south side of Chicago and after gaining support from the Regional Trauma and EMS Advisory Boards, the application for a new Level 1 Trauma Center was submitted to IDPH. After a site visit, IDPH designated the University of Chicago as a Level 1 Trauma Center in 2018.

Regional EMS Systems

EMS Resource Hospitals

Once the University of Chicago was designated by IDPH as a Level 1 Trauma Center, the next step was integration into the current EMS System. In Illinois, the Resource Hospital has the authority and responsibility for an EMS System as outlined in an EMS System Plan. The System Plan includes all the documents that define EMS patient care as defined by EMS Protocols, Policies, and Procedures. The Resource Hospital, through the EMS Medical Director, assumes responsibility for the entire EMS System, including clinical aspects, operations, and education. The University of Chicago had been a Resource Hospital for the Chicago South EMS System since 1976. In the State of Illinois, most of the Resource Hospitals were also Trauma Centers. Therefore, the new trauma status was embraced and welcomed by EMS leadership at the University of Chicago. Additionally, one of the roles of a Resource Hospital was to review and approve renewal of EMS licenses based on continuing education for IDPH. The new Trauma Center designation also brought more ambulance transports to the University of Chicago from licensed EMS personnel that operated under the Chicago South EMS System which strengthened the connection between EMS personnel and their Resource Hospital.

EMS Region 11

The purpose of defined EMS Regions within the State of Illinois is to promote standardization between geographically close EMS Systems. Most of the Regions are defined by county boundaries, however the city of Chicago defines the boundaries for Region 11 [2]. There are 4 EMS Resource Hospitals with 4 separate EMS Systems that together make up Region 11. This unique situation was needed to provide a unified set of EMS Protocols, Policies, and Procedures for the agency that responded to all 9-1-1 calls throughout the city of Chicago, the Chicago Fire Department. Within this structure, the EMS Medical Directors at each of the four Resource Hospitals formed the EMS Medical Directors Consortium in order to work collaboratively as Region 11. Each of the other Resource Hospitals was also a current Trauma Center and when the University of Chicago added this designation, it was an opportunity to take an active role in redefining prehospital trauma care on the south side of Chicago. Additionally, at the regional level, the hospital and EMS representatives on the EMS Advisory Board and the Trauma Advisory Board work collaboratively to discuss issues and facilitate solutions regarding EMS and trauma.

EMS Protocols, Policies, and Procedures

Protocols

Prehospital trauma patient care in Region 11 was defined by EMS Protocols, Policies, and Procedures. EMS Protocols are written documents by the EMS Medical Directors that provide clinical guidelines for patient care categories that all licensed EMS personnel follow for patient care. The prehospital trauma protocols included General Trauma Management, Blast Injury, Crush Injury, Extremity Trauma/External Hemorrhage Management, Facial/Dental Injury, Head Injury, High Threat Considerations, Spinal Care, and Traumatic Arrest. EMTs and Paramedics working in Region 11 had already received education and training for these prehospital trauma protocols, which was a benefit of adding University of Chicago as a Trauma Center site into a currently operating EMS System. Maintaining

EMS Protocols, Policies, and Procedures that are up to date with consensus or evidence based prehospital care is an important job of the EMS Medical Director as it defines the medical care in the out of hospital environment prior to handoff at the Trauma Center.

Policies

EMS Policies are written documents that provide guidance on prehospital communication, documentation, and destination of patients. Region 11 defined the criteria for a trauma patient to be transported by EMS to a Level 1 Trauma Center or Level 1 Pediatric Trauma Center. The "Trauma Patient Destination Policy" defined the four steps of physiologic criteria, anatomic criteria, mechanism of injury criteria and special circumstances criteria. This was evidence and consensus-based trauma field triage criteria published by the Center for Disease Control (CDC) that was adapted and implemented for Region 11. The policy also defined each Level 1 Trauma Center and Level 1 Pediatric Trauma Center which served as destinations for EMS to transport trauma patients. Comer Children's Hospital had been designated as a Level 1 Pediatric Trauma Center since 1986. When the University of Chicago was added to the list of Region 11 Trauma Centers, the Trauma Patient Destination Policy was updated and a memo was distributed to all Region 11 participants which documented the date and time of the official start of EMS transports to the newly designated facility.

Procedures

EMS Procedures that are performed for trauma patients are defined by the EMS Medical Director. Each procedure is listed by the level of EMS personnel that are educated, trained, and credentialed to perform that procedure. This is based on scope of practice for the EMT or Paramedic working in an EMS System. Trauma management skills are generally at the basic life support (BLS) level, which emphasizes the importance of basic trauma interventions. Defined trauma procedures for the EMT level are also performed by paramedics and include cervical collar application, chest seal application, hemorrhage control (using direct pressure, pressure dressing, wound packing, or tourniquet), joint splinting, long bone splinting, spinal motion restriction (SMR), START/JumpSTART triage, and traction splinting. Trauma procedures for the paramedic or advanced life support (ALS) level included pleural (chest) decompression for suspected tension pneumothorax after chest trauma.

Local EMS Systems

EMS Agencies

With the new Level 1 Trauma Center designation, multiple EMS agencies began transporting trauma patients to the University of Chicago. There were local 9-1-1 transports by Chicago Fire Department, interfacility transports of patients from non-trauma hospitals by private EMS services, and other emergency transports from outside of Chicago including the south suburbs and northwest Indiana. Some of these EMS agencies operated outside of Region 11 and had their own local protocols and policies regarding trauma care, but still transported trauma patients to the University of Chicago as their closest trauma center.

EMS Personnel

There were over 5000 EMTs and Paramedics that are licensed to provide prehospital care in Region 11. This large amount of EMS personnel is needed to provide prehospital and interfacility transport services to a city the size of Chicago—however it limits the rate at which change can occur. Notification of the new Level 1 Trauma Center was positive news to EMS personnel as it was an additional resource for critical trauma patients and would reduce their driving distance to a further hospital. Given the presence of multiple other Level 1 Trauma Centers in the city and the established EMS Protocols, Policies, and Procedures related to trauma care, there was no need for an additional surge of EMS education to accompany the opening of the trauma center.

Emergency Communication Registered Nurse (ECRN)

In Illinois, registered nurses that successfully completed a 40-hour course on EMS System Protocols and Policies can be licensed to answer the EMS radio as an Emergency Communication Registered Nurse (ECRN). Most EMS calls consist of pre-notification for a patient enroute to that facility—but there are also questions about prehospital care or appropriate destination for a patient. For complex situations or questions, the ECRN can consult an ED physician. When University of Chicago started receiving trauma patients by EMS, the role of the ECRN was critical to determine patients that may need a Trauma Center level of care if not defined in the Region 11 EMS Policy. Additionally, the ECRNs had additional tasks including creating an electronic chart for the incoming patient, sending out the trauma activation pages, and printing registration documents. This streamlined the transition from the prehospital to the hospital setting with this transfer of information for the incoming trauma patient by EMS.

EMS Incidents and Disaster Planning

In Chicago, incidents such as motor vehicle accidents, mass shootings, building collapses or explosions with multiple trauma patients that require triage, treatment, and transport is a frequent occurrence. After a major incident, EMS contacts the Resource Hospital as the "Command Hospital" to manage the distribution of patients based on acuity and criteria for destination as defined in the Region 11 "Multiple Patient Incident Policy". For those incidents that occur geographically on the south side of Chicago, the University of Chicago was now able to accept patients that met trauma criteria for transportation. This new designation and integration within the EMS system for managing incidents and providing trauma care established the Trauma Center as a major resource with capacity to treat multiple patients as part of a mass casualty incident. Additionally, hospital disaster planning needed to accommodate a surge of trauma patients and proper resource allocation in the resuscitation bay and the operating rooms.

Emergency Department

The University of Chicago opened a new Emergency Department (ED) at the end of 2017. The planning for this space included the anticipated trauma center services and additional patients. Highlights of the new ED included more physical space, central resuscitation bays for critical patients, and on-location radiology services (x-ray and CT scan). Integration of trauma patients in mid-2018 increased the patient volume, but also changed the type of conditions and complexity of the patients that received emergency care at the University of Chicago. There were other changes including internal public safety expansion and a constant presence of law enforcement officers at the hospital. The trauma patients were prioritized in their emergency care, and this led to delays for other medical patients and in ED throughput given waits in obtaining required CT scans or consultation by surgical services.

EMS Fellowship

In 2019, the University of Chicago matched the first fellow to the EMS fellowship program. This program was a one-year training program for post-residency physicians on all aspects of EMS Medicine. Physicians had completed an Emergency Medicine or Pediatric Emergency Medicine Residency and elected to complete EMS training focused on education and experiences to become an EMS Medical Director or leader in the subspeciality of EMS. Curriculum included ground and helicopter EMS programs, prehospital medical and trauma patient care, disaster medicine, tactical EMS, hazardous materials response, confined space rescue, and urban search and rescue. By functioning as a Trauma Center, the University of Chicago became positioned to host the fellowship and recruit qualified residents into the position. The high volume of EMS transports to the University of Chicago with patients requiring specialty services made the Emergency Department a rich clinical environment to practice both Emergency Medicine and EMS Medicine. The EMS Fellowship expanded to two fellows per year and formed a Division of EMS Medicine within Emergency Medicine.

Conclusions

Early planning stages for the University of Chicago Trauma Center required integration with state, regional, and local level EMS frameworks. Successful opening of a new Level 1 Trauma Center was the result of coordination and collaboration with EMS stakeholders in both the prehospital and the hospital settings.

Clinical Pearls

- Emergency Medical Services (EMS) is a critical partner to developing a new trauma center as most patients receive their initial medical care in the field by EMTs and Paramedics and are then transported to the Trauma Center to continue resuscitation.
- Collaboration with EMS at the state, regional, and local level is part of a successful implementation plan for a new Level 1 Trauma Center.

References

1. Illinois Department of Public Health, Emergency Medical Services website. https://dph.illinois.gov/topics-services/emergency-preparedness-response/ems.html. Accessed 14 Dec 2023.
2. Illinois Department of Public Health, EMS Region Map. https://dph.illinois.gov/content/dam/soi/en/web/idph/files/publications/emsjuly2016small.pdf. Accessed 14 Dec 2023.

UCAN: Air Medical Transport and the Transfer of the Trauma Patient

Ira J. Blumen, Michael McCartin, Caitlin Kilcoyne, and Candice Schaper

Introduction

Given the proximity of healthcare facilities and trauma centers in a place like Chicago, the value Helicopter Emergency Medical Services (HEMS) adds to an urban trauma center may not be immediately apparent. However, having an Air Medical Transport (AMT) program can be a valuable addition to any comprehensive trauma and emergency medical services (EMS) system. Any physician who interacts with trauma patients will likely find themselves interacting with HEMS teams at some point either to send or receive patients. HEMS, also referred to as HAA (Helicopter Air Ambulance), acts as the vital link for rural communities and critical access hospitals to distant emergency and trauma care. In fact, in the United States, HEMS represents the only modality by which nearly 28% of residents have access to level I or level II trauma centers within 60 minutes [1]. Rapid transfer of injured patients to a trauma center is important for patient survival. For trauma centers wishing to extend their reach beyond their immediate catchment area, HEMS plays a vital role. With an AMT program available, trauma centers can now receive patients from distances requiring a flight by medical helicopter (e.g., >20–25 minutes by ground ambulance), and in some geographic areas by medical airplane.

UCAN (University of Chicago Aeromedical Network), the hospital-based air medical program at UChicago Medicine, staffs a single aircraft (EC-145) with one

I. J. Blumen (✉) · M. McCartin
UCAN, UChicago Medicine, Chicago, IL, USA

Section of Emergency Medicine, Department of Medicine, University of Chicago, Chicago, IL, USA
e-mail: Ira.Blumen@bsd.uchicago.edu; Michael.Mccartin@bsd.uchicago.edu

C. Kilcoyne · C. Schaper
UCAN, UChicago Medicine, Chicago, IL, USA
e-mail: Caitlin.Kilcoyne@uchicagomedicine.org; Candice.Schaper@uchicagomedicine.org

S. O. Rogers, Jr (ed.), *Creating a Modern Trauma Center*,
https://doi.org/10.1007/978-3-031-66524-0_15

pilot and two flight nurses. UCAN coordinates and performs the transport of trauma patients from both local area hospitals by ground as well as distant referring facility locations by helicopter. UCAN is also capable of responding directly to the scene of injury (i.e., to the side of the highway for a motor vehicle collision) in so-called 'scene transports'. If the distance is short or the weather is not safe for flight, UCAN will perform transports by sending flight nurses via ground ambulance. While this chapter focuses on trauma, UCAN is a specialty transport team that transports all patient populations including patients on mechanical circulatory support (e.g., ECMO, intra-aortic balloon pump), pediatrics, neonates, high-risk obstetrics, cardiac, medical, cerebral vascular accidents and more.

To have a clear appreciation as to how an AMT program can contribute to the development and success of a trauma center, it is important to have a general understanding of AMT, interfacility transfers, and scene transports. The focus of this chapter is on HEMS but will also address some aspects of critical care ground transport of the trauma patient, a service that the UCAN program also provides. This chapter will also explain and highlight some of the significant considerations when utilizing air medical transport that is fully integrated into the UCAN program. Trauma centers and hospitals considering the development of a trauma center should be aware of the different options available to provide this critical service and the various responsibilities during trauma transfers and transports. Ideally, the trauma center itself would have the necessary personnel to facilitate both the acceptance and performance of the patient transport. With the right policies, procedures, and personnel in place, a trauma center will be able to facilitate the timely transfer of patients from outside hospitals, as well as direct from-the-scene transports.

Air Medical Transport of the Trauma Victim

Following the enactment of the 1966 National Highway Safety Act, the attention of the United States (US) government shifted toward highway-related accidents and fatalities. Drawing on experience from the military, in 1969 the first hospital-sponsored fixed-wing air medical program was introduced. The inaugural civilian HEMS program was instituted in 1972, offering prehospital transport for trauma victims and facilitating interhospital transport for critically ill and injured patients. Since its inception in the early 1970s, HEMS in the US has experienced significant growth, expanding in both scope and scale to become a vital component of the country's emergency medical response system. By the end of 2022, there were over 950 dedicated medical helicopters as well as an additional 120 dual-purpose (fire department, law enforcement, etc.) and military helicopters transporting civilian patients in the US [2].

When compared to ground emergency medical services (GEMS), HEMS transport is most beneficial for time-sensitive medical conditions (e.g., cerebral vascular accident (CVA), ST Elevation Myocardial Infarction (STEMI), and trauma) [3, 4]. Of these three major diagnostic categories, trauma has been the most studied.

Research has shown a mortality benefit for trauma patients when transported by HEMS [5–10], especially those transported from rural areas [11–13]. In a study of over 469,000 trauma patients transferred by air or ground, patients who were transferred by helicopter were 57.0% less likely to die than those transferred by ground ambulance after adjusting for age, Injury Severity Score (ISS), and gender [14]. Intuitively, a shorter time to definitive care (e.g., percutaneous coronary intervention (PCI), mechanical thrombectomy, surgery) should denote improved patient outcomes. However, it is possible that some of the mortality benefit of HEMS over GEMS is due to the crews responding, not just the receiving facility's definitive care. HEMS crews are typically highly trained and experienced EMS clinicians with a more advanced scope of practice than their GEMS counterparts. HEMS clinicians are usually capable of performing rapid sequence intubation, carry blood products, and have extensive critical care experience. Some crews can perform field amputations in the setting of entrapped patients which is beyond the scope of the typical Advanced Life Support (ALS) clinician.

Transport Environment

The transport environment is much different than the trauma bay or emergency department. While technology makes it possible to nearly replicate the inpatient critical care environment during transport, it remains a resource-austere environment. Limited space, personnel, equipment, and sometimes lighting, contribute to making the transport environment a challenge and can significantly hinder the provision of optimal patient care. Compared to a ground ambulance, the cabin of a helicopter is significantly smaller. Aircraft weight restrictions may also prevent the transport of some obese patients. Despite appropriate planning, patient monitoring may be difficult, and the capability to manage emergencies is restricted.

For interfacility transport of trauma patients, crews will typically respond to another hospital's emergency department. Varying levels of care will have been initiated, depending on the resources and capabilities of the transferring hospital. Blood products may not be available, imaging may not have been performed, and patients may not yet be stabilized for transport. A hand-off occurs at the bedside, flight crews perform their history and physical and package the patient as quickly as possible for transfer (provided the patient is stable). Before departing, crews may elect to intubate a trauma patient with an altered mental status, hang more blood products, obtain additional IV access, adjust ET tubes, repeat a chest x-ray, or initiate an additional pressor. During take-off and landing, crews must be fastened in their seatbelts and will not be able to provide emergent patient care should the patient suddenly decompensate during these phases of flight (e.g., start vomiting, go into cardiac arrest, become hypoxic). This is an important point to keep in mind if trauma center personnel find themselves providing online medical consultation to their AMT during a transfer.

For scene transports, if the trauma patient is not entrapped, a flight program might typically rendezvous in the back of the ambulance of the EMS agency that called. Similarly to interfacility, a hand-off will occur, and the HEMS crew will perform a brief history and physical. Some programs, including UCAN, will initiate the necessary life-saving treatments prior to loading into the aircraft. Other programs may prefer to immediately load the patient into their helicopter and do procedures in the aircraft either before takeoff or while in flight. In the case of traumatic arrest or impending traumatic arrest, UCAN will transfer to the nearest comprehensive emergency department and not load that patient into the aircraft. Some programs, however, may have procedures to terminate resuscitative efforts in the field while others may elect to take off with the traumatic arrest and continue to "code" the patient enroute to the trauma center

Options for HEMS Operations

There are several business models available to provide HEMS service to a trauma center. Understanding these options may be beneficial to existing trauma centers or to facilities planning to develop a new trauma center to serve a large geographic footprint.

While UChicago Medicine and many other hospitals and trauma centers across the country have a medical helicopter program based at their facility, the original non-profit hospital-based operation, sponsored by a single hospital or a consortium of institutions is now less common than the for-profit community-based programs or hybrid programs. Public service agencies may also sponsor HEMS services or partner with private companies.

A hospital-sponsored program typically contracts with and pays an aviation operator to provide all aviation personnel, services, and aircraft to comply with Federal Aviation Administration (FAA) regulations. A smaller percentage of hospital sponsor programs may opt to keep everything in-house and provide their own aviation services. In both options, the medical personnel are employed by the hospital. The branding of the HEMS program and the paint scheme of the helicopter are typically consistent with the hospital branding. In this business model, the hospital assumes the greatest financial risk and is responsible for patient billing and collection.

In a hybrid or alternate delivery model, there is still a contractual relationship between a hospital and an aviation operator. Medical personnel are employed by the hospital, but more financial risk is assumed by the aviation operator who now does the patient billing and collection. The branding is typically similar to the hospital-sponsored program. In this model, the aviation company reimburses the hospital for medical personnel, supplies, and other services. UCAN is currently a hybrid program.

Both the hospital-sponsored program and hybrid program may offer significant benefits to the hospital, the trauma center, and the HEMS program itself. Training of the medical personnel, development of medical protocols, medical control, program leadership, and coordination with other hospital services may all be enhanced. In addition, these programs are more apt to incorporate critical care ground transport within their service line for close facilities, or when the helicopter is not able to fly. Personnel to coordinate the air medical transport, as well as physician-to-physician contact for transfers, are more likely to be in-house service providing a more streamlined, one-call service to get a patient accepted, mobilize helicopter transport, and coordinate all communications.

Having a HEMS based at the trauma center represents an opportunity for the receiving trauma center to alter the course of a trauma patient's care more directly and avoid potentially redundant efforts. For instance, if a receiving trauma surgeon knows and trusts the assessment of a familiar AMT crew, they might feel more comfortable bypassing the trauma bay and going directly to the operating room based on the AMT crew assessment. Our trauma center has a close working relationship with UCAN. It is not uncommon for trauma surgeons to meet our crews on the helipad if requested and proceed directly to the operating room. Without such familiarity or trust, such innovation is unlikely to be possible.

In a community-based model, the independent aviation company owns and operates the entire program. The aviation and medical personnel are all employed by the aviation operator who is responsible for all aspects of the program. While a hospital may contract with the aviation operator for HEMS services, the program name and branding typically reflect the aviation company and not a hospital or medical system. The helicopter is typically based off-site at an airport or other location and their communication center is often located in a central location in a different state.

Financial considerations can be one of many factors when a trauma center or other tertiary care facility considers its options for helicopter services. The cost of a medical-configured helicopter can range from under \$1 M for a used single-engine aircraft to over \$16 M for a new large twin-engine helicopter with a medical interior. A new popular medium-sized twin-engine aircraft can cost \$8.5 M to \$12 M. Annual operating expenses for a typical hospital-based program could range from \$2.5 M to \$4 M, not taking into account the costs to either purchase or lease the aircraft directly or pay the aviation operator monthly. The hospital would be able to generate direct revenue by billing for the transports to offset their expense. If a hospital chose the hybrid model, they might average a savings of \$1.5 M to \$2 M over the hospital-sponsored model. While there would typically be some level of reimbursement from the aviation operator to the hospital for medical personnel and supplies, the hospital would not have the benefit of direct revenue for flights to offset their costs. In a community-based model, the hospital may have no annual expenses. While this may seem appealing at first, the hospital must consider all the benefits of a branded helicopter program and the input and control they might have over the medical care provided to their patients.

Components of an Air Medical Transport Program

Numerous associations and publications have developed standards, guidelines, and position statements to ensure the appropriate and safe transfer of critically ill and injured patients [15–24]. These guidelines typically address transport personnel, medical equipment and supplies, and in some cases vehicle options and configuration.

Air Medical Transport Vehicles

Helicopters

UCAN provides HEMS transport to over 250 trauma patients each year. While HEMS has unique risks when compared to GEMS, research shows that critically ill or injured patients can be transported safely without adverse impact on clinical outcomes [25–34]. With speeds ranging from 120 to 180 mph, HEMS can significantly reduce transport time, often by 75% compared to ground transportation over the same distance. This makes helicopter transport particularly important in situations where minimizing out-of-hospital time is essential.

Helicopter programs typically operate within 150 to 200 miles from their base, but the distances covered in transports are often considerably shorter. Rotor-wing aircraft can navigate around common traffic delays and ground obstacles, providing access to rural and remote locations, including coastal islands, where other modes of travel may be impractical. Helicopters often represent the fastest means of transport for distances ranging from 25 to 150 miles. Additionally, helicopters can practically go "door-to-door" or "direct to scene" when on-site helipads or landing areas are available at both the sending and receiving locations.

Downsides of helicopters include issues like noise, vibrations, changes in temperature, and other factors that can cause stress for both patients and the crew. Weather conditions can occasionally pose significant limitations on the availability of helicopter transport. While certain medical helicopters have the capacity to transport two patients, the majority are designed to accommodate only one. Additionally, smaller helicopters, confined spaces (see Fig. 1), and weight restrictions might constrain the number of transport personnel or medical equipment that can be carried, making it more difficult to perform procedures.

Many helicopter programs operate only under visual flight rules (VFR). Essentially, the weather is clear enough for the pilot to be able to see where they are going. With VFR, pilots navigate and control the aircraft by visual reference to the ground as opposed to relying solely on instruments. When the weather conditions (ceiling and visibility) fall below established program minimums, a flight request may be declined for safety reasons. However, an increasing number of programs are

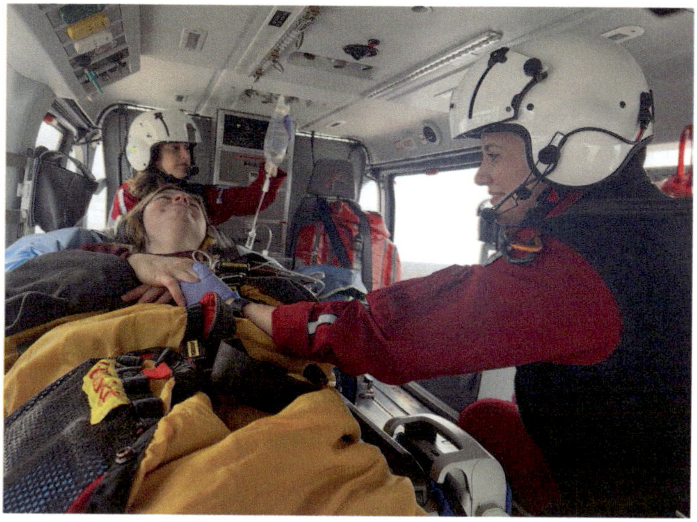

Fig. 1 Medical helicopters may be limited by cabin size and weight restrictions. This could limit the number of medical crew or amount of medical equipment that can be carried. and may present some challenges with patient care while in flight. (Courtesy UCAN (University of Chicago Aeromedical Network), UChicago Medicine, 2024)

equipping their helicopters and training their pilots for instrument flight rules (IFR) to allow safe travel in less favorable weather conditions. With IFR, pilots rely on instruments to navigate and control the aircraft. IFR flight may be facilitated to fixed locations such as hospital helipads that have developed IFR approaches, but it does not facilitate travel to the scene of illness or injury. Other weather considerations such as winds, precipitation, and temperature could affect both VFR and IFR flight availability.

HEMS may be categorized as primary or secondary response and both can make a significant contribution to the trauma center and the trauma region. Primary responses ("scene flights") are when the helicopter responds directly to the scene of an accident and transports the patient directly to an appropriate trauma center. Aircraft involved in secondary responses (interfacility transport) move patients from distant outlying hospitals to regional trauma centers.

The UCAN helicopter is a twin-engine Airbus EC-145 capable of a cruise flight of 120 to 130 miles per hour. The aircraft can accommodate three to four medical crew members, depending on total weight, weather considerations, and fuel capacity. The aircraft can accommodate two patients—one on the routine collapsible litter and the second secured on a flat litter to the floor of the aircraft. However, we have never done this and would likely only do it in the case of a mass casualty event. If two critically ill or injured patients require HEMS, we would request a second helicopter from one of our mutual aid partners. Doing this would provide each patient with a dedicated two-member critical care transport team.

Airplanes

Although HEMS are crucial for transporting patients in many trauma situations, medical airplanes (fixed-wing aircraft) become advantageous when transporting patients over long distances, spanning hundreds or even thousands of miles to reach definitive trauma care. These airplanes not only provide an extended range but also offer higher speed and greater capacity for patients, crew, and equipment compared to most helicopter transports. The reduced cabin noise and turbulence contribute to smoother patient management, while cabin pressurization helps counteract the physiological effects of altitude and gas laws. However, fixed-wing operations are constrained to areas with suitable airports featuring adequate runways and refueling facilities. In fixed-wing transports, transferring patients involves using multiple vehicles for each segment of the journey, such as from the hospital to a ground ambulance to the airplane. UCAN does not provide fixed-wing air medical transport.

Ground Ambulances

While HEMS is the main focus of this chapter, every clinician needs to have an understanding of ground ambulances and the role they play in patient transport and the UCAN program. On an annual basis, critical care ground transport accounts for approximately 40–45% of all UCAN transports.

Across urban, suburban, and rural communities the availability of ground ambulances makes them the most frequently used vehicle for interfacility transport and the primary mode of transport in the prehospital setting. They can provide door-to-door service (see Fig. 2) without the need for a helipad, temporary landing zone, or runway. Once the patient is secured to the stretcher and placed in the ambulance, the patient can be transported directly to the receiving facility without the inherent hazards of moving from one vehicle to another.

A ground ambulance patient compartment is typically more spacious than what can be found in helicopters and airplanes (see Fig. 3). Some ground ambulances may be able to transport as many as four medical crewmembers and one to two patients while offering greater flexibility with fewer restrictions on the size, weight, and amount of equipment that can be carried. Another advantage is the ability of the ambulance to easily "pull over" to facilitate patient assessment and intervention or to divert to an alternate destination if necessary. This is in stark contrast to a helicopter, where patient care could be affected during takeoff or landing due to the requirement for crews to have seatbelts on and fastened. Lastly, ground ambulances can operate in variable weather conditions that may limit safe HEMS operations, providing a dependable mode of transport for a wide range of weather scenarios.

Despite its advantages, the use of ground ambulances comes with notable disadvantages, the foremost being the increased time necessary to transfer patients between distant facilities compared to air transport. Construction, traffic congestion, poorly maintained roads, and inclement weather can all delay ground transport. Additionally, remote areas may have limited road access and a scarcity of

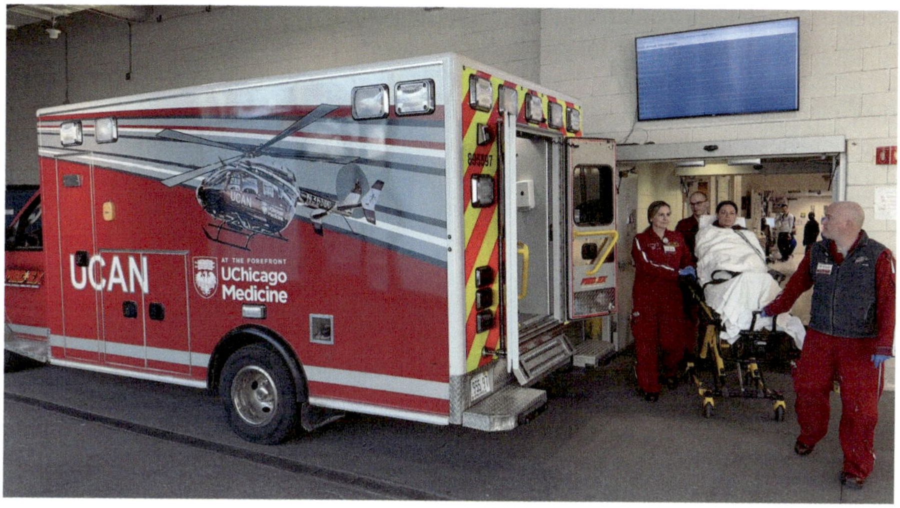

Fig. 2 With a ground ambulance the patient can be transported directly to or from a facility's ambulance bay without the need to move from one vehicle to another, reducing the potential for an adverse event during the transfer between vehicles. (Courtesy UCAN (University of Chicago Aeromedical Network), UChicago Medicine, 2024)

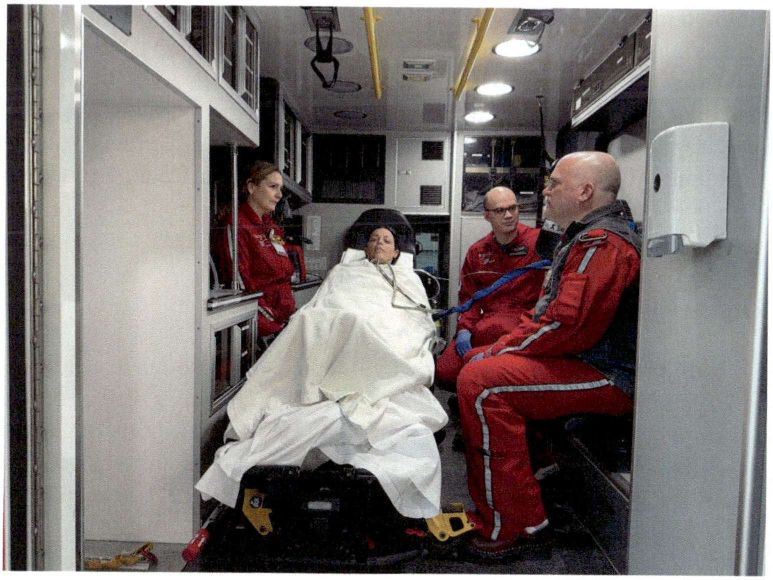

Fig. 3 Ground ambulance typically offer larger cabin space and greater flexibility with fewer restrictions on the size, weight, and amount of equipment that can be carried when compared to helicopters and airplanes. (Courtesy UCAN (University of Chicago Aeromedical Network), UChicago Medicine, 2024)

ground ambulances available to serve a large geographic area. In addition, the use of a ground ambulance for long-distance transport may leave a service area without an ambulance available for the next emergency. Finally, ground ambulances and their patients may be subject to rough and turbulent rides. This may be particularly problematic or excessively painful to trauma patients with orthopedic injuries, spinal cord injuries, and more.

Transport Team Personnel

The air medical transport team is made up of many different professionals who are highly trained, highly skilled, and highly motivated. While individual air medical programs may differ in the patient populations they might transport, it is common for the crews to provide medical care at a critical care level.

Medical Crew

Healthcare professionals involved in air medical transport come from a diverse range of backgrounds. In the United States for both fixed-wing and rotor-wing, the most common medical crew configuration is nurse/paramedic. The next most common is nurse/nurse. Team combinations such as RN/EMT, RN/MD, EMT-P/EMT-P, and RN/RT make up a relatively small remaining percentage [35, 36]. Flight nurses contribute their significant clinical experience by working in intensive care units or emergency departments. Paramedics, on the other hand, play a crucial role in transporting critically ill patients from accident scenes, as their training predominantly focuses on being first responders.

UCAN Flight Nurses

UCAN's staffing currently consists of two dedicated nurse-nurse team members working 24-hour shifts to allow concurrent HEMS transport as well as critical care ground transport. With the spectrum of patients UCAN transports (e.g., neonates, pediatrics, adults, high-risk obstetrics), UCAN flight nurses are required to have a minimum of five years of registered nursing experience, with time working in both critical care pediatrics and critical care adults.

Once hired, the UCAN flight nurse will go through an orientation phase that can last upward of six months and is dependent on transport call volume (40–60 transports) and value. This would include exposure to all patient populations and experience with skill sets and procedures. UCAN nurses are trained to intubate using rapid sequence intubation (RSI), place chest tubes, perform finger thoracostomies, cricothyroidotomies, eFAST (extended focused assessment with sonography for trauma) exams, field amputations, administer blood products, mechanical ventilation management, manage cardiac devices (impella, left ventricular assist device (LVAD), intra-aortic balloon pump (IABP), pacemakers, and extracorporeal membrane oxygenation (ECMO)), deliver inhaled nitric oxide (iNO), initiate and maintain therapeutic hypothermia, and high flow nasal cannula (HFNC). Though intense, this process has ensured that all UCAN flight nurses are ready to meet the demands of the air and ground medical transport environment.

Communications Specialists

Other key members of the transport team are the communications specialists (CS). They are often referred to as "dispatchers" but this title would be incorrect. The in-house UCAN Communication Center (CommCenter) is staffed 24/7, typically with two CSs on duty. In addition to providing a critical role for the adult and pediatric trauma services, they play a role for all patient populations including those going to an intensive care unit, emergency department. operating room, labor and delivery, cath lab, or interventional radiology. Specifics regarding the important role the UCAN CS plays are detailed later in this chapter.

Aviation Personnel

The aviation personnel (pilots and maintenance technicians) round out the air medical transport team and it's imperative that all individuals who interact with the flight program understand the critical role they play. All aviation-related aspects of the air medical program are the responsibility of the aviation operator. In accordance with FAA regulations, the pilot on duty has complete authority to make all decisions concerning the suitability of weather conditions, landing areas, condition of the helicopter for flight, loading of the helicopter, and all other factors affecting flight safety.

Program Leadership and Medical Control

Out-of-hospital medical transport is regulated on a state-by-state basis. While most air medical programs may have a program manager and clinical manager, some aspects of medical direction and medical control are necessary for all interhospital and prehospital patient transports. Public service and private ground ambulances are commonly under the direction and control of an EMS System, their EMS resource hospital(s), and written Standing Medical Orders (SMOs). Air medical services typically have their own medical direction and medical control physicians. These air medical directors are responsible for overseeing, evaluating, and ensuring the quality of medical care provided by the service. The National Association of EMS Physicians (NAEMSP) and the Air Medical Physician Association (AMPA) have established guidelines for the medical director of an air medical service.

Transport Equipment

AMTs require the necessary equipment and adequate training on that equipment to deliver optimal care to critically ill trauma patients. The level of monitoring during transport should be similar to the ER or ICU. Transport equipment must be portable, durable, lightweight, and battery-powered, but also capable of being directly plugged into a power source to prevent unnecessary battery drain. Audible and visible alarms for monitors, infusion pumps, and ventilators are crucial for promptly identifying significant patient changes or equipment malfunctions during transit. Crews should have enough batteries on hand to support the entire transport duration and handle unexpected delays. It is also vital to ensure that transport equipment is compatible with the lines, fittings, and power outlets at both the destination and in the transport vehicle.

All transport equipment should easily fit into elevators and transport vehicles, providing space for transport personnel to perform their duties. Securing the equipment within the transport vehicle not only enhances visibility but also safeguards it from accidental damage.

In addition to monitoring and physiologic support equipment, airway (intubation) and intravenous equipment, along with medications, must be accessible and transportable. Transport medications should encompass standard resuscitation drugs, analgesics, sedative/hypnotic agents, and neuromuscular blocking agents as needed.

Increasingly common for trauma transports is the availability of HEMS programs to carry blood products. UCAN currently carries packed red blood cells (PRBCs), whole blood (WB), and fresh frozen plasma (FFP). Importantly, if a trauma center works regularly with a transport team, it is helpful to know if they use blood products and what kind they use. UCAN can give RhD-negative whole blood and RhD-negative packed red blood cells first line to females of childbearing potential, but more commonly HEMS programs are rolling out RhD-positive whole blood programs. Receiving trauma centers will need to have systems of care in place to offer the appropriate alloimmunization prophylaxis for females of childbearing potential who have received RhD-positive products in the transport environment.

Portable ultrasound has gained popularity in the critical care transport environment and is available to the UCAN medical crew. Point-of-care ultrasound has numerous advantages that include assessment for pericardial effusions and tamponade physiology, the presence of lung sliding to evaluate for pneumothoraces, and FAST exams to assess for hemoperitoneum in trauma patients. In addition to assisting in patient assessment, UCAN crews can relay FAST exam findings to receiving trauma surgeons to aid in making 'direct to OR' decisions.

Safety of Transport

Accidents occur with all modes of patient transport. While ground ambulances have a higher probability of being involved in an accident, they offer a better chance of survival than aircraft mishaps. As a result, safety is the foremost concern of air medical operations, and ensuring a safe flight is a fundamental responsibility of every HEMS program. Safety must also be an overriding consideration in weighing the risks and benefits of HEMS.

Many factors go into the safety of operations, including, but not limited to the airworthiness of the aircraft, situational awareness, decision-making, fatigue, and the pressure to fly from peers, program leadership or others. Weather requirements ("minimums") must be strictly enforced. When there is a flight request, the pilot must verify the weather conditions and the condition of the aircraft. To ensure objectivity, the pilot should not be informed of any patient information. The pilot maintains the unquestioned authority to accept, turndown, or abort a flight because of aircraft or weather considerations or any other safety concern. These decisions should not be questioned or influenced in any way by administrators, flight crew, or other parties.

Flight crews must not be the only ones concerned about transport safety. This responsibility extends to the trauma service, hospital staff, and EMS agencies that rely on HEMS programs to transport their patients. The practice of "helicopter shopping" can be a serious problem and has been a factor in several fatal HEMS accidents. Helicopter shopping occurs when a requesting party calls numerous HEMS programs sequentially until one agrees to accept a flight—without revealing that other programs turned down the flight due to bad weather or other safety concerns [37, 38]. The practice was such a concern that in 2006 the FAA issued a letter to all state EMS directors describing helicopter shopping and urging them to take action to prohibit this practice [39].

Interhospital Transport

Interhospital transfer is needed when a referring facility lacks the necessary resources, equipment, personnel, or expertise to address the needs of a critically ill trauma patient. These patients often require further diagnosis, specialized care, or a timely treatment (i.e., surgery, mechanical thrombectomy, or percutaneous coronary intervention) that the referring hospital cannot provide. Some physicians hold misconceptions about certain patients being "too sick" to transfer, often due to a lack of awareness about advanced patient transport teams and systems.

A successful interfacility transport relies on a "transfer triangle" involving three key participants. The referring and receiving physicians/facilities form the bottom corners, laying the foundation for the patient transfer. While direct physician-to-physician communication is ideal, in many cases, physicians may delegate transfer coordination to a representative. At the apex of the triangle are the transport personnel, including communication and medical teams, serving as a vital link between the referring and receiving facilities. Collaborating effectively, these stakeholders ensure that each patient transfer optimally utilizes available resources, such as vehicles, personnel, and equipment. At the UChicago Medicine Trauma Center, UCAN takes on the role of the apex in the transfer triangle. Interfacility transports account for approximately 85% of all UCAN flights,

A myriad of factors must be considered when planning patient transport, including the availability of local resources (e.g., referring and receiving hospitals, ambulance services), mode of transport (ground vs. air), weather considerations (e.g., inclement weather, snow, fog), ground traffic, construction, or the accessibility of roads and landing areas (helipads or airports). Travel to deliver the patient (one-way vs. round trip or two legs of a three-legged transport). A vehicle dispatched directly from the referring hospital to the receiving hospital constitutes a one-way transport. A two-way transport has the vehicle and crew being sent from the receiving hospital to the referring hospital to pick up the patient. This represents the most common UCAN transport. Three-legged transports describe those in which a third party (hospital-sponsored program or independent ambulance company) provides the vehicle and team from a location other than the receiving or referring hospital. Hospital-sponsored flight programs and independent ambulance companies (air and ground) often do third-party transfers under terms of an established transport agreement but can also be on-demand.

Role of the UCAN Team in the Interfacility Transfer and Transport

The ideal critical care transport program would have the capabilities of providing comprehensive communications and different modes of transport – for air and ground transport. UCAN has the resources to provide these services and different vehicle options to support our trauma center based on the geographic, logistical, and clinical needs of each trauma victim. It's important to note that for some trauma centers, this part of the transfer may be accomplished by an independent third party that only does air medical transport. Coordination and communications regarding patient acceptance typically are not done by these independent providers and will usually be done internally through a hospital transfer center or other method of communication.

UCAN Communications Specialists

For the trauma transfer, the UCAN CS performs three separate functions: coordination of the transfer process, transport triage, and coordination of the air or ground transport.

Coordination of the Transfer

The communication and coordination for the transfer of a trauma patient from an outside facility can be handled in many different ways. For many trauma centers, this responsibility may be incorporated into a dedicated in-house transfer center that coordinates all patient transfers to that receiving hospital. For some facilities, this task may be an added function of the admissions office. Some trauma centers may outsource this vital function to a third party. For the UChicago Medicine Trauma Center, the UCAN CommCenter coordinates the transfer of all pediatric and adult trauma patients. Over the past four years, the UCAN CommCenter has averaged nearly 850 calls for adult trauma transfer requests each year and more than 300 pediatric trauma transfer requests annually.

In addition to the trauma transfers, the UCAN CommCenter is the point of contact for transfers to other UChicago Medicine service lines including acute strokes, burns, and all pediatric transfers. In 2022 alone, our communication specialists fielded nearly 6,500 patient transfer requests, with our numbers only projected to increase in subsequent years. It is important to note that a single patient transfer/transport can result in dozens of phone calls between the referring and receiving hospitals, transfer centers, physicians, transport services, and more.

To initiate the transfer process, the referring physician or their designee, will call the UCAN communications center, provide their name, easy access call back number (e.g., hospital telephone number, pager, mobile phone), the name of the referring hospital and referring unit to facilitate follow-up phone calls. On a pre-made transfer sheet, all this provided information will be documented by the CS. The patient's name, date of birth, weight, nature of illness or injury, and vital signs are then reported. If the trauma transfer request is to UChicago Medicine, the CS will page the trauma attending on call and conference the referring physician directly to the trauma attending. Once the trauma attending is on the phone, patient physical findings, results of any pertinent diagnostic studies, treatment provided, current condition, and reason for transfer are described in detail.

Once the patient is accepted for transfer, the accepting trauma attending may make recommendations regarding ongoing patient management. Ideally, both the referring and receiving physicians would document these recommendations. Of note, no receiving hospital can insist that their transport team undertake a transport for them to accept the patient in transfer, as that would be a violation of the Emergency Medical Treatment and Active Labor Act (EMTALA).

Transport Triage

All transfers to UChicago Medicine are triaged by a UCAN CS in an effort to utilize the appropriate transport resources for each patient. After the patient is accepted for transfer to our facility, the CS will make a recommendation to the referring physician regarding patient transport. These recommendations are based upon an established UCAN triage tool that is used for interfacility transports. For distant referring facilities, the first question is whether the patient meets the criteria for air medical transport. Appropriate utilization of air medical transport can be found in Table 1. If HEMS is not indicated or the patient is at a close referring facility, the second triage question is whether the UCAN critical care team is needed for the patient transport. The triage recommendations are merely that -- recommendations. Per EMTALA, the final decision rests with the referring physician. Utilizing the triage tool and working closely with referring physicians, less than 20% of the nearly 1,200 annual pediatric and adult trauma transfers result in a UCAN air transport.

Coordination of Air and Ground Transport

When the referring physician decides on the mode of patient transport, the CS then coordinates the transport. If a flight is requested and the UCAN helicopter is available, the CS contacts the on-duty pilot and informs them of the flight request without providing any patient information. If the pilot accepts the flight based on weather, weight capacity, and any other safety of flight considerations, the CS will

Table 1 Appropriate Utilization of Air Medical Transport

Distance: When the closest appropriate facility is too far for safe and timely ground ambulance transport
Avoiding Delays: When ground transport-related delays could compromise the patient's condition
Clinical Condition: The clinical condition of the patient necessitates that the transport time be as short as possible
Critical Care Support: Patient transport requires critical care life support that is not available from local ground ambulance services
Time-Critical Treatment: The patient requires time-critical or specific medical care that is not available at the referring hospital
Inaccessible Areas: The location of the patient is inaccessible to regular ground traffic, preventing ambulance access or egress
Long Distance Ground Transport: When local ground EMS is not available or appropriate for long-distance transport
EMS Coverage: When transport by local ground EMS would leave their service area without adequate EMS coverage for an extended period
For **Interfacility Transport:** the requesting physician determines the need for air medical transport based on their best medical judgment and available information at that time
For **Transport Direct from the Scene:** Utilizing best judgment, applicable procedures, and information available, the requesting prehospital provider or agency determines that the patient might benefit from air medical transport directly from the scene to an appropriate receiving facility

Courtesy UCAN (University of Chicago Aeromedical Network), UChicago Medicine, 2024. Originally based on: Association of Air Medical Services: Position paper on the appropriate use of emergency air medical services. *J Air Med Transp* 9:29, 1990; and Determination of medical necessity for air and critical care medical transportation. Position statement of the Air Medical Physician Association. Revised April 13, 2002. In: Blumen IJ (ed): Principles and direction of air medical transport. second edition. Salt Lake City, Utah, 2015, Air Medical Physician Association communicate relative ETA's with the referring facility. If UCAN is unable to fly, the CS will immediately discuss alternatives with the referring facility.

If conditions are suitable for flight but the UCAN helicopter is not available due to maintenance or being on a simultaneous flight, the CS will contact another HEMS program in the Chicagoland area for mutual aid to undertake the flight. When simultaneous flights do occur into UChicago Medicine, the CS must maintain communication with our UCAN crews, but also with the visiting HEMS programs as well. With four designated areas to land aircraft (two rooftop helipads and two alternate ground landing areas), these multiple helicopter situations show how proficient the UCAN CSs are in the communication and collaborative skills to coordinate these multi-aircraft landing and take-offs safely and efficiently.

Offering both air and ground transport, UCAN may undertake critical care ground transports for trauma patients when the pilot turns down a flight for any of the previously mentioned reasons or when the aircraft is unavailable and a UCAN flight nurse team is immediately available. In addition, the UCAN team can go by ground when the referring facility is in close proximity to our hospital, or to referring hospitals without an on-site helipad or a nearby landing area.

For non-UCAN ground transports, the CS will offer to call our partnering ambulance service to set up a ground ambulance (basic life support [BLS], advanced life support [ALS], Critical Care) for transport. By offering to make these calls, the referring physician and staff can return to their patients and other responsibilities sooner.

Regardless of the mode of transport, while the UCAN crew is out on transport, the CS will remain available in the event the crew needs to be put in contact with either the accepting physician, UCAN medical control, or the receiving unit. Along with maintaining communication with the crew on transport, it is also the CS's responsibility to "track" the aircraft or ambulance utilizing computer-based software and mapping. These maps provide the current location of the crew and provide an additional safety measure in the event an emergency arises.

UCAN Flight Nurse Role on Transports

The UCAN nurses have two important roles in transport – safety and patient care. When a flight or ground request is a "go" the CS notifies the flight nurses with the basic information that is available (e.g., patient's age, weight, mechanism of injury, diagnosis, if intubated, on any intravenous (IV) drips, etc.). For the trauma patient, this is generally all the UCAN team needs to know before an immediate departure. However, for other patient populations, the UCAN nurses may decide to talk with the referring physician or nurse or receiving physician to retrieve more patient information to be better prepared for transport. This is an important consideration in transporting the patient safely to assure that appropriate therapies are continued (or initiated by UCAN) since certain medical equipment (e.g., high-flow nasal cannula, intra-aortic balloon pump, Impella) is not routinely kept on the aircraft or ambulance.

While the pilots have the ultimate authority on all factors affecting flight safety, the UCAN nurses (and communication specialists) also have significant responsibility concerning UCAN safety. The entire UCAN team will do a safety assessment ("4 to go, 1 to say no") before a transport begins. If there is a concern, it is discussed, resolved or an alternate method of transport will be determined. Once a flight is confirmed, other safety-related responsibilities begin for the flight nurses including an aircraft walkaround looking for any abnormalities before entering the helicopter and the use of pre-flight checklists prior to takeoff. During takeoff and landing and at all times in flight when not directly involved in patient care, the flight nurses scan the airspace for obstacles and potential hazards. At nighttime, the pilot and one flight nurse will be wearing night vision goggles (NVGs) to facilitate this situational awareness.

As the flight crew arrives at the referring hospital, one flight nurse will obtain an updated or full report from the referring nurse while the other flight nurse starts their primary and secondary assessments. It is at this time that it is determined by the flight crew whether the patient needs further stabilization prior to transport. The flight nurses utilize and operate under the UCAN patient care guidelines (PCGs), which is a series of standardized guidelines developed by the UCAN flight nurse team and their medical directors, with the input of specialty physicians. Despite having these PCGs, while at a referring hospital, the flight nurses do not provide patient care in a bubble and will frequently discuss plans with the referring physician. If a question, or disagreement regarding patient care does arise, the UCAN crew would contact their medical control physician or the receiving attending in an attempt to help resolve the patient care issue.

Enroute to the receiving facility, the patient is continuously monitored and managed for any changes in condition.

At the referring hospital or in transport, the UCAN crew can contact the trauma attending through the UCAN CommCenter if they have additional information about the patient (e.g., a positive FAST exam) or if the patient's condition has changed dramatically. It is often during these discussions, that a decision may be made by the trauma attending to meet the crew on the helipad to determine if they should bypass the trauma bay and go directly to the operating room. On an annual basis, approximately 2% of our trauma flights end up going directly to the operating room.

Upon arrival at the receiving hospital, the patient is offloaded from the aircraft and transported to the appropriate unit. Before undoing the patient seat belts, a standardized report is given to the receiving team (e.g., nurse, physician, respiratory therapist). This ensures patient information is appropriately being distributed and allows for questions pertinent to patient care. Once the patient is transferred to the hospital bed, the care of the patient is complete for the UCAN crew. However, the "transport" is not complete until the aircraft is ready for the next transport. The flight nurses decontaminate the litter, gear bags, and non-disposable equipment that was used and restock supplies and blood if used. Additional post-transport duties include debriefing with the entire crew, and charting.

Referring Physician and Referring Hospital Responsibilities

When a referring (sending) physician recognizes that their hospital capabilities are inadequate to meet the needs of a critically ill trauma patient, or if specialized treatment or expertise is required but not available, the patient must be transferred to a facility capable of providing these services. This is especially true for trauma patients. To assist in this decision-making, hospitals can proactively outline their facility's capabilities in policies that are easily accessible to physicians, administrators, and staff. In this section, we discuss the logistical and legal aspects that referring physicians and hospitals need to consider when transferring a patient to another hospital and when considering HEMS transport.

Both emergency departments and in-patient units can initiate the interfacility transport of a patient. In the United States, if the transfer is from an emergency department, the Emergency Medical Treatment and Active Labor Act (EMTALA) [40] applies. EMTALA requires that all unstable patients be transported by qualified personnel with the appropriate transportation equipment.

Established in 1986, EMTALA introduced federal requirements for patient stabilization and transfer, setting guidelines for hospitals and physicians. Initially applying to individuals arriving at the emergency department, the Centers for Medicare and Medicaid Services (CMS) has broadened its interpretation to encompass various areas of the hospital campus. The original EMTALA regulations did not specifically address the interfacility transfer of unstable patients from inpatient units. Consequently, different interpretations were reached across federal courts and regional CMS offices. However, in September 2003, CMS published new regulations to resolve this issue. CMS concluded that "the transfer and stability issues for a patient, once he or she is admitted, are governed by the Medicare hospital conditions of participation, State law, and professional considerations, not EMTALA requirements" [41]. So while the CMS position is that EMTALA does not apply to inpatient units, EMTALA transfer provisions may still in the best interest of the patient and warrant careful consideration.

When a patient presents to the emergency department with an "emergency medical condition," specific requirements must be met prior to initiating an interfacility transfer. The referring hospital must examine the patient and "provide the medical treatment within its capacity which minimizes the risks to the individual's health". Should the hospital be unable to stabilize a patient, an "appropriate transfer" under EMTALA is permissible only after adhering to the remaining provisions of the law. In 2009, the CMS Interpretive Guidelines [42] established that hospitals may transfer a patient prior to the referring hospital exhausting available resources if the patient requests the transfer to another hospital and refuses treatment at the referring hospital.

EMTALA prohibits an "automatic transfer" based on referral patterns or affiliations, including managed care, trauma systems, and perinatal networks. The referring physician determines the appropriate facility and physician for the patient. The most appropriate facility for a patient is not always the closest, though it may be difficult to transport a critically ill patient to a distant facility without a specialty transport team or by ground ambulance. This is often a consideration when decisions are made to call UCAN to transfer distant trauma patients to our facility. Once an appropriate facility has been identified, the referring physician will consult a receiving trauma physician, confirm the trauma center receiving facility has available bed space, and consent to accept the transfer.

EMTALA regulations state "the transfer is effected through qualified personnel and transportation equipment, as required, including the use of necessary and medically appropriate life support measures during the transfer". Unfortunately, the law does not define "qualified." The 2009 Interpretative Guidelines [42] clarified responsibilities by stating that "The physician at the sending hospital (not at the receiving hospital) has the responsibility to determine the appropriate mode, equipment, and attendants for transfer." While the guidelines state that the referring hospital is ultimately responsible for ensuring the transport is carried out appropriately, referring hospitals are afforded some degree of flexibility in determining how to fulfill this obligation. For instance, the guidelines do not mandate that a hospital operate its own EMS transport service.

There are several key decisions the referring physician should consider when making arrangements for patient transport. Defining the personnel and the level of care that will accompany the patient during the transport is crucial (BLS, ALS, or Critical Care/Specialty Care Transport Team). Critically injured trauma patients require highly skilled teams capable of managing these often difficult and complex patients during transport. Choosing the type of vehicle, or mode of transport is another important decision.

A final consideration rests with selecting a transport team with the proper equipment, medications, and in many cases blood products to have "on--hand" during transport. Not all critical care transport or ALS teams are the same. It is advisable for referring facilities and physicians to have a reasonable understanding of the capabilities of HEMS programs and other transport services within their service area, even if that service is provided by the receiving hospital or a third party.

The patient's clinical condition defines each of these decisions. Although it's impossible to predict all potential complications during any transfer, the referring physician must accurately assess the patient's actual and potential injuries and anticipate complications that might arise during transport. They must also estimate the serious nature of the injuries to judge whether "team or time" represents the greater opportunity to improve the patient's outcome. This is a major role where UCAN communications specialists who are experienced in transport medicine, aided by their triage tools, can greatly assist in recommending the most appropriate mode of transport and personnel to optimize the patient transfer.

It is the responsibility of the referring physician to explain to the patient (or family) the reasons for transfer, the receiving facility, the receiving physician, and the method of transport. This discussion should take place early in the transfer process. Considerable time may be lost if a transfer is set into motion only to have the family refuse the selected receiving hospital or mode of transport. Written, signed consent for transfer is to be obtained by the referring hospital. Many transport teams, like UCAN, use their own supplemental consent forms as well.

A comprehensive overview of the risks and benefits of a transfer must be documented in the patient's records. EMTALA mandates that specific risks and benefits be considered and explained to the patient or the "legally responsible person acting on the individual's behalf." A generic statement asserting that the benefits of transfer outweigh the risks is not sufficient. Hospitals that are frequently involved in patient transfers may find it helpful to have prepared forms with checklists to facilitate the completion of the necessary transfer documents. The referring facility is obligated to send all medical records, or copies of them, related to the present emergency condition including imaging, preliminary diagnosis, treatment provided, results of any tests, and the informed written consent for transfer are to be sent by the referring facility to the receiving facility. Patients coming from an inpatient unit will likely have additional records accompanying them including physicians' and nurses' notes, consultations, medication sheets, order sheets, flow sheets, EKGs, radiology reports, lab results, and pertinent imaging (x-rays, CTs, MRIs). Whenever possible, a discharge summary or transfer note is also included.

From a logical and logistical perspective, hospitals that may benefit from the rapid transport of patients by HEMS should have or explore the establishment of an on-site helipad or landing zone. The helicopter's efficiency may be compromised if an appropriate landing area is not readily available. In the absence of a suitable landing area, the time required for locating and securing a landing zone may gradually undermine the helicopter's speed advantage. Furthermore, if the chosen landing zone is situated far from the sending facility, it may necessitate the arrival of a ground ambulance at the landing zone to complete the remainder of the journey.

Landing zones need only be small (100 × 100 feet), flat, and devoid of obstructions for takeoff and landing. An ideal location would be a ground-based helipad in close proximity to the emergency room. Alternatively, if there is not enough open land for a helipad that would be clear of obstructions, a rooftop helipad should be considered. (see Fig. 4) All helistops whether on the ground or rooftop should file with the FAA or state agency to ensure there are clear flight paths in and out of the location. This will help verify that it is a safe location for helicopter operations. Also, the FAA recommends perimeter lights and a lighted windsock when night operations are expected to take place. To construct a concrete ground helipad that would meet the FAA requirements, it might cost in the range of $150,000 to $200,000. For a rooftop helipad, there are a great many variables, and the cost could be anywhere from $750,000 to $1,500,000.

Responsibilities of the Receiving Physician and Facility

Trauma centers looking to become regional resources and major receiving centers for critically ill trauma patients must have an effective system to facilitate communications, transfers, and transports. Communications can be improved through

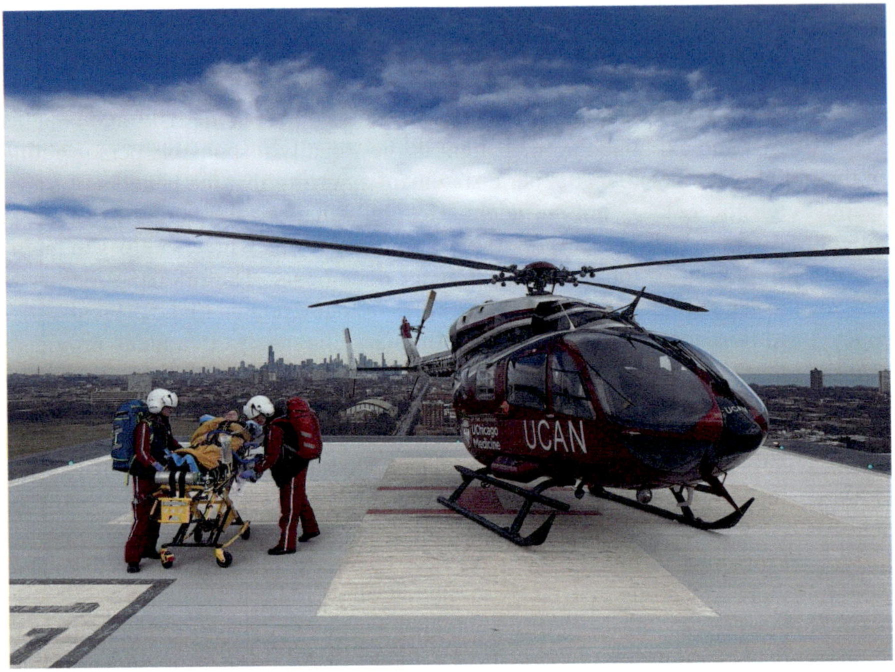

Fig. 4 A rooftop helipad with clear flight paths in and out of the location would be ideal when a ground level helipad is not feasible at a hospital. (Courtesy UCAN (University of Chicago Aeromedical Network), UChicago Medicine, 2024)

designated communications or transfer centers, setting up dedicated telephone lines, or collaborating with the hospital operator. The most efficient trauma tertiary care centers have dedicated communications or transfer centers and trauma consulting/receiving physicians available 24 hours a day with the authority to accept transfers. These trauma tertiary care centers are also familiar with off-site patient management and can provide clinical guidance to the referring physician during the transfer process. As previously described, at UChicago Medicine, the UCAN Communications Center fulfills all of these essential functions for the transfer of trauma patients.

Trauma centers that plan on accepting transfers or scene response by helicopter should have a designated and secure rooftop or ground-level helipad that is appropriately lit (Fig. 5), with fixed coordinates and predesignated liftoff and approach patterns.

Receiving centers that stay current on bed availability, hospital resources, and transport options can make prompt and well-informed transport decisions. Once a patient is accepted for transfer, the referring and receiving physicians can discuss the mode of transport, the transport team composition, and the equipment needed for transport. This discussion could also include or be deferred to the transport team. While EMTALA leaves these decisions with the referring physician for unstable patients in the emergency department, the basic transfer decisions for inpatient

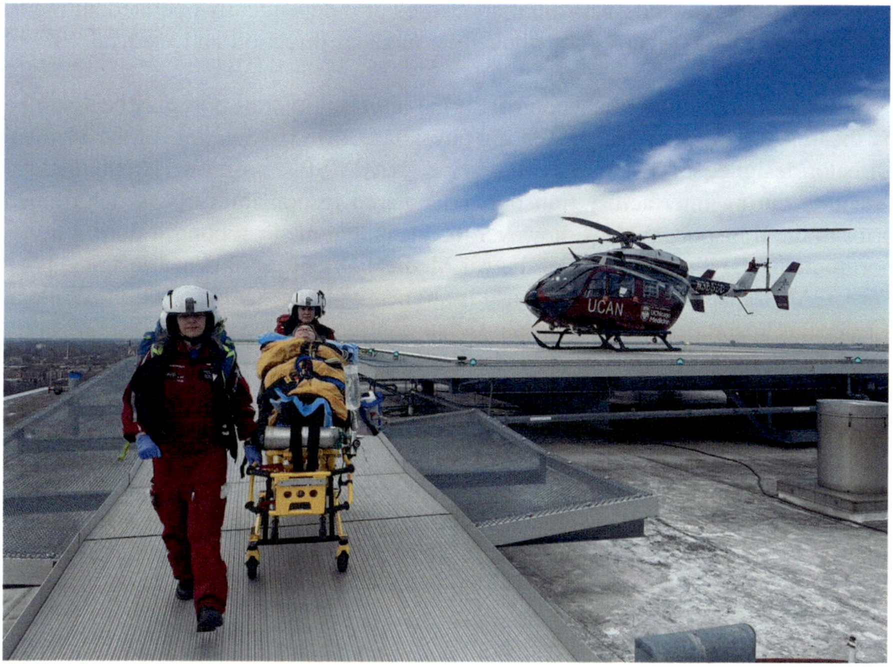

Fig. 5 A designated rooftop or ground-level helipad with proper lighting, a lighted windsock and perimeter security is essential for safe, timely and efficient operations. (Courtesy UCAN (University of Chicago Aeromedical Network), UChicago Medicine, 2024)

transfers should be made by the physician present and caring for the patient at the referring facility.

In the United States, federal law also establishes mandates outlining the responsibilities of receiving facilities. EMTALA identifies "obligations of hospitals with specialized services," and specifies that "participating hospitals with specialized facilities shall not refuse to accept an appropriate transfer if they have the capacity to treat the individual." Receiving hospitals should document in hospital policy which of their services are "specialized," addressing the capabilities and capacities of these services. Under EMTALA, a receiving hospital cannot refuse to accept the transfer of a patient who is unstable or has an emergency medical condition if they have the capacity and ability to care for a patient.

Medical Direction and Medical Control

For interfacility transfers, EMTALA has determined that the transferring physician is responsible for patient transport decisions. However, the law does not make any reference to the transport service, its medical director, or medical control. If these transports are conducted by hospital-sponsored or independently operated air medical services, they typically have their own medical direction and medical control physicians.

In some situations, medical control during interfacility transport may be assumed by the transferring physician, receiving physician, EMS base station, or the Medical Director/designee of the transport service. NAEMSP's position is that medical direction during interfacility transport is a shared responsibility [43], determined prior to the transport. AMPA, however, believes that medical control during transport remains the responsibility of the Air Medical Director or his/her designee [44]. For UCAN transports, medical control is aligned with the AMPA position. While at a referring hospital, the referring physician continues to have some responsibility while the transport team is at the referring facility. The air medical control physician, however, is responsible for the care provided by the transport team during patient stabilization and preparation for transport. In situations when a difference of opinion occurs regarding patient care, the referring physician and the medical control physician must reach an agreement. This is when knowledge and experience regarding the transport environment are crucial to ensure the quality of medical care and the safety of transport. Once the UCAN team leaves the referring facility, a UCAN medical director is responsible for medical control for the duration of the transport.

Scene Response Transports and Integration with EMS

Rapid access to scene victims that are well beyond the reach of local ground EMS can be a valuable resource for a trauma center. Such is the case for the UChicago Medicine Trauma Center and UCAN. At the same time, having access to a regional trauma center can be an invaluable resource to EMS agencies and trauma victims located many miles away. Trauma physicians, EMS medical directors, and physicians who may encounter trauma victims should have a general understanding of how HEMS can be integrated into the prehospital environment.

Indications for Scene Response

Mobilization of HEMS services to a prehospital or scene response generally starts with a determination of appropriateness from first responders. First responders such as police, fire, and EMS professionals may determine whether an air medical team should respond to the scene of an incident due to the speed of HEMS transport, the expertise provided by an air medical team, or a mass casualty incident requiring additional support. A scene response is most commonly requested from first responders for a traumatic injury, but in recent years, flights for medical emergencies in areas far from an appropriate hospital (or any hospital) have increased.

Different EMS systems and/or trauma regions across the country may establish indications for the appropriate use of HEMS at the scene of an accident. While the mechanism of injury and injury patterns (identified or suspected) are often used for field triage to a trauma center, situational or geographic considerations are often added when considering the benefit of HEMS. One of the considerations might be if the estimated transport time to the trauma center is greater than "X" minutes by ground ambulance. For some systems, 20 minutes may be used, while other regions could use a different time frame. Another indication to call HEMS for a traumatic injury would include a patient who is entrapped in a vehicle requiring prolonged extrication by EMS, which delays transport to and definitive treatment at the trauma center. The dispatch time for HEMS and flight time to the scene are often canceled out by the time required for extrication. In addition, entrapped victims have a high probability of serious injury. The use of HEMS will then reduce the transport time to the trauma center team as much as possible after patient extrication. When the transport time from the "scene" to a local hospital by ground ambulance is greater than the transport time to a trauma center by helicopter represents another good use of HEMS. Another possible indication would be a patient who is hemorrhaging and would benefit from the speed of helicopter transport as well as blood administration en route to the trauma center.

Air medical teams are trained in life-saving skills such as rapid sequence intubation, surgical cricothyrotomy, needle decompression thoracostomy, finger thoracostomy, and chest tube insertion. Many air medical teams have access to blood products, with the UCAN team carrying whole blood, packed red blood cells, and plasma. In these examples, HEMS can offer speed or clinical expertise that may improve patient outcomes.

Building Relationships

Air medical team collaboration with EMS should start well before the team is needed in an emergency and should include educational components such as landing zone classes as well as trauma and medical classes as requested.

HEMS providers should be proactive in developing strong relationships with public safety, police, fire, and EMS, as well as industry providers such as steel mills, chemical plants, farming, oil refineries, factories, and more. These relationships are important to encourage safe landing zone preparation and encourage the use of the HEMS when appropriate; ultimately providing efficient care to the patient in need. The air medical team is responsible to initiate and offer training to community providers to ensure the safety of all involved when landing at unimproved or temporary landing sites. The air medical team is the experts in their aircraft and what they need to operate efficiently and safely. The air medical team can also benefit from these relationships in that they can be better informed of the needs of the patients in their communities. For example, when partnering with EMS and industry providers, the air medical team may learn about specific hazardous chemicals or potentially dangerous operations occurring within their service area. This may better inform an approach the air medical team may have for a specific injury or exposure as well as team educational goals for low frequency and high-risk situations.

The UCAN team strives to maintain strong partnerships with the public safety, police, fire, EMS, and industry providers in our area. UCAN works with the Chicago Police Department SWAT as well as FBI SWAT teams which serves as another opportunity to promote UChicago Medicine and its trauma program as well as provide trauma education to these groups. Providing education on STOP THE BLEED[R] for these professionals could prove to be life-saving as they may have to treat themselves or each other in an emergency situation, as well as victims of violent crime. The UCAN team often provides lectures as requested by our prehospital partners, beyond what is covered in a landing zone class. Training these providers helps to educate them on priorities in patient management for cases we collaborate on, and also provides an opportunity for the UCAN team to learn from them.

When a trauma center can establish a strong relationship with HEMS and EMS, this in turn provides an opportunity to extend the trauma center's reach further into the community and at earlier points in patient management. At UChicago Medicine, the UCAN program enjoys an excellent collegial relationship with our trauma team which allows us to represent the great care provided.

Prehospital and Temporary Landing Zones

Most primary (scene) responses occur at temporary landing zones. Therefore, an important consideration for HEMS and EMS with regard to scene operations includes landing zone (LZ) safety. Scene calls can be more dangerous for HEMS simply because they are often landing at improvised LZs, sometimes at night, where surrounding hazards (e.g., wires, radio antennae) may not be known. Ground personnel must be trained to designate and secure a safe LZ for helicopter operations. These landing sites for scene responses may include lanes of an expressway, a rural road, an open field, a parking lot, or even a residential or industrial area.

Helicopter LZs can be inherently hazardous places. The risk of injury may come from the main blades that dip lower to the ground during engine start-up and shutdown or from the tail rotor blades which can be virtually invisible when moving at full speed. Debris propelled through the air by "rotor wash" may also cause injuries.

HEMS programs have an obligation to help train ground personnel on proper landing zone setup, operations, and safety. See Tables 2 and 3.

This landing zone education for EMTs, paramedics, firefighters, law enforcement, and industrial safety personnel can be done in a classroom setting or may be more effective "in the field" with the helicopter present. See Fig. 6. Ideally, this education is provided as continuing education for referring providers annually.

HEMS response directly to the scene of an accident may pose unique risks from hazards near the landing zone and the risk may be heightened at night. In addition, it may not always be possible to identify a safe and secure LZ near the scene of an

Table 2 Landing zone (LZ) identification and coordination

The Landing Zone (LZ)
Should be as close as possible to the hospital entrance or scene of an incident, but not so close that it may interfere with ground operations or patient care
Should be at least 100 × 100 feet (30 × 30 meters) in size
The surface should be as level and flat as possible
Must be clear of debris
Approach and Departure Path
Should not pass over treatment areas, command posts, or congested areas on the ground
Should point into the wind and be free of obstruction to an altitude of 500 feet (152 meters) above the surface
Obstructions and Hazards
All potential hazards on the ground or near the approach/departure path of LZ should be identified and removed if possible
The LZ must be clear of wires, poles, trees, buildings, vehicles, and spectators
Avoid the use of road cones, ropes, tape, and barricades near the LZ
Maintain a **50-foot distance** from potential obstructions and hazards
Position the LZ **upwind** from any hazardous material incidents
Daylight Operations
Utilize both radio and hand signals for communications
Stand with your back to the wind
Night Operations and Light Sources
Use lighting and radio communications to identify the LZ
Illuminate the top of potential hazards with spotlights
Never point lights toward an approaching or departing helicopter
Place a light source (portable light, vehicle headlights, emergency vehicle flashing lights, or chemical stick) at each corner of the LZ, with an additional light upwind
Flares should not be used
If portable lights are used, they *must* be well secured
Lights *must* be clear of the LZ
Turn off nonessential lights
Wind Indicator
Use a windsock, flag, or smoke to indicate wind direction
Position the indicator away from the LZ
If portable, the indicator must be well secured

Courtesy UCAN (University of Chicago Aeromedical Network), UChicago Medicine, 2024

accident. Some prehospital providers and HEMS programs have found it beneficial and safer to use a hospital helipad to rendezvous with ground EMS and the patient. Initially, this practice raised concerns concerning EMTALA responsibilities for the hospital to provide a medical screening examination for these patients. In May 2004, the Centers for Medicare and Medicaid Services (CMS) addressed this concern, noting that the use of a helipad on hospital property does not trigger EMTALA provisions as long as the helipad is being used only as a stopping place for EMS personnel to rendezvous with AMT, to facilitate transport of a patient to the closest appropriate facility.

Table 3 Safety in and around the landing zone (LZ)

General LZ Safety Procedures
Vehicles and personnel should be at least 100 feet (30 meters) from the LZ
Spectators should maintain a distance of at least 200 feet (61 meters) from the LZ
No smoking or running within 50 feet (15 meters) of the helicopter
Keep all items (such as intravenous lines and poles) below shoulder height
Keep the LZ clear or secure of all loose articles (e.g., hats, scarves, sheets, pillows)
Protect the patient from dust and debris
Flight Crew Responsibilities
Opening and closing aircraft doors
Directs and supervises the loading and unloading of the patient and equipment
Ground Personnel Safety
Should wear eye and ear protection
Approach the helicopter *only* when signaled to do so by the pilot or an onboard crew member
Approach and depart the helicopter forward of the rear cabin door maintaining a crouched position with your head down
Never approach or depart from the rear of the helicopter
Stay clear of the tail rotor—it is virtually invisible and extremely dangerous
If the LZ is on a slope, approach and depart the helicopter on the downhill side for the greatest clearance under the blades
Always follow the instructions given by the flight crew
If you do not know if an action is safe, ask before you act
Special Considerations in Disaster Situations and Mass Casualty Incidents
Victims, witnesses, and spectators may become hysterical or exhibit signs of an acute situational reaction
These individuals must be kept clear of the LZ and helicopter
Injured victims who display such behavior should not be triaged for helicopter transport unless adequate physical or chemical restraints are used.

Courtesy UCAN (University of Chicago Aeromedical Network), UChicago Medicine, 2024

Moving Forward

UCAN is a critical partner with the UChicago Medicine Trauma Center as well as all the critical care service lines. The ongoing relationship with the trauma service allows us to reflect on our current practices, and through our diligent quality assurance programs, continue to improve the care we extend to our patients. Open and honest communication between the trauma surgeons and the UCAN team allows us to understand our capabilities and identify opportunities for improvement. Our goal is simple: to always improve our processes, to never stop learning, and to help educate others—and to always provide critical care transport in the most efficient and safest transport environment possible.

At UCAN, we are continuously trying to better the patient transfer process for our time-sensitive patients and prevent prolonged out-of-tertiary care center times. Total quality management is an important part of monitoring and improving our program. All calls to the UCAN CommCenter are recorded to ensure that quality assurance is being met and to identify any areas needing improvement. UCAN utilizes "Protean", a web-based platform that allows the communication specialists, flight nurses, pilots, and medical directors to collaborate and communicate

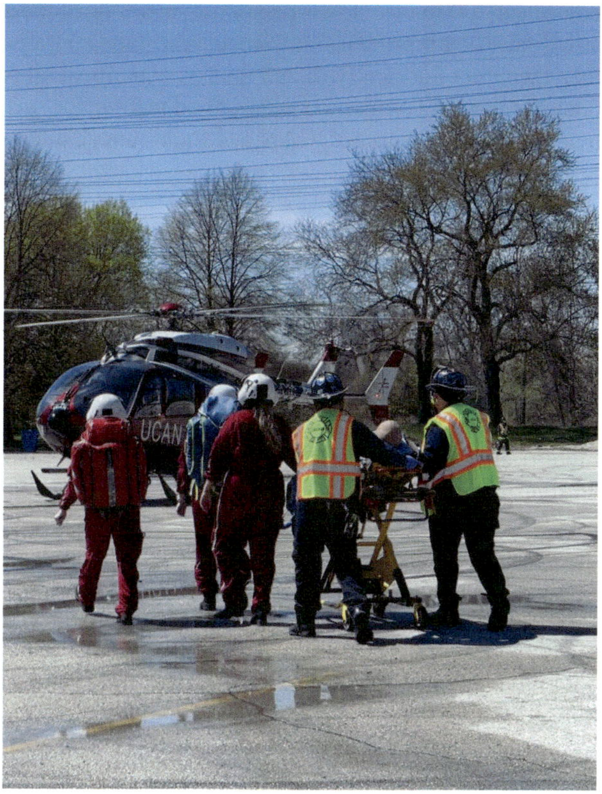

Fig. 6 Training on HEMS Landing Zone requirements and safety for field personnel may be most effective "in the field" with the helicopter present. (Courtesy UCAN (University of Chicago Aeromedical Network), UChicago Medicine, 2024)

effectively to audit 100% of our patient charts, track quality markers and identify any opportunities for improvement (OFIs) regarding safety and/or therapy/patient management. UCAN maintains and practices a "Just Culture" with the goal of improving patient safety and enhanced decision-making amongst the entire crew. By practicing a "Just Culture" in our peer review of charts, case presentations, and transport debriefing, we create a safe learning space and foster growth amongst the entire team including our pilots and UCAN communication specialists.

Continuing education will always remain a key focus and responsibility for UCAN. Not only in our own education but the opportunity to bring training and continuing education to the communities that we serve. In addition to the prehospital landing zone classes already mentioned, UCAN personnel provide teaching on requested topics (e.g., pediatric trach care, basic pediatric care, burn care) to local EMS departments, as well as emergency departments and ICU nurses at referring institutions. UCAN will provide these classes for free continuing education credits for EMS personnel and nurses.

Many of the UCAN nurses are also invited speakers to local, regional, and national conferences or at our own *"UCAN Make a Difference" Critical Care and Trauma Conference*. This full-day Indiana and Illinois event now attracts nearly a combined 700 nurses, EMS personnel, respiratory therapists, nursing students, and allied healthcare professionals each year. Our conference focuses on the care and management of critically ill and injured patients of all patient populations. Not only does the annual conference promote education for surrounding healthcare personnel, but it also promotes UCAN and the trauma center at UChicago Medicine.

Summary

The introduction of a HEMS program into a trauma system brings the benefits of shortened transport time to definitive care and the delivery of advanced prehospital interventions to the scene of injury. HEMS represents the only mechanism by which more than 90 million American citizens have timely access to mortality-improving high-level trauma center care. As a result, it would seem obvious that some form of air transport is a "must-have" for some EMS regions. Such is the case for UChicago Medicine Trauma Center and UCAN with some of the geographic areas surrounding the metropolitan Chicagoland area and extending into neighboring Indiana.

UCAN's contribution goes far beyond the transport of trauma patients by helicopter. The integration of UCAN into the Trauma Center represents the ideal coordination of HEMS, critical care ground transport, and comprehensive communications. Our fully integrated system benefits all aspects of the transfer and transport of critical trauma patients and ensures the appropriate utilization of resources for each patient.

Our on-site 24/7 communication center provides referring facilities with one phone number to speak directly with a trauma attending, coordinate acceptance, and manage all aspects of the air or ground transport. These in-house services support the trauma center to attract and easily accept transfers from facilities that lack the necessary resources for trauma patients – both local area hospitals, and more distant facilities. The system also enables the trauma center to extend its service area to scene trauma patients who are well beyond the reach of local ground EMS.

Across the country, HEMS and critical care ground transport may offer various medical crew configurations. However, the UCAN nurse-nurse team has proven to be ideal for the most complicated and critically injured patient from a scene accident, emergency department, or referring hospital's operating room.

Acknowledgment This chapter is dedicated to the memory of our dear friend and colleague Kelley Holdren, UCAN's Administrative Director and Chief Flight Nurse. Kelley had agreed to be a co-author for this chapter, but sadly never had the chance to participate. In November 2023, Kelley passed away after a hard-fought battle with cancer. UCAN's success and our exceptionally strong relationship and integration with our trauma center are largely due to Kelley's leadership, passion, and expertise. Her commitment to collaboration, patient care, education, and safety were always her top priorities. #ForeverFlySafe

References

1. Branas CC, MacKenzie EJ, Williams JC, Schwab CW, Teter HM, Flanigan MC, et al. Access to trauma centers in the United States. JAMA. 2005;293(21):2626–33.
2. Blumen I. A statistical analysis of HEMS accidents and risk. Presented at the air medical transport conference. Columbus, October 2023.
3. Thomas SH, Arthur AO. Helicopter EMS: research endpoints and potential benefits. Emerg Med Int. 2012;2012:698562.
4. Fritz CL, Thomas SA, Galvagno SM Jr, Thomas SH. Survival benefit of helicopter scene response for patients with an injury severity score of at least nine: a systematic review and meta-analysis. Prehosp Emerg Care. 2023;18:1–10.
5. Werman HA, Darbha S, Cudnik M, Caterino J. Do trauma patients aged 55 and older benefit from air medical transport? Prehosp Emerg Care. 2017;21(4):461–5.
6. Tsuchiya A, Tsutsumi Y, Yasunaga H. Outcomes after helicopter versus ground emergency medical services for major trauma – propensity score and instrumental variable analyses: a retrospective nationwide cohort study. Scand J Trauma Resusc Emerg Med. 2016;24(1):140.
7. Kim OH, Roh YI, Kim HI, et al. Reduced mortality in severely injured patients using hospital-based helicopter emergency medical services in interhospital transport. J Korean Med Sci. 2017;32(7):1187–94.
8. Weinlich M, Martus P, Blau MB, et al. Competitive advantage gained from the use of helicopter emergency medical services (HEMS) for trauma patients: Evaluation of 1724 patients. Injury. 2019;50(5):1028–35.
9. Jung K, Huh Y, Lee JC, et al. Reduced mortality by physician-staffed HEMS dispatch for adult blunt trauma patients in Korea [published correction appears in J Korean Med Sci. 2018;33(14):e118]. J Korean Med Sci. 2016;31(10):1656–61.
10. Funder KS, Rasmussen LS, Hesselfeldt R, et al. Quality of life following trauma before and after implementation of a physician-staffed helicopter. Acta Anaesthesiol Scand. 2017;61(1):111–20.
11. Malekpour M, Younus JM, Jaap K, et al. Mode of transport and clinical outcome in rural trauma: a helicopter versus ambulance comparison. Am Surg. 2017;83(12):1413–7.
12. Zhu TH, Hollister L, Opoku D, Galvagno SM Jr. Improved Survival for Rural Trauma Patients Transported by Helicopter to a Verified Trauma Center: A Propensity Score Analysis. Acad Emerg Med. 2018;25(1):44–53.
13. Urdaneta LF, et al. Evaluation of an emergency air transport service as a component of a rural EMS system. Am Surg. 1984;50(4):183.
14. Michaels D, Pham H, Puckett Y, Dissanaike S. Helicopter versus ground ambulance: review of national database for outcomes in survival in transferred trauma patients in the USA. Trauma Surg Acute Care Open. 2019;4(1):e000211.
15. 2022 Accreditation Standards, 12th ed. Commission on Accreditation of Medical Transport Systems (CAMTS). Anderson; 2022.
16. Insoft RM, Schwartz HP. American academy of pediatrics, subcommittee for revision of interhospital transport guidelines, section on transport medicine. In: Guidelines for air and ground transport of neonatal and pediatric patients. 4th ed. Elk Grove Village; 2015.
17. Treadwell D, Santiago J, editors. Standards for critical care and specialty transport. 2nd ed. Aurora: Air & Surface Transport Nurses Association; 2019.
18. Guidelines for the Use and Availability of Helicopter Emergency Medical Transport (HEMS). United States Department of Transportation, April 2015. https://www.transportation.gov/sites/dot.gov/files/docs/Guidelines%20for%20the%20Use%20and%20Availability%20of%20Helicopter%20Emergency%20Medical%20Transport%20%28HEMS%29.pdf. Accessed 3 Jan 2024.
19. Lyng JW, Braithwaite S, Abraham H, Brent CM, Meurer DA, Torres A, Bui PV, Floccare DJ, Hogan AN, Fairless J, Larrimore A. Appropriate air medical services utilization and recommendations for integration of air medical services resources into the EMS system of care:

a joint position statement and resource document of NAEMSP, ACEP, and AMPA. Prehosp Emerg Care. 2021;25(6):854–73.
20. American College of Emergency Physicians. Appropriate and safe utilization of helicopter emergency medical services. Policy statement. Ann Emerg Med. 2014;63(5):627.
21. Critical Care Transport Standards. Association of Critical Care Transport, ACCT for Patients. https://nasemso.org/wp-content/uploads/ACCT-Standards-Version1-Oct2016.pdf. Accessed 3 Jan 2024.
22. Critical Care Paramedic Position Statement, International Association of Flight and Critical Care Paramedics, July 2009. https://cdn.ymaws.com/www.iafccp.org/resource/resmgr/docs/critical_care_paramedic_posi.pdf. Accessed 30 Apr 2022.
23. Guidelines Committee of the American College of Critical Care Medicine; Society of Critical Care Medicine and American Association of Critical-Care Nurses Transfer Guidelines Task Force. Guidelines for the transfer of critically ill patients. Crit Care Med. 1993;21:931–7.
24. Warren J, Fromm RE Jr, Orr RA, Rotello LC, Horst HM, American College of Critical Care Medicine. Guidelines for the inter- and intrahospital transport of critically ill patients. Crit Care Med. 2004;32(1):256–62.
25. Szem JW, Hydo LJ, Fischer E, et al. High-risk intrahospital transport of critically ill patients: Safety and outcome of the necessary "road trip". Crit Care Med. 1995;23:1660–6.
26. Stenbach G, Sumchai AP. Is aeromedical transport of patients during acute myocardial infarction safe? J Emerg Med. 1989;7:73–7.
27. Selevan JS, Fields WW, Chen W, et al. Critical care transport: outcome evaluation after interfacility transfer and hospitalization. Ann Emerg Med. 1999;33:33–43.
28. Gebremichael M, Borg U, Habashi N, et al. Interhospital transport of the extremely ill patient: the mobile intensive care unit. Crit Care Med. 2000;28(1):79–85.
29. Broman LM, Frenckner B. Transportation of critically ill patients on extracorporeal membrane oxygenation. Front Pediatr. 2016;13(4):63.
30. Kang TS, Ko BS, Drakos SG, Stehlik J, Bott SI, Koliopoulou A, Tonna JE, Bowen ME, Stoddard K, Selzman CH, McKellar SH. Safety of long-distance transfers of patients on acute mechanical circulatory support. J Surg Res. 2018;224:18–22.
31. Muramatsu KI, Omori K, Kushida Y, Nagasawa H, Takeuchi I, Jitsuiki K, Shitara J, Ohsaka H, Oode Y, Yanagawa Y. An analysis of patients with acute aortic dissection who were transported by physician-staffed helicopter. Am J Emerg Med. 2021;44:330–2. https://doi.org/10.1016/j.ajem.2020.04.034.
32. Pan A, Peddle M, Auger P, Parfeniuk D, MacDonald RD. Interfacility transport of mechanically ventilated patients with suspected COVID-19 in the prone position. Prehosp Emerg Care. 2022;2:1–6.
33. Trojanowski J, MacDonald RD. Safe transport of patients with acute coronary syndrome or cardiogenic shock by skilled air medical crews. Prehosp Emerg Care. 2011;15(2):240–5.
34. Aggarwal B, Raymond C, Jacob J, Kralovic D, Kormos K, Holloway D, Menon V. Transfer of patients with suspected acute aortic syndrome. Am J Cardiol. 2013;112(3):430–5.
35. Data compiled from the Atlas and Database of Air Medical Services. Center for Transportation Injury Research in alliance with the Association of Air Medical Services and the air medical industry, 2018.
36. Stocking JC. Crew configuration. In: Blumen IJ, editor. Principles and direction of air medical transport. 2nd ed. Salt Lake City: Air Medical Physician Association; 2015. p. 50–6.
37. Shaffer T. EMS helicopter shopping: dead wrong. FlightSafetyNeet. https://flightsafetynet.com/helicopter-shopping-price-worth-paying/. Accessed 3 Jan 2024.
38. Responsible "Helicopter Shopping" Through Selective Resource Management. Air & Surface Transport Nurses Association, Emergency Nurses Association, International Association of Flight and Critical Care Paramedics Joint Position Statement. https://cdn.ymaws.com/www.astna.org/resource/collection/4392B20B-D0DB-4E76-959C-6989214920E9/Joint_Position_Statement_Selective_Resource_Mgmt_FINAL_11.12.18.pdf. Accessed 3 Jan 2024.

39. Federal Aviation Administration: FAA letter to state EMS Director on helicopter shopping, August 2006. Available at http://www.oacct.org/safety/FAA-State-Letter.pdf. Accessed 3 Jan 2024.
40. Congressional Omnibus Budget Reconciliation Act (COBRA) of 1985 (42 USCA 1395 DD), as amended by the Omnibus Budget Reconciliation Acts (OBRA) of 1987, 1989, and 1990.
41. 42 CFR Parts 413, 482, and 489. Medicare Program; Clarifying Policics Related to the Responsibilities of Medicare-Participating Hospitals in Treating Individuals With Emergency Medical Conditions; Final Rule. Centers for Medicare & Medicaid Services (CMS), Department of Health And Human Services (DHHS), Federal Register, September, 9, 2003. https://www.govinfo.gov/content/pkg/FR-2003-09-09/pdf/03-22594.pdf. Accessed 3 Jan 2024.
42. Revisions to Appendix V, "Emergency Medical Treatment and Labor Act (EMTALA) Interpretive Guidelines". CMS Manual System, Pub. 100-07 State Operations Provider Certification, Centers for Medicare & Medicaid Services (CMS), Department of Health & Human Services (DHHS), Transmittal 46, May 29, 2009. https://www.hhs.gov/guidance/sites/default/files/hhs-guidance-documents/R46SOMA.pdf. Accessed 3 Jan 2004.
43. Shelton SL, Swor RA, Domeier RM, Lucas R. Medical direction of interfacility transports: National Association of EMS Physicians Standards and Clinical Practice Committee. Prehosp Emerg Care. 2000;4(4):361–4
44. Air Medical Physician Association. Medical direction and medical control of air medical services. Position statement of the Air Medical Physician Association. Prehosp Emerg Care. 2002;6(4):461–3.

Trauma Chaplaincy an Integration of Care

Julian A. Bond

> Isn't there something more impressive about what the weed has achieved through perseverance compared to what the flower accomplished through ease? Those weeds are people who have had environmental risk factors stacked against them. They are survivors. Imagine how they could flourish and flower, if we could just get them into a lush garden with nourishing soil and unlimited sunlight. (Nzinga Harrison, MD) [1]

The formation at the University of Chicago Medical Center Emergency department is unique and consists of a unit that involves a team of trauma surgeons to environmental services workers that are impacted by traumas and what they clean, observe, and prepare for in the next trauma and or medical patient. During a recent observation visit by a human resource representative of the University of Chicago Medical Center, they noted that the operation truly depends and impacts every skill set of each service that fulfills an obligation in the emergency department. For example, if a room is not cleaned it takes away from the nurses productivity, who at times may have to stop and clean a room for the next patient versus the environmental service personnel cleaning so that a patient can claim and access the room for treatment and care. The same is reflected for those patients that come into our trauma bay area and are examined for the injury or immediate emergency that requires attention. Information taken back from our HR representative's 10 hour shadowing and observation shined that light and empathetic importance for this community that resides where this care is so desperately needed. The insight gained from this experience, forced a realignment and stabilized the care necessary for this population of patients and care providers. As much as care is provided to our patients, the HR representative also expressed how important it is to have a chaplain that can provide spiritual care not only to the patients but certainly for the staff. Enduring the impact of the trauma seen is trauma experienced. The presence of the

J. A. Bond (✉)
Trauma Chaplain, Spiritual Care, UChicago Medicine, Chicago, IL, USA
e-mail: Julian.Bond@uchicagomedicine.org

S. O. Rogers, Jr (ed.), *Creating a Modern Trauma Center*,
https://doi.org/10.1007/978-3-031-66524-0_16

trauma chaplain in the emergency room adds accessibility to caring for the soul which is necessary and beneficial. An art of collaboration was witnessed by the intentional investment and observation of emergency room operations, that is not grasped in a walk through, it takes sitting and witnessing like others in the community that we serve in the emergency room.

As a spiritual care provider I partner with a team of physicians, nurses, security guards, respiratory therapists, environmental services men and women, medical residents, fellows, social workers and violence recovery specialists. When I am consulted to visit a patient and when I need to make a consultation, there are three vehicles that are accessible twenty four hours a day and seven days a week through channels of our EPIC software system, paging, and cisco phone system that operate with direct lines to services in need. I often consult with service providers via EPIC to record requests and then by phone. However, what has become essential is being visible and making rounds with each service during a shift so that an offer of reassurance is available, just call, text, or overhead page, the trauma chaplain is available. I have found often that when providers know that I am serving that specific shift, I am told "so glad you are here Rev", then I get their request. Building this relationship takes time and effective integration. Each month in the monthly newsletter for the emergency department, there is space in the newsletter for a Spiritual Care note to provide a reflection that speaks to their area of focus of trauma from neuro, plasma, cardiac, and self care. I attempt to engage the readers of the newsletter and motivate how they are important and the banner of stewardship that they uphold and are obligated too.

The format of our consultation and or referral process requires that it is documented in a provider note or by selection in EPIC. At times this can be overlooked if the providers are not reading existing notations in patient charts and or in auxiliary request. Mostly, I have direct access to mental health providers and send email communication to those that can accelerate care for a patient. This request requires a conversation and or is discussed in interdisciplinary team meetings that occur various times a week. For example, during our overnight shifts a mental health provider is not always physically available but accessible by phone at all times. However, social workers are present in the ER during both day and night shifts, and they assists with immediate referrals and care coordination or as we call them to provide proper discharge resources. Upon intake it coordinates how proper discharges includes evaluation of psychosocial needs along with medical care follow up necessary for each patient. As each patient is discussed in interdisciplinary meetings we also have a database that houses psychosocial needs called RedCap that tracks how we are impacting the whole health of our patients. In this private database we discuss outcomes/goals and proceed with utilizing this information to possibly outsource if necessary care for specialists that at times are necessary. I am quite comfortable with discussing cases and case loads with mental health providers and providing context for each patient or situation. This collaboration is an opportunity for me to say it well and touch others with my words. Charles Swindoll once wrote "a good illustration not only helps to clarify the mysterious or obscure, it also helps the listener appreciate the relevance of a particular point". [2] Therefore, I am confident in my ability to share my recommendation and navigate confidentiality. Each time I share it sparks how continuity of care can proceed and informs my colleagues how to approach the situation in their own discipline. In the event that a case discusses harm to oneself and or another, I am to report or escalate to a medical professional immediately to relevant agents. As a method of establishing trust with my patients and interdiscipline teams, I practice equality, live it out in front of my colleagues, to demonstrate the leadership and stewardship required of a trauma chaplain specialist in my trauma informed spiritual care.

As a chaplain of a grant study called the violence recovery program also known as the BHC collaborative, The Violence Recovery Program is the backbone of the BHC Collaborative. The VRP provides adults, children, and families with a holistic intervention aimed at sustainable, long-term recovery, including the following core components:

- In-hospital crisis intervention
- Trauma-specific interventions
- Reinjury risk assessment
- Violence interventions, including access to violence interruption and street outreach services
- Health care navigation and assistance with Medicaid or other programs
- Long-term planning and access to community service providers
- Bereavement support
- Family support services including medication management, legal and victim advocacy, and help with housing, child care, employment, or educational needs [3].

Achieving a proper intervention is the aim for each patient over the time of patients' care in house. Once a patient arrives at our Emergency Room, my role as a chaplain begins to assess the needs of the patient as medical care providers are evaluating the injuries, physical and moral, that come into our trauma bay as level one and or level two traumas. As I engage from observation initially and interact with a patient as a source of comfort and calm I directed to offer counsel that is advocating for their concerns, I reinforce what is happening in the moment to and by medical staff and offer reassurance that I will contact whomever they wish, as the moment is often scary or traumatic. And when patients are requesting that a friend and or love one be contacted to inform of their new medical status, provided by medical staff I facilitate updates or coordinate efforts for them to see their family member. This typically happens in a short period of time within fifteen minutes of evaluation and impacted by CT scans, X-Ray, Radiology reads and or sudden medical status change that requires that the patient goes to the operating room. In this time, I work with violence recovery specialists to coordinate updates and identify persons who can receive proper health care information deemed via HIPAA. Our team understands each role and provides each other necessary information or details that can assist in the endeavor. I am offering my priestly duties and pastoral presence immediately, and upon completion of a medical evaluation I am able to assist in delivering what type of assistance can be useful to our patients. I understand my role as a non anxious presence and to uphold confidentiality of the patient and establish parameters that fit within a care provider capacity as chaplain. As a member of the community and homeowner that lives amongst the people we serve, this knowledge of the neighborhood and being a leader that is visible, strikes a balance between trust and distrust for healthcare providers as I serve as a bridge that dispels myth of medical treatment. Often this opportunity builds up health awareness and deescalates fear, and healthcare legends that patients come in with. As a skilled provider I utilize the spiritual assessment tools FICA, OARS and PST mostly. This variation of modalities allows a spiritual care provider to ask open ended questions that begin or ignite the goals and objectives of the patient. This has become a favorable tool kit for both religious and non religious patients or staff members cared for. When addressing patient centered care, a chaplain is instrumental in understanding spiritual and mental health to reach desired patient goals. I invite the patient to imagine what further exploration with another professional can do to benefit adding balance to their traumatic experience or situation that requires a pivot. Providing the invitation is instrumental and creates a linkage so that when a mental health provider sees the patient, the patient is not apprehensive but yet somewhat prepared for the journey. As a practice of my effectiveness I am aware of my boundaries, " and have a good sense of what that walk feels like, looks like, sounds like and tastes like" [4]. Having the opportunity to practice emotional awareness has informed me of my own triggers and therefore has provided the necessary outlet to express my own past experiences and traumas. Therefore, when I engage with patients my story is not used as an example nor does it dominate if at all become a part of the narrative of chaplain and patient encounter Laura van Dernoot Lipsky reminds me in her writing of Trauma Stewardship that "we can sustain our work with trauma only if we combine our capacity for empathy with a dedication to personal insight and mindfulness. This is difficult terrain to navigate" [5]. However, owning my story assists in helping others and knowing when to collaborate with mental health professionals. For each of my patients that I care for that have experienced a sudden death, and or motor vehicle accident I do well guiding them to express their feelings, as I recall what I felt and how and what was not made available in my personal experience with trauma. In my effort I am effective and attribute my experience to assisting my patients and am truly considerate of their space and time as they reflect. It is never about me in the encounters with my patients.

As I further learn to understand the variety of moral injuries that occur in a person, I've learned to apply reflective listening qualities such as OARS. When I attempt to close the loop in communication, I believe I am doing so in the required medical treatment that is apparent that a patient will have to follow upon discharge. When rounding with an advanced practice provider and or physician, the opportunity to follow up and explain how to address wound care, or how often a certain medication needs to be taken etc., engages the patient with best care practices after a discharge. During these visits some patients will rely on the chaplain to champion their care and ask for clarity from the practitioners to speak in elementary terms. This requirement softens the load and produces a patient that is cooperative. This clarification and greater exploration increases the probability and participation of the patient. When this opportunity is not struck between a patient and provider it increases or produces a gap in service. I have deemed it a disparity in health care but try to eliminate it if at all possible.

Evidence based practice is the sum of all parts in our Emergency Room for each discipline. For example, metrics are a critical element of what we do as a trauma center. The data we collect gives us deeper insights into the nature of trauma on the SouthSide of Chicago and helps us improve our interventions. It forms the basis for evaluation of our programs and development of a national model. Data collection for this initiative is complex. It requires gathering information from different sources that historically did not communicate with one another, and developing new systems capable of acquiring and organizing it. Among the metrics being tracked:

- Patient demographics
- Type of injury: gunshot wound, stab wound, domestic violence or assault
- Number of patients engaged with VRP, by age
- Number of engagements with family/friends during VRP crisis intervention
- Number of patients at imminent risk
- Number and types of VRP imminent risk interventions
- Number of staff trainings in trauma-informed care, and number of attendees
- Numbers of patients served by REACT clinic and numbers receiving psychiatric services, child-parent psychotherapy, and individual psychotherapy
- Number of patients engaged by Child Life [3].

As a part of a certified body of chaplains that is capable and are training more about crisis interventions, moral injury and the work of pluralistic and non religious capacities, it is stretching the field in a great way and asking more chaplains to expound our capabilities. As a commonality I believe that it's psychosocial as a whole that's adjusting to better ways to perform duties to reach humankind and the human condition. Our disciplines are somewhat alike as we desire holistic outcomes for patients, it's navigating how and utilizing similar language that builds trust.

To illustrate how effectively building out the language of spiritual care is important, I suggest charting has highlighted a pattern of worth in the conversation of medical record keeping for patients. Our discipline's effort to build out a method of telling the story of our patient encounter has become critical for how patients are approached and references when engaging that patient. With such a practice we are demonstrating our worth and creating additional dialogue for how we can be further utilized. In the world of Covid-19, tele chaplaincy has advanced and thanks to our adaptation we have stretched interdisciplinary customs to include our input. Therefore, I practice using a formulated outline for my notes that inform myself and the team, so that collectively we capture information that is pertinent to everyone including the patient.

As a trauma chaplain, I have learned how to practice neuroplasticity and engage the patient to rewire a function that has not been performed. In other words, often when a trauma patient comes into our trauma bay and returns from a CT after having a full evaluation by our trauma medical team, they have a moment to pause and reflect. Typically, this is the moment I am able to come along the bedside and begin to explore that space. Upon invitation we engage and with good guidance we go as deep as the patient is willing. At times this can go theological and also can expound on a cognitive exercise that is consistent with what outcome they have been meaning to tap into but have yet to do so. In this time I along with the patient's help can guide goals and passions that a patient has articulated through mindfulness. As a patient fights through the pain it becomes healing and redirecting their injury, too intentionally engaging in only principles that get them closer to their goals. Once identified goals are named, I have encouraged patients to begin making alerts on their phones to set reminders that it's time to value and practice and or pursue their goal. This healthy direction is pastoral and demonstrates the strength and presence of a trauma chaplain attentive to the needs of a patient holistically. Secondly, when I have had the chance to work with a patient from an initial meeting and or during a follow up have begun to utilize mobile applications such as the Trauma Resource Institute that improves the skill set of patients to become more resilient and learning to understand what is going on in the body which include tracking, resourcing, grounding, gesturing, and lastly shift and stay. This app has become incorporated in my care and is profound as it is lasting and connects the patient with forms of practicing improving their condition. This community resilience model has met the needs of victims, injured in a vehicle crash and overall those suffering moral injury. It is a great conversation starter that creates moments of further dialogue. When I chart this experience I am finding other disciplines are downloading the iChill [5] app and utilizing it to manage themselves and engage with patients at their level of resiliency.

The Encounter

It was a Saturday night, I was located in the Emergency Room (ER) trauma bay when my pager signaled a level 1 trauma activation for a 17 year old, Gunshot Wound (GSW) to head, estimated time of arrival 5 minutes. As I sat in the ER bay, I observed Nurse technicians, Registered Nurses RN's, medical students, x ray technicians, and respiratory specialists prepare for the incoming trauma. It was spoken by someone "Shouldn't this trauma go to Comer? Since he is a minor." I recall one of the education training RN's articulating that trauma's typically of 16 year olds and older youth come to the adult ER versus Comer, due to policy. The bay is prepared, medical apparel on and charge RN brings into Trauma bay, what detail is known from Ambulance before arrival. The trauma MD arrives to trauma bay through one door and the patient arrives in another. As the medical staff prepare for hand off from ambulatory service they discuss assignments for focus, and begin to evaluate patient. If you've ever observed an assembly line, the ER works much like it. Everyone has a purpose and works toward the main goal in providing the best possible care for patients. I remain as an observer, and listener that documents details such as if the patient is alert and oriented, able to communicate name, reaction to trauma endured, capability of passing assessment questions, and if needed ability to calm patient by holding hands and or reminding them of a supportive presence is with them as they are medically evaluated. It can be overwhelming for many patients as none of them planned on this experience to happen.

At this time we receive a 17 year old African American Male, that has an obvious injury to his head as blood is dripping and is noticeable on the floor. However, the patient is calm, very calm and able to answer all questions asked of him as the assessment is being conducted. As the evaluation continues it is learned this victim, who is a high school student that lives at home with his family and was in the family home sitting on the couch playing video games was impacted, when a gunshot came through the living room window that faces the street. struck the young man in the head. As he felt and heard the shot he did not notice that he was struck not until he saw blood on the floor. It is noticeable that this young man has a lot of hair and the style is known as dreadlocks, for which upon assessment the bullet grazes the skin, then lodges into one of his many dreadlocks. The bullet/fragments were found as an RN looked thoroughly through his scalp and hair and saw the evidence in the victims hairs. The young man was surprised as was the staff. As this assessment was nearing an end everyone was grateful and the patient went for a CT scan and returned for additional X Rays. As the patient is transported to the CT scanner, I engage the patient and gather his name, mothers information to contact, and encourage the young man that he has the best medical support on hand to assist with his injury and affirm what he is feeling. My time with patients is often minimal, but I've learned how to be effective and navigate to provide solid care that benefits all. Upon coming out of the CT scan, I contacted the number that the patient provided and notified the family that the patient is in our care and encouraged them to come to the hospital as soon as possible to be supportive and a presence. As the patient returns to the bay more X-rays have been ordered and I begin to get more time to talk with him and learn that he was at home with other siblings and that his mother was not home at the time of the incident but was made aware. I wondered how? It was communicated to the patient that I made contact with his family and that they were en route and coming to the hospital. He was assured that support was on the way from his family and that he would soon see his mother. During our exchange, I learned where he went to highschool, that he was interested in engineering and programming. Also, I gathered he was aware of shootings that happened on his block. Therefore, it can be noted that he is a victim of his own community that has had multiple gun shootings that have marked his neighborhood and block. As he explained, this is why he does not play outside and focuses on playing video games when in the house to escape and utilize his imagination. However, the impact of he becoming a victim, his imagination I note will be forever changed and identifying a safe space will be a challenge as he was in his own home and shot from someone outside, as the bullet was not meant for him, and is regarded as a student not involved in any gang or gang activity. Additionally, he stated that no one in his family is a part of a gang and that just gangs are simply active in his neighborhood. As we further conversed, he appeared a bit skinny and malnourished and that for a 17 year old young man his hygiene was not up to par, as made evident from his clothes, molded socks and odor. It is not typical that someone living in a home has such challenges and clothes that are kept up with. As I further assess he had only ate once that day and it was not a meal, and I asked if and when he was able to if he would like some food. He said no to food but yes to something to drink. I informed him of what to expect next and that once it was ok'd by medical staff that I would get him something to drink.

Upon completion of eval, I shared my insight with a trauma nurse and she noted that she had the same assessment and began orders to give an iv drip for dehydration. We were quite concerned and wondered if he had any pre-existing medical conditions that we were not aware of. As we awaited family to arrive I noted that this was a question we needed to ask so that the medical staff could be aware of. An hour goes by and family still has not arrived and is a caution for concern, as the home address of the young man is 15 minutes away from the hospital. The results from the CT scan and Xray come back and he is cleared from concern but has a need to have his wound cleaned sutured. One of the medical students begins to wash out his wounds and I sit next to him bedside and converse as he is sutured. This care is to assist and keep the patient calm, lower any anxiety that can come during such a procedure with needles etc. The suturing is completed and he reminds me of the drink that he requested and identifies what we have available but more importantly what he wants so that we can be as hospitable to the patient as possible. He wants a soda and juice. I ask the medical staff if he has been cleared and upon the ok, I get his drinks. The emergency room is very busy and no rooms are available for the patient. As we are still awaiting the patient's mother to arrive, I raise a concern to the emergency room nurse that has been charting on the patient and collaborate if it is appropriate to get child life involved and a social worker on board as the encounter is entering a case that needs further attention. She agreed and soon after I was made aware by security that the mother had arrived, its midnight and the trauma bay is filled with patients from other trauma incidents and mom is not going to be allowed into the bay due to policies in place. I informed the trauma surgeon that mom is present and that we need to meet with her in the consultation room to update and learn of any pre-existing medical information. We meet with mom and an older sister, they updated on the patient's medical status, informed of next steps, observation etc. They want to see the patient and we arrange for the patient to go to a hallway. As we begin to transport patients into the hallway the charge RN informs that an exam room has opened and that he can have visitors. The mom was instructed to wait in the consultation room and she noted that if it took too long she may have to leave to get back home to her other children at home. I asked and was unable to gather an updated phone number for mom during the consultation and learned that the best contact was the older sister. When I came back to the consult room ten minutes later to inform mother and sister that they could visit, I observed they had left. Also I noticed that the police arrived and were looking to speak with mom. I asked security if they were in the waiting room and was told that they had to leave? Upon this detail I called the number that was provided and attempted to learn where they were. I reached the sister and began to learn they had to leave and parked on the street illegally and were concerned about the other children at home? I asked her to remain on the phone so that she could speak to her brother and handed the phone to the patient so that he could make a connection with family. They spoke and minutes later he hung up and expressed to me that they want a call once he is discharged. I explained to him that I will contact them and explained that mom has to return in order to be discharged. He understood and we concluded that he would be with us in the hospital until she returns. I share what happened with trauma RN and escalate this information to Social Worker and page them to get involved asap. Additionally, we inform the trauma MD and we agree that the patient should be admitted and followed by all our services that can assist in the manner.

This incident was reviewed by child life, social work, violence recovery and medical staff as it was concluded that the patient was experiencing abandonment possibly, and in need of additional social resources for mom. Upon moms return she met with each discipline and was provided with resources that could assist with the care of her family and self.

Typically, as a chaplain, my assessment consists of a tool used known in our industry as FICA. This is where one learns the faith or beliefs, interest, importance, influence, community and ways to address in the care of patients. I believe I accomplished this in the matter, and collaborated with other disciplines to assist in the needs of patients and family. I am glad that I continued to pay attention to some of what was not being said by the patient but further engaged and built trust as I learned more about him through his stay in ER. I later was able to order the patient food and he was surprised by the amount of options that he had, to satisfy his hunger. In all I served a young man that was a victim of community violence as he occupied his home and a bullet found him. The bullet led to challenges that his family had been dealing with for some time and I hope that it has provided aid, and direction for their future. I pray that he has a trusted meaning of a chaplain and what good medical assistance can do in an emergent care situation. Lastly, one day I trust, he will pass along the caring presence that was provided to him.

References

1. Harrision N. Un-addiction, 6 mind-changing conversations that could save a life. Union Square & Co. LLC; 2024. p. 116.
2. Swindoll C. Saying it well: touching others with your words; February 02, 2012.
3. The Block Hassenfeld Casdin Collaborative: building childhood and family resilience – a status report prepared for Ellie Block; November 2019.
4. Lipsky LVD. Trauma Stewardship: an everyday guide to caring for self while caring for others. ©2009 Laura Van Dernoot Lipsky (P); 2017.
5. The trauma resiliency model and the community resiliency model via the Trauma Resource Institute; 2015.

Part IV
Protocol Development

Transfusion Support for a New Adult Level 1 Trauma Center: Evolution of a Blood Bank

Mihir Chaudhary, Oloruntoba Bolaji, Fatima A. Aldarweesh, Geoffrey D. Wool, and David A. Hampton

Introduction

Death from hemorrhagic shock is the leading cause of preventable death following traumatic injury. Civilian and military literature support early blood resuscitation in severely injured patients. During the recent Middle East conflicts, injured military personnel who received packed red blood cells (pRBCs) demonstrated increased 24-hour and 30-day survival compared to those who did not receive a transfusion [1]. While pre-hospital pRBC transfusion has not yet shown a mortality benefit in the civilian population there is increasing evidence that pre-hospital plasma administration is associated with a mortality benefit in systems with prolonged transport times [2, 3]. This growing body of evidence suggests that earlier blood product resuscitation in patients with traumatic hemorrhagic shock improves survival.

Prior to the University of Chicago Medicine (UCM) re-opening an adult Level 1 trauma program, the UCM Blood Bank's adult massive transfusion protocol (MTP)

M. Chaudhary (✉) · O. Bolaji · D. A. Hampton
Department of Surgery, Section of Trauma and Acute Care Surgery, University of Chicago Medicine, Chicago, IL, USA
e-mail: Mihir.Chaudhary@uchicagomedicine.org; Oloruntoba.bolaji@uchicagomedicine.org; dhampton2@bsd.uchicago.edu

F. A. Aldarweesh
Department of Pathology, Section of Transfusion, Hemostasis, and Apheresis (THAM), University of Chicago, Chicago, IL, USA
e-mail: faldarweesh@bsd.uchicago.edu

G. D. Wool
Department of Pathology, Section of Transfusion, Hemostasis, and Apheresis Medicine (THAM), Transfusion Medicine Fellowship Program, University of Chicago, Chicago, IL, USA
e-mail: geoffrey.wool@uchicagomedicine.org

S. O. Rogers, Jr (ed.), *Creating a Modern Trauma Center*,
https://doi.org/10.1007/978-3-031-66524-0_17

consisted of 6 pRBC units, 4 plasma, and 1 plateletpheresis product. The MTP was generally transported through the pneumatic tube system, with a significant possibility of wastage due to improper storage if not used prior to expiration or secondary to temperature constraints. While the Level 1 pediatric trauma center had been supported by the blood bank, the establishment of the adult trauma center meant a significantly increased patient volume with a high potential for significant blood product consumption. Increasing the blood product supply was not the solution. A logistical paradigm shift to ensure efficient delivery occurred. There were several approaches and innovations implemented in adapting to the adult trauma patients' needs. This included updating the content of an MTP pack, staffing changes and delivery and utilization protocols.

History of Massive Transfusion

A massive transfusion is defined as a patient requiring ten or more units of pRBCs within a 24-hour period [4]. Emergency physician, Dr. Robert Dailey, described the first MTP for patients presenting in hemorrhagic shock secondary to a traumatic event. His protocol consisted of two phases: (1) rapid large bore femoral vein central line cannulation with the initiation of crystalloid infusion, and (2) blood product transfusion [5]. Since Dailey's time, further clinical evidence supporting balanced blood product resuscitation has emerged [6]. Aggressive, early, and balanced blood product resuscitation of traumatically injured patients in hemorrhagic shock has a demonstrated survival benefit [1–3]. This finding has resulted in nearly every major trauma center developing a MTP [6].

Prior to May 1st 2018, the UCM Trauma Center's opening day, there were approximately 20–50 MTP activations per year. Subsequently, this number increased to over 600 activations annually with over two-thirds received by trauma patients. Additionally, the operating rooms and trauma resuscitation areas accounted for nearly 80% of the MTP activation sites. This demand and shift in location results from the increasing number of trauma activations the UCM receives. In 2023, the UCM trauma center will have received approximately 5000 trauma patients. In 2022, 7001 MTP blood products were transfused. This included 3418 pRBCs (11% of all transfused pRBCs), 3198 plasma (26.5% of all transfused plasma) and 360 platelets (4.1% of all transfused platelets). While UCM obtains the majority of blood products from third-party vendors, our Blood Donation Center (BDC) contributed 4.5% of pRBCs (1399 units), 10.7% of plasma (1293 units) and 2.4% of platelets (214 units) in 2022.

Defining an "MTP pack"

The MTP pack is the standard set of blood products that are delivered. The original UCM trauma center's MTP pack consisted of 6 units of pRBCs, 4 units of thawed plasma and 1 plateletpheresis pack. The current UCM Trauma MTP pack is based on the Pragmatic, Randomized Optimal Platelet and Plasma Ratios (PROPPR) trial. This study found improved hemostasis in patients receiving a 1:1:1 ratio of plasma, platelets and packed red blood cells versus a 1:1:2 ratio [7]. Thus, while a 1.5:1:1 ratio has never been proven inferior, the current MTP pack was modified to 6 units of pRBCs, 6 units of thawed plasma, and 1 plateletpheresis pack. Our pediatric MTP pack, intended for patients less than 40 kg, consists of 3 units of FFP and 3 units of pRBCs. To decrease waste, a partial MTP pack (2 units of pRBCs and 2 units of FFP) is also available in the trauma bay for less severely injured patients.

Blood Bank Staffing

Due to the significantly increased supply of blood products requiring processing, storage, compatibility testing, and dispensing, the blood bank hired additional employees to meet the hospital's heightened transfusion needs. While the training, onboarding, and roles and responsibilities of the blood bank staff is beyond this chapter's scope, those logistical and operational elements were critical to the blood bank's successfully transition.

Delivery Protocols

Prior to receiving adult trauma patients, the hospital's pneumatic tube system was utilized to deliver blood products. Given the potential for lost or damaged shipments and the immediate need for a potential large volume delivery, the UCM blood bank switched to a runner based system. The clinical areas that frequently activated MTPs identified and trained runners to utilize the most efficient routes from their respective clinical units to the blood bank. Once an MTP is activated, the clinical unit's blood runner presents to the blood bank with the patient's information. The blood bank confirms the patient and dispenses the initial MTP pack, which the runner delivers to the patient's nurse. To expedite movement, blood runners are provided special MTP badges to facilitate priority elevator access. The runners return the MTP cooler when the MTP order is deactivated, the cooler has 15 minutes until expiration, or the cooler is empty. The MTP pack's expiration time is written on top of the cooler, allowing for clear communication with the transfusing team. High MTP activating units were involved in training staff and conducting time trials to ensure efficient MTP delivery.

To improve blood product storage following dispensing, the original commercial coolers were transitioned to dedicated multi-compartment blood coolers (MaxPlus MTP coolers, see Fig. 1). The multiple compartment coolers consists of: (1) a "payload" container with plasma and pRBCs, (2) a separate container for cooled gel packs, and (3) an anterior platelet container separated from the "payload" container with blue foam to prevent platelet cooling (se Fig. 1). This cooler design was advantageous in protecting blood products from direct contact with cold packs thus

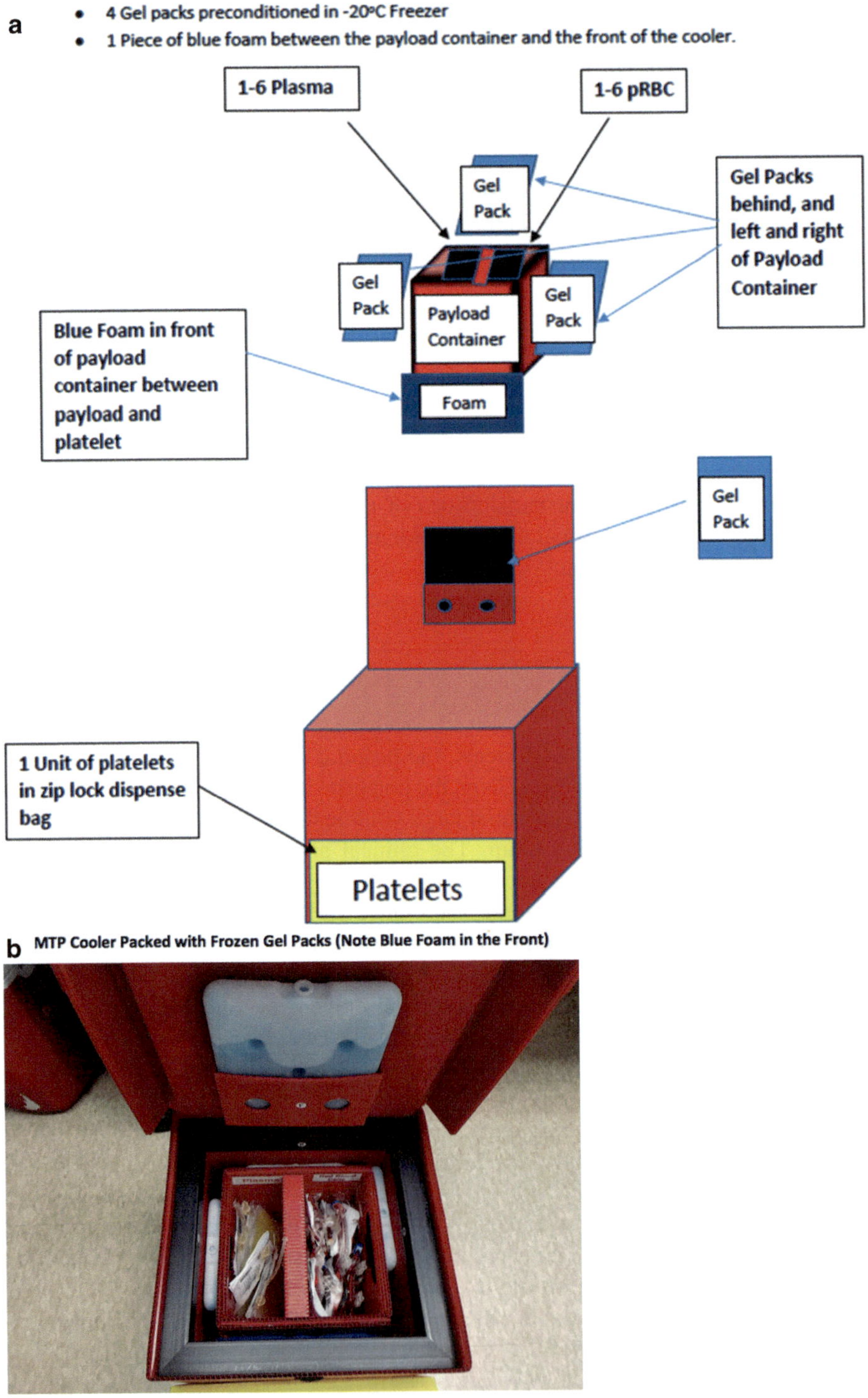

Fig. 1 Schematic (**a**) and picture (**b**) demonstrating the multi-compartment cooler used to transport pRBC, FFP and platelets in MTP packs

decreasing the risk of hemolysis and also allowing for more intuitive storage of blood products in clinical units. A limited supply of MTP packs and emergency release blood products were placed in the ED, trauma bay and main OR—spaces which highly utilize MTPs. During the inaugural year, the runner based system resulted in 94% of initial blood products being delivered within 5 minutes of ordering.

MTP Cooler Validation

The MaxPlus MTP cooler's introduction required a rigorous validation protocol to ensure the cooler was able to maintain the various blood products at the recommended temperature. The validation protocol involved assessing pRBC, plasma and platelet temperature after transfer from the blood bank to the cooler. To validate the MaxPlus MTP cooler the pRBC and plasma compartments must demonstrate rapid cooling within 30 minutes and maintain a temperature between 1 and 6 °C for at least 4 hours at minimum and maximum capacity. Additionally, the platelet compartment must be able to maintain a temperature between 20 and 24 °C for at least 4 hours. Electronic data loggers contained in the MaxPlus MTP coolers were used to assess the temperature in the coolers after loading and with minimum and maximum loads. The MaxPlus MTP coolers successfully passed the validation process. Switching to this cooler design has allowed for longer storage times in clinical units and may have contributed to minimizing blood product wastage.

Blood Product Utilization Protocols

MTP packs and emergency release blood products are locally stored in locked refrigerators in the trauma bay and OR and can be immediately used once an MTP is activated. Following exhaustion of these supplies, additional MTP packs come from the UCM blood bank. An MTP pack consists of:

- O-positive pRBCs and group A plasma for patients 55 years or older
- O-negative pRBCs and group A plasma for females ≤55 years old
- O-negative pRBCs and group AB plasma for pediatric patients ≤40 kg

Platelets and cryoprecipitate are issued without regard to ABO type. Group A plasma has been shown to be safe for emergency use in hemorrhaging patients [8]. Once the patient's type and screen and ABO verification are complete, the standard MTP can be transitioned to type-specific blood products.

Once delivered, a rapid transfusing system administers the blood products based on the clinical context and intravenous access. After each MTP pack is exhausted, labs, including a complete blood count, coagulation labs, and chemistry, are obtained. Once the clinical team activates an MTP, they maintain a high level of communication with the blood bank regarding their patient's additional needs. Upon MTP deactivation, any unused blood product is promptly returned to the blood bank in the validated MTP cooler. This current system has resulted in less than a 1% blood product wastage rate, which exceeds national quality standards.

Utilizing Whole Blood Resuscitation

Military literature continues to support the use of whole blood [4, 5]. This literature has since been reproduced in the civilian population [6]. In the military settings, Spinella's group retrospectively found combat casualties from Afghanistan and Iraq who received warm fresh whole blood had an improved 30-day survival compared to those receiving standard component therapy [9]. Similarly, Nessen's group found the same in Afghanistan combat casualties [10]. Likewise, in the civilian setting, Brill et al., in a prospective observational cohort study of 1377 trauma patients found that patients receiving whole blood had improved survival and decreased overall blood utilization [11].

Given the emerging safety data and potential mortality benefit, whole blood was incorporated into our trauma resuscitation protocols. Starting in August 2020, 6 units of low-titer group (anti-A titer less than 1:200) O-positive whole blood were stocked in the trauma center for use in patients 55 years and older. These units have lower levels of anti-A antibodies making them safer for universal transfusion even to group A and AB individuals [12]. It is the UCM trauma center's policy to utilize whole blood without leukoreduction or that have been leukoreduced using platelet-sparing filters to maintain platelet counts and function. Generally whole blood without leukoreduction has a higher chance of maintaining platelet count and function [13].

Whole blood has a 21-day shelf life from the point of collection. Whole blood products are obtained from the American Red Cross (leukoreduced with platelet-sparing filter). The UCM Blood Bank processes low-titer group O whole blood approaching expiry into components and collects the red blood cells for longer-term use. At any given time, there are 6 units of whole blood available in the trauma bay refrigerator and an additional 6 units of whole blood in the blood bank. Indeed recent evidence suggests that including whole blood in MTPs improves survival. Torres et al. demonstrated in a cohort of 2785 trauma patients from US and Canadian adult civilian trauma centers that those who received whole blood as an adjunct to MTP had lower 24-hour and 30-day mortality [14]. This survival benefit was found as early as 5 hours after emergency department arrival. Additionally, the UCM trauma center helicopter critical care transport service, University of Chicago Medicine Aeromedical Network (UCAN), carries low-titer O whole blood, pRBCs and plasma. Aerially transported adult patients greater than 40 kilograms in weight who require blood transfusion preferentially get whole blood initially while those less than 40 kilograms receive component pRBCs and thawed plasma. Women of childbearing age preferentially receive Rh-negative blood product.

Future Directions

To efficiently and effectively resuscitate trauma patients, our blood bank routinely evaluates its staffing and evidence-based transfusion protocols. However, there remain areas of ongoing improvement. This includes the role of thromboelastography (TEG) testing. This test assesses the kinetics and viscoelastic properties of a patient's whole blood providing a hemostasis profile. The information allows for real-time adjustment of blood product transfusions to meet the needs of specific patients. While TEG has a clear diagnostic and prognostic role in trauma-induced coagulopathy, further studies to define its ability to improve patient outcomes remain ongoing [14]. Other areas of improvement include determining the role of tranexamic acid (TXA) in our MTP, protocols for calcium repletion, automated coagulation parameter laboratory orders, and possible expansion of the role of our hospital-based blood donation center in maintaining blood product supply. Building upon the various discussed organizational and technical innovations, our blood bank and trauma center continually seek to decrease time to transfusion for our trauma patients ensuring the highest potential for survival.

References

1. Shackelford SA, Del Junco DJ, Powell-Dunford N, Mazuchowski EL, Howard JT, Kotwal RS, Gurney J, Butler FK Jr, Gross K, Stockinger ZT. Association of prehospital blood product transfusion during medical evacuation of combat casualties in Afghanistan with acute and 30-day survival. JAMA. 2017;318(16):1581–91. https://doi.org/10.1001/jama.2017.15097. PMID: 29067429; PMCID: PMC5818807.
2. Crombie N, Doughty HA, JRB B, Desai A, Dixon EF, Hancox JM, Herbert MJ, Leech C, Lewis SJ, Nash MR, Naumann DN, Slinn G, Smith H, Smith IM, Wale RK, Wilson A, Ives N, Perkins GD, RePHILL Collaborative Group. Resuscitation with blood products in patients with trauma-related haemorrhagic shock receiving prehospital care (RePHILL): a multicentre, open-label, randomised, controlled, phase 3 trial. Lancet Haematol. 2022;9(4):e250–61. https://doi.org/10.1016/S2352-3026(22)00040-0. Epub 2022 Mar 7. PMID: 35271808; PMCID: PMC8960285.
3. Sperry JL, Guyette FX, Brown JB, Yazer MH, Triulzi DJ, Early-Young BJ, Adams PW, Daley BJ, Miller RS, Harbrecht BG, Claridge JA, Phelan HA, Witham WR, Putnam AT, Duane TM, Alarcon LH, Callaway CW, Zuckerbraun BS, Neal MD, Rosengart MR, Forsythe RM, Billiar TR, Yealy DM, Peitzman AB, Zenati MS, PAMPer Study Group. Prehospital plasma during air medical transport in trauma patients at risk for hemorrhagic shock. N Engl J Med. 2018;379(4):315–26. https://doi.org/10.1056/NEJMoa1802345. PMID: 30044935.
4. Dailey RH. "Code Red" protocol for resuscitation of the exsanguinated patient. J Emerg Med. 1985;2(5):373–8. https://doi.org/10.1016/0736-4679(85)90293-8. PMID: 4086774.
5. Moore SA, Raval JS. Massive transfusion: a review. Ann Blood. 2022;7. https://doi.org/10.21037/aob-22-3.
6. Holcomb JB, Tilley BC, Baraniuk S, Fox EE, Wade CE, Podbielski JM, del Junco DJ, Brasel KJ, Bulger EM, Callcut RA, Cohen MJ, Cotton BA, Fabian TC, Inaba K, Kerby JD, Muskat P, O'Keeffe T, Rizoli S, Robinson BR, Scalea TM, Schreiber MA, Stein DM, Weinberg JA, Callum JL, Hess JR, Matijevic N, Miller CN, Pittet JF, Hoyt DB, Pearson GD, Leroux B, van Belle G; PROPPR Study Group. Transfusion of plasma, platelets, and red blood cells in a 1:1:1

vs a 1:1:2 ratio and mortality in patients with severe trauma: the PROPPR randomized clinical trial. JAMA. 2015;313(5):471–82. https://doi.org/10.1001/jama.2015.12. PMID: 25647203; PMCID: PMC4374744.
7. de Roulet A, Kerby JD, Weinberg JA, Lewis RH Jr, Hudgins JP, Shulman IA, Fox EE, Holcomb JB, Brasel KJ, Bulger EM, Cohen MJ, Cotton BA, Fabian TC, O'Keeffe T, Rizoli S, Scalea TM, Schreiber MA, Inaba K; PROPPR Study Group. Group A emergency-release plasma in trauma patients requiring massive transfusion. J Trauma Acute Care Surg. 2020;89(6):1061–7. https://doi.org/10.1097/TA.0000000000002903. PMID: 32890339; PMCID: PMC7830815.
8. Spinella PC, Perkins JG, Grathwohl KW, Beekley AC, Holcomb JB. Warm fresh whole blood is independently associated with improved survival for patients with combat-related traumatic injuries. J Trauma. 2009;66:S69–76.
9. Nessen SC, Eastridge BJ, Cronk D, et al. Fresh whole blood use by forward surgical teams in Afghanistan is associated with improved survival compared to component therapy without platelets. Transfusion. 2013;53:S107–13.
10. Brill J, Tang B, Hatton G, Mueck K, McCoy C, Kao L, Cotton B. Impact of incorporating whole blood into Hemorrhagic shock resuscitation: analysis of 1,377 consecutive trauma patients receiving emergency-release uncrossmatched blood products. J Am Coll Surg. 2022;234(4):408–18. https://doi.org/10.1097/XCS.0000000000000086.
11. Spinella PC, Pidcoke HF, Strandenes G, et al. Whole blood for hemostatic resuscitation of major bleeding. Transfusion. 2016;56(suppl 2):S190–202.
12. Morris MC, Veile R, Friend LA, Oh D, Pritts TA, Dorlac WC, Spinella PC, Goodman MD. Effects of whole blood leukoreduction on platelet function and hemostatic parameters. Transfus Med. 2019;29(5):351–7. https://doi.org/10.1111/tme.12622. Epub 2019 Aug 5. PMID: 31382318; PMCID: PMC6863083.
13. Torres CM, Kent A, Scantling D, Joseph B, Haut ER, Sakran JV. Association of whole blood with survival among patients presenting with severe hemorrhage in US and Canadian Adult Civilian Trauma Centers. JAMA Surg. 2023;158(5):532–40. https://doi.org/10.1001/jamasurg.2022.6978. Erratum in: JAMA Surg. 2023 Apr 5: PMID: 36652255; PMCID: PMC9857728.
14. Da Luz LT, Nascimento B, Shankarakutty AK, Rizoli S, Adhikari NK. Effect of thromboelastography (TEG®) and rotational thromboelastometry (ROTEM®) on diagnosis of coagulopathy, transfusion guidance and mortality in trauma: descriptive systematic review. Crit Care. 2014;18(5):518. https://doi.org/10.1186/s13054-014-0518-9. PMID: 25261079; PMCID: PMC4206701.

Mass Casualty Events: Preparedness and Response for Trauma Centers and Institutions

Jackquelin Loera and Priya S. Prakash

Introduction

In recent years, the landscape of public safety has been marred by a concerning increase in mass casualty incidents (MCI), both on a large scale and, notably, on a smaller scale known as mini-mass casualty events [1]. Many current-day MCIs are intentional acts of violence, such as mass shootings, improvised explosions, driving vehicles into crowds of people, and other similar assault tactics [1]. The staggering statistic that there have been more mass shootings than days in the year 2023 [2] speaks to the national crisis our country currently faces, while still not capturing the lived reality of many urban communities who live with "mass causality events" that are not captured and reported on by the media [3].

The Gun Violence Archive has defined mass shootings as an incident in which four or more victims are shot or killed, not including any shooter who may also have been killed or injured in the incident [2]. This type of incident is all too common in many urban Level 1 trauma centers and a level of daily preparedness is to support a system of care for these patients. But mini-mass casualty events are of course not limited to shootings and can range anywhere from farming accidents to workplace disasters to multi-vehicle accidents [4]. In addition, a cluster of victims from various events can also present within a short period, also placing a strain on system resources, similar to mass casualty events [5]. This chapter seeks to explore the distinct challenges posed by smaller-scale mass casualty events, with a specific focus on mass shootings, and elucidate the critical preparedness measures that trauma centers and institutions must undertake to effectively respond to these evolving threats.

J. Loera · P. S. Prakash (✉)
University of Chicago Department of Surgery, Chicago, IL, USA
e-mail: jackquelin.loera@uchicagomedicine.org; pprakash@bsd.uchicago.edu

S. O. Rogers, Jr (ed.), *Creating a Modern Trauma Center*,
https://doi.org/10.1007/978-3-031-66524-0_18

Understanding Mass Casualty Events and Mini Mass Casualty Events

Mass casualty events encompass incidents where the number of victims overwhelms the resources and capabilities of the local response system [1, 4]. Traditionally associated with large-scale disasters or acts of terrorism, mass casualty events have taken on a new dimension with the emergence of mini-mass casualty events. These smaller-scale incidents, though involving fewer casualties, place a strain on a single institution's resources and capabilities and present unique challenges due to their often unpredictable nature and rapid onset. Examples of such incidences may be a multi-vehicle collision, a house fire with multiple victims, a workplace accident, a house-party shooting, or a clustered arrival of firearm-injured patients [5]. Institutions with Level 1 trauma centers must be resourced and prepared to deal with multiple mini-mass casualty events on a day-to-day basis, with many incidences often presenting within a short time frame of one another, placing real-time stress on institutional resources and capabilities.

Defining Mass Shootings

Within the spectrum of mini-mass casualty events, mass shootings represent a particularly alarming subset. Mass shootings are defined as events in which four or more people are shot and wounded or killed [6]. Mass shootings are not just limited to the high-profile public events reported on by the media but also encompass clustered arrival of firearm-injured patients [5]. These incidents can involve targeted acts of violence resulting in a limited number of casualties, yet their impact can be disproportionately devastating. Often victims arrive over a short period, depending on the circumstances and location of the incident. Thus trauma centers should be prepared to receive and care for these patients rapidly and efficiently and with experience.

Preparedness Measures for Trauma Centers and Institutions

Trauma centers and institutions play a pivotal role in the treatment, management, and aftermath of mass shootings, mass casualty events, and clustered events. A trauma center must be prepared to respond to multiple patients rapidly presenting over a short duration of time and often with limited pre-notification. Below are listed some of the key elements of trauma center preparedness, including personnel training, resource allocation, and communication strategies [7, 8].

1. **Training and Simulation:** Developing and regularly conducting realistic drills and simulations to ensure that staff is well-prepared to handle the unique challenges posed by mini-mass shootings or events.
2. **Resource Allocation:** Allocating resources strategically to meet the immediate and long-term needs of victims, including medical supplies, personnel, and mental health support.
3. **Interagency Collaboration:** Establishing strong collaborations with law enforcement, emergency medical services, and local authorities to streamline communication and coordination during crises.
4. **Community Engagement:** Working closely with the community to foster awareness, communication, and a collective commitment to preventing and responding to mini-mass shootings and mass casualty events.
5. **Mental Health Support:** Recognizing the psychological toll on both victims and healthcare providers, and implementing comprehensive mental health support systems to facilitate healing and resilience.

Medical Surge Planning

MCIs challenge a community's ability to care for patients and have the potential to exhaust available local resources. We must acknowledge that training and equipment between different medical systems can vary considerably. Tertiary hospitals may be better prepared to care for large numbers of patients as they routinely see high patient volume; a disaster that stresses the staffing and resources of one medical facility may feel like a "busy day" for another.

Regardless of the setting, hospital management of a sudden surge of patients presents a logistically difficult yet imperative responsibility to rapidly process, treat, and determine the disposition of several casualties. Each hospital should have a comprehensive mass casualty management plan [7, 8] (i.e. medical surge plan) to ensure an existing level of preparedness before catastrophe strikes. Plans should detail a chain of communication, key personnel, community partnerships available for additional support, traditional and non-traditional treatment areas such as hallways or treatment tents, decontamination, and a triaging system with anticipated staffing and supply needs based on patient acuity and the MCI scenario [8]. For example, a response to anthrax poisoning will require supplies and protective gear that differ from that of a mass shooting.

Leadership

Personnel should understand their roles and responsibilities during an MCI well before one occurs [8]. Key leadership includes the medical director, administrative director, head nurse, and EMS coordinator. Though the specific roles and responsibilities of each leadership individual may vary from institution to institution, there should be clearly defined roles and responsibilities for each individual. For example, the medical director is often an experienced trauma surgeon or general surgeon with trauma experience. They establish teams, assign clinical roles and responsibilities, triage patients, prioritize surgeries, and determine admissions to ICUs and wards. The administrative director is often the director of the Emergency Department. They manage logistics and use of imaging, ensure blood bank availability and relay information to hospital administration. The head nurse manages transfers out of the ER, directs floor nurses recruited to help while additional nursing support arrives, collects information regarding patient status and disposition, and determines the ER's need for special equipment or resources. The EMS coordinator updates hospital leadership on the type of MCI, location, expected casualty number, and severity of injuries. Overall, key leadership personnel should know their role and responsibilities well before an MCI occurs and be ready and prepared to step into those roles when called upon.

Training and Simulation

Periodic drills enhance a team's ability to respond to challenges encountered during a disaster and are pivotal to disaster preparedness [9, 10]. Given the structure of hospital systems and postgraduate training programs, residents are an essential component of the frontline response in an MCI [4]. In disasters such as Hurricane Katrina, the Orlando nightclub shooting, and the Boston Marathon bombing, emergency medicine and general surgery residents were responsible for treating several injured patients [11]. Inherent to general surgery training, trauma exposure aids the development of key skills such as patient triage, rapid assessment, and trauma team organization. In preparation for MCI, it is recommended that residents receive dedicated training for disaster management [12]. While several emergency medicine residency programs include MCI training, most general surgery residency programs have not implemented dedicated MCI training into their GME curriculum [11]. This is an area for improvement in MCI preparedness that should be considered in general surgery training.

Scripting and routine rehearsing of various trauma scenarios with varying degrees of stress on the existing system is important in training and preparing personnel for how to respond and manage an MCI if and when it occurs. Regular and repetitive training and simulation exercises help enhance the preparedness of emergency response teams and healthcare professionals [13]. Practice scenarios enable better coordination among different agencies involved in responding to mass casualty events. Training enhances decision-making skills in high-stress situations, allowing professionals to make critical choices efficiently. Simulations provide an opportunity to test and refine resource management strategies, ensuring that medical resources are used effectively during a crisis [14]. Training allows different stakeholders, including medical personnel, law enforcement, and emergency services, to practice working together seamlessly. Simulation exercises allow teams to adapt and refine response strategies based on lessons learned, ensuring continuous improvement [14].

The importance of training and simulation cannot be overstated. Preparedness, coordination, and effective resource management are critical elements in mitigating the impact of such incidents on both a local and systemic level.

Resource Allocation

Mass casualty events can strain local healthcare systems and trauma centers, leading to a sudden influx of patients. Limited resources, such as hospital beds and medical staff, may be overwhelmed. Trauma centers may face challenges in coordinating with emergency services and managing the surge of patients efficiently. Existing protocols need to be adapted to handle unexpected scenarios. Mass casualty events can prompt a reassessment of resource allocation strategies. Institutions must ensure that protocols are in place to allocate resources during MCIs, ensuring that emergency medical resources are distributed effectively.

Interagency Collaboration and Partnership

Hospitals should establish working relationships with public and private community health and medical partners. Examples include non-profit groups, other hospitals, primary care providers, and support services such as laboratories, pharmacies, and blood banks. Partnerships exist to provide additional support when patient volume and needs exceed the capacity of a single hospital.

Mass casualty events and mass shootings require a coordinated response from various institutions, including law enforcement, emergency medical services, and public health agencies [8]. The importance of cross-disciplinary collaboration is important in establishing effective communication channels and response protocols [8]. By fostering strong partnerships between trauma centers and relevant institutions, the overall community resilience can be strengthened.

Community Engagement and Education

Preventing MCIs and mass shootings involves not only addressing immediate threats but also implementing proactive measures within the community. Empowering individuals to recognize warning signs and participate in prevention efforts can contribute to a more resilient and prepared society. Exploring the contributing factors behind mass shootings is crucial for developing targeted intervention and prevention strategies. Multifaceted elements influencing these events, including mental health considerations, social determinants of health, and access to firearms should be examined and addressed at a public policy level. By examining the intersection of these factors, trauma centers, and institutions can better anticipate the challenges posed by mass shootings and tailor their preparedness plans accordingly with an overall mission to eliminate such events.

Mental Health Support

The importance of mental health support for individuals affected by mass casualty events, including shootings, cannot be overstated. Such incidents can have profound and lasting psychological impacts on survivors, witnesses, first responders, and the broader community [15, 16]. Mass casualty events, especially violent ones like shootings, can result in acute trauma and post-traumatic stress disorder (PTSD) [16, 17] for those directly involved or even those who witnessed the incident. Prompt mental health support is essential to help individuals process their experiences and cope with the psychological aftermath.

Mental health professionals play a critical role in providing support and counseling to help individuals navigate the complex emotions associated with these experiences [15, 17]. Mass casualty events can create a collective sense of fear, anxiety, and grief within the community. Mental health services contribute to community healing by providing resources and support to those affected on a broader scale. Timely mental health intervention can help prevent the development of long-term mental health issues, including chronic anxiety, depression, and substance abuse disorders. Mental health support helps reduce the stigma associated with seeking help for psychological distress. Encouraging open dialogue about mental health can contribute to a more supportive community environment.

Emergency responders and healthcare professionals who witness and respond to mass casualty events may also experience significant mental health challenges. Providing mental health resources and support is crucial for the well-being of these individuals who play a critical role in the immediate aftermath of such events. Mental health services contribute to the overall recovery and resilience of individuals and communities. Establishing a comprehensive mental health support system ensures continuity of care, addressing both immediate needs and long-term recovery. Follow-up support is crucial for monitoring and addressing evolving mental health needs.

Mental health support is a critical component of the overall response to mass casualty events and shootings. It plays a pivotal role in promoting healing, resilience, and recovery for individuals and communities impacted by these traumatic incidents. Early and ongoing intervention is essential to address the multifaceted mental health challenges that may arise.

Conclusion

Mass casualty events, mass shootings, and clustered events present a complex and evolving challenge, demanding a proactive and multifaceted response from trauma centers and institutions. By leveraging data, understanding contributing factors, and enhancing preparedness measures, healthcare providers and community leaders can work collaboratively to mitigate the impact of MCIs and the impact of mass shootings and clustered shootings in our communities. In summary, preparedness is a comprehensive and proactive approach that saves lives and enhances communities' overall resilience in the face of mass casualty events. It involves strategic planning, training, coordination, and ongoing assessment to ensure an effective response to the diverse challenges posed by such incidents.

References

1. Hodgson L. How violent attacks are changing the demands of mass casualty incidents: a review of the challenges associated with intentional mass casualty incidents. Homeland Security Affairs. 2021;17
2. Gun Violence Archive. Mass Shootings. https://www.gunviolencearchive.org; 2024.
3. Kaufman EJ, et al. Making the news: victim characteristics associated with media reporting on firearm injury. Prev Med. 2020;141:106275.
4. Lomaglio L, et al. Mass casualty incident: definitions and current reality. In: WSES handbook of mass casualties incidents management; 2020. p. 1–10.
5. Beard JH, et al. Clustered arrivals of firearm-injured patients in an urban trauma system: a silent epidemic. J Am Coll Surg. 2019;229(3):236–43.
6. General Methodology—Gun Violence Archive. www.gunviolencearchive.org
7. American College of Surgeons, Committee on Trauma. Resources for Optimal Care of the Injured Patient 2022 Standard. https://www.facs.org/quality-programs/trauma/quality/verification-review-and-consultation-program/standards/. Chicago: American College of Surgeons; 2022.
8. Borgohain B, Khonglah T. Developing and organizing a trauma system and mass casualty management: some useful observations from the Israeli trauma model. Ann Med Health Sci Res. 2013;3(1):85–9.
9. Sarin RR, et al. Disaster education: a survey study to analyze disaster medicine training in emergency medicine residency programs in the United States. Prehosp Disaster Med. 2017;32(4):368–73.
10. Albert E, Bullard T. Training, drills pivotal in mounting response to Orlando shooting. ED Manage: Monthly Update Emerg Depart Manage. 2016;28(8):85–9.
11. Joshi A, et al. Incorporating mass casualty incidents training in surgical education program. Global Surg Educ-J Assocr Surg Educ. 2022;1(1):17.
12. Uddin SG, et al. Emergency preparedness: addressing a residency training gap. Acad Med. 2008;83(3):298–304.
13. Klima DA, et al. Full-scale regional exercises: closing the gaps in disaster preparedness. J Trauma Acute Care Surg. 2012;73(3):592–8.
14. Biddinger PD, et al. On linkages using exercises to identify systems-level preparedness challenges. Public Health Rep. 2008;123(1):96–101.

15. Gabbe BJ, et al. Review of the requirements for effective mass casualty preparedness for trauma systems. A disaster waiting to happen? Br J Anaesth. 2022;128(2):e158–67.
16. Lowe SR, Galea S. The mental health consequences of mass shootings. Trauma Violence Abuse. 2017;18(1):62–82.
17. Roudini J, Khankeh HR, Witruk E. Disaster mental health preparedness in the community: a systematic review study. Health Psychol Open. 2017;4(1):2055102917711307.

Navigating Roadblocks: Challenges of Opening a New Surgical Intensive Care Unit

Mary Noory, Samuel Osei, Michael O'Connor, Gary An, David A. Hampton, and Susan Rowell

Introduction

Renovating an existing Surgical Intensive Care Unit (ICU) to support a new trauma center is a complex endeavor that involves numerous challenges and considerations. In this chapter, we will explore the various obstacles that we overcame including: (1) assessing publicly available data to determine the volume of anticipated patients, (2) estimating the number of operative cases that would be additional to our routine scheduled procedures, (3) preparing the Emergency Department (ED) and its staff, (4) establishing protocols to ensure timely transitions between the ED, the operating room (OR), the ICU, and the floor, (5) developing relationships with outside facilities, and (6) ensuring patient safety.

M. Noory (✉) · S. Osei · D. A. Hampton · S. Rowell
Department of Surgery, Section of Trauma and Acute Care Surgery, University of Chicago Medicine, Chicago, IL, USA
e-mail: dhampton2@bsd.uchicago.edu; susanrowell@bsd.uchicago.edu

M. O'Connor
Department of Anesthesia, University of Chicago Medicine, Chicago, IL, USA
e-mail: moc5@bsd.uchicago.edu

G. An
Department of Surgery, University of Vermont Medical Center, Burlington, VT, USA

S. O. Rogers, Jr (ed.), *Creating a Modern Trauma Center*,
https://doi.org/10.1007/978-3-031-66524-0_19

Assessing the Volume of Anticipated Patients

Accurately assessing the anticipated patient volume allows for appropriate resource allocation, staffing, and infrastructure planning [1]. To achieve this, we conducted a comprehensive analysis of historical data from citywide and National trauma registry databases, to gain insights into the patterns and trends of traumatic injuries in the region. Chicago trauma is localized by neighborhood. Proximity to a Level-1 trauma center and transit time can potentially equate to a loss of life [2]. Therefore, we collaborated with local Emergency Medical Services (EMS) providers to estimate the frequency and severity of trauma cases in our surrounding area. Recognizing EMS patterns helped develop the models assessing the likelihood a patient will present at our facility. These data sets previously demonstrated that Chicago's South Side is a trauma desert [2]. The establishment of a Level 1 Trauma Center would decrease transit times by 15 minutes.

Our anticipated annual trauma patient volumes were based upon publicly available information. We utilized data from Mt. Sinai Hospital—a large trauma center on Chicago's West side -, the Chicago Police Department's (PD) publicly available information, and data from local crime watch organizations [3]. The local organization data was derived from news sources, the Chicago PD, and the Cook County medical examiner office. These estimates were utilized to understand injury patterns and the subsequent surgical demands for subspecialty support such as: neurosurgery, orthopedics, plastic surgery, or critical care services. The derived patient volume numbers underestimated the actual numbers upon opening. They did not account for the number of outside hospital transfers. Given its proximity, these trauma transfers were primarily from Northwest Indiana. These "feeder" or "referral hospitals" were incorporated into our future estimations.

Preparing for Mechanism of Injury- Blunt Vs. Penetrating Trauma

Our understanding of the regional trauma patterns and mechanisms of injury helped tailor hospital resources and expertise. Naturally, regions with higher rates of penetrating trauma may necessitate different needs compared to those with a higher incidence of blunt trauma [5]. For instance, increased amounts of penetrating and operative trauma will require greater access to operating rooms and a higher demand for blood products. As such, our blood banks preemptively increased the blood product supply and re-evaluated the delivery methods. Also, blood products were prepositioned in the trauma bays for immediate use. Finally, our OR developed a staffing schedule to ensure a high level of redundancy in the event multiple operative trauma cases were activated.

Estimating Operative Volume and Postoperative Disposition

Accurately estimating our trauma patient volume for an expanding SICU enabled us to plan resource utilization and staffing allocations in other clinical areas such as the Emergency Department (ED) and OR [1]. We created predictive models, utilizing national databases such as Trauma Quality Improvement Program (TQIP) and National Surgical Quality Improvement Program (NSQIP) to estimate a patient's likelihood of requiring care in the surgical ICU, PACU, or general floors. Additionally, we calculated the estimated trauma volume, accounting for the injury severity and mechanism (blunt vs penetrating) of traumas. This was then used to project an estimated ED bed utilization, OR capacity, and subsequent SICU census. Our pre-assessment evaluation anticipated the need to develop six trauma bays with the capacity to expand to eight. In addition, we anticipated the need to utilize six trauma ORs simultaneously. These data were then applied to our anticipated personnel logistics accounting for the in-house and on-call OR staff, surgical subspecialty availability, and ICU staffing. We also projected the hospital discharge needs for a Skilled Nursing Facilities (SNF), Long-Term Acute Care (LTAC) centers, and rehabilitation facilities. Overall, optimal outcomes were achievable through collaborative care planning, effective communication, and clear protocols for patient transfers within the hospital itself, and the development of appropriate staffing models.

Staffing- Over or Under Staffing Issues

Determining the optimal staffing levels for a new trauma center and surgical ICU constitutes a critical consideration. Inadequate staffing compromises patient safety and quality of care, while excessive staffing can lead to unnecessary costs [4]. We applied the data sources previously mentioned to determine anticipated volume to estimate high and low seasons and staff accordingly during designated "trauma seasons" [1]. Again, our specific needs were unique and required adjustments in various departments specifically to facilitate our higher level of penetrating operative trauma and its translation into ICU staffing, OR staff, nursing, technician, and physician needs, as well as back up coverage.

Moreover, professional organizations like the American Association of Critical-Care Nurses (AACN) have developed evidence-based guidelines that can serve as a foundation for determining nurse-to-patient ratios and optimizing staffing levels. Overall, determining peak trauma seasons, estimating the volume of operative trauma, and translating these numbers to clinical needs is critical in the pre-planning of staffing with the goal of preventing over or under staffing.

Ensuring Patient Safety

Our Violence Recovery Program (VRP) consists of social workers, chaplains, and specialists who interface with our patients and their families. They have training to identify environmental factors which could result in recidivism. Their ultimate goal is to disrupt the cycle of violence which brought the patient to our facility. Aside from the continued local social support, our VRP will assist with relocation services, educational or occupational opportunities, and social support.

Conclusion

Re-inventing our SICU resulted in challenges related to assessing patient volume, estimating admitting and operative volume, developing external relationships, and increasing preventative services. Healthcare institutions can establish successful trauma centers with associated ICUs that provide high-quality care to their communities by utilizing evidence-based practices, collaborating with multidisciplinary teams, and proactively addressing these challenges by preparing themselves to the best of their ability.

References

1. Stonko DP, Dennis BM, Callcut RA, Betzold RD, Smith MC, Medvecz AJ, Guillamondegui OD. Identifying temporal patterns in trauma admissions: informing resource allocation. PLoS One. 2018;13(12):e0207766. https://doi.org/10.1371/journal.pone.0207766. PMID: 30507930; PMCID: PMC6277067.
2. Crandall M, Sharp D, Unger E, Straus D, Brasel K, Hsia R, Esposito T. Trauma deserts: distance from a trauma center, transport times, and mortality from gunshot wounds in Chicago. Am J Public Health. 2013;103(6):1103–9. https://doi.org/10.2105/AJPH.2013.301223. Epub 2013 Apr 18. PMID: 23597339; PMCID: PMC3698742.
3. Chicago Crime 2022 Archives – Criminal Infographics – Heyjackass!, heyjackass.com/category/chicago-crime-2022/
4. Mihalj M, Corona A, Andereggen L, Urman RD, Luedi MM, Bello C. Managing bottlenecks in the perioperative setting: optimizing patient care and reducing costs. Best Pract Res Clin Anaesthesiol. 2022;36(2):299–310. https://doi.org/10.1016/j.bpa.2022.05.005. Epub 2022 Jun 3. PMID: 36116911.
5. Fitch CDR, Jamie L, et al. Blunt versus penetrating trauma: is there a resource intensity discrepancy? Am J Surg. 2019;218(6):1201–5. https://doi.org/10.1016/j.amjsurg.2019.08.018. Elsevier BV.

Examining the Hospital as a Complex Dynamical System: Using Agent-Based Modeling to Gain Insight into Potential Process Bottlenecks

Samuel Osei, Mary Noory, Michael O'Connor, Gary An, David A. Hampton, and Susan Rowell

Introduction

Over the past three decades, Traumatic injury has become the leading cause of death in the United States among patients younger than 45 years [1]. The type of trauma varies based on the geographical area; penetrating trauma is disproportionately high among the urban areas [2]. A multitude of research have demonstrated that designated state, regional or national designated trauma centers improve survival in trauma related injuries [3]. Timely transport of injured patients to a designated trauma centers is crucial in providing optimal care to trauma patients [3]. Appropriate prehospital care and prehospital triage of trauma patients plays significant role in patient survival. Longer prehospital transport times can contribute to higher mortality rates among severely injured trauma patients [1, 4, 5]. The city of Chicago is one of the metropolitan areas that have been devastated with gun violence in recent years. Unfortunately, not all neighborhoods in the greater Chicago area have equal access to trauma centers. As in most socioeconomically disadvantaged communities, Chicago's south side has one of the highest homicide rates. The city of Chicago prior to University of Chicago medical center becoming a level 1 trauma center, there were seven Illinois verified level 1 adult trauma center and four level 1

S. Osei (✉) · M. Noory · D. A. Hampton · S. Rowell
Department of Surgery, Section of Trauma and Acute Care Surgery, University of Chicago Medicine, Chicago, IL, USA
e-mail: dhampton2@bsd.uchicago.edu; susanrowell@bsd.uchicago.edu

M. O'Connor
Department of Anesthesia, University of Chicago Medicine, Chicago, IL, USA
e-mail: moc5@bsd.uchicago.edu

G. An
Department of Surgery, University of Vermont Medical Center, Burlington, VT, USA

S. O. Rogers, Jr (ed.), *Creating a Modern Trauma Center*,
https://doi.org/10.1007/978-3-031-66524-0_20

pediatric trauma centers. Though with the highest concentration of penetrating trauma, the southside of Chicago did not have any centrally located Level 1 trauma center [3]. These left victims of gun violence and other penetrating trauma in the south side of Chicago a considerably greater travel distance to a level 1 trauma center.

A study done by Marie Crandall et al. 2013 investigated the correlation between the distance from a trauma center, transport times and mortality in victims of gun violence in Chicago. They concluded that victims of gun violence in the south side of Chicago were on average 5 miles away from a nearby level 1 trauma center, this led to a longer prehospital time and increased mortality in this patient population [1]. With the increase in gun violence in the south side of Chicago and virtually no trauma center to serve this population, the university of Chicago medical center on the southside of Chicago became the latest level 1 trauma center to meet the needs of the community and fill the void of trauma desert.

Before becoming a level one trauma center, the university of Chicago medical center was already a renowned institution known for its excellence in patient cate specifically in performing complex oncological surgery, cardiovascular surgery, and research. The hospital offered comprehensive care for various medical conditions. The hospital had well-structured departments including the emergency department, the surgical and medical intensive care units, the regular patient floors and well ran operating rooms. As renowned and well established the university of Chicago medical center is, for over 25 years, the hospital was not a trauma center. It was not equipped to handle the level of severe and complex trauma patients; the intensive care units were not built to handle the patient population and the census that a level 1 trauma center requires. It was therefore necessary to reengineer the surgical intensive care unit to accommodate the new patient population.

Hospitals as Complex Systems

A hospital is a complex system that incorporates multiple scales of organization in its operational structure, spanning the activities of individual patients and healthcare delivery personnel, which are organized into a series of interacting and often overlapping functional units/teams, often with specific geographical locations (that impact operational flow) to an intersecting modular organizational structure that seeks to optimize both outcomes, delivery efficiency and economic viability (Fig. 1). Since it is a complex system the specific dynamics of a hospital are determined by the interactions and behaviors of its components (i.e. individuals). However, the fact is that hospitals are also "top-down" management structures, with decisions being made at an administrative level that purports to govern the direction and function of the overall system. This is a structural distinction that can be made between "human" multi-component systems and "biological/multicellular" systems: the latter are generated by evolutionary and Darwinian forces that act as constraints on the forms of the resulting systems, whereas human organizations operate with "intentional" governance and planning. The constraints on the human system are often cast in terms

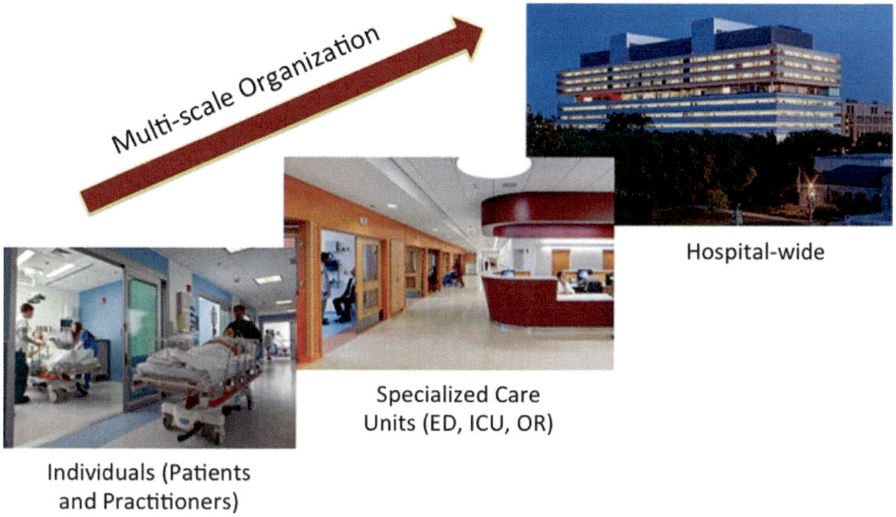

Fig. 1 Multiscale nature of a hospital. Individuals with define roles (e.g. patients, specialized healthcare professionals) interact within function modules (care units) that are then linked hospital-wide

of economic forces with pseudo-evolutionary terminology: e.g. "competition," "survival of the fittest," etc. The difficulty with those analogies is that there is a very real, and generally unacceptable, human cost as those "selective dynamics" play out. This is not to imply malice, but rather points out a limit on the predictive, projective, and planning capabilities of the administrative level. Thus, there exist an additional multi-scale component to hospital operations related to the classes of decisions that need to be made. These directly pertain to the predictive horizons associated with different types of decisions: "Strategic/Policy" (such as location of specific resources and structural factors), "Tactical/Management" (such as composition of various care modules and how they interact) and "Operational/Logistics" (such as specific care pathways or care delivery processes).

With increasing recognition of the complexity of interactions between the various components of hospital operations there has been a desire to apply more quantitative and rigorous methods to QI activities. This has prompted the application of tools and methods drawn from the areas of operations research and industrial/systems engineering. These methods have been applied to various aspects of the business and manufacturing domains, and many of these processes can be readily mapped to components of a healthcare system and hospital operations. The International Society for Pharmacoeconomics and Healthcare (ISPOR) published a series of papers discussing the application of modeling and simulation to healthcare systems [6, 7], including a description of methods most commonly used, including agent-based modeling [7].

Agent-Based Model and Simulation (ABMS)

Agent-based models (ABMs) are object-oriented, discrete-event, rule-based, interaction-space-explicit computational models that represent systems as sets of interacting components, termed *Agents*. ABMs are by their very nature multi-scale, linking together generative-behavioral rules (lowest scale) to define the behavior of agents (middle scale) that interact to produce agent-population level dynamics (highest scale). In ABMS, active components or decision makers are conceptualized as agents being modeled and implemented using agent-related concepts. There have been several ABMs applied to hospital operations. These include models of specific areas of the hospital, such as the emergency department [8–11] or the intensive care unit [12]. Others have examined the longitudinal care of specific types of patients [13], or patient throughput for an entire hospital [14]. One of the primary benefits of using ABMs is that they are intuitive to non-computational people, and thus facilitate interactivity in terms of their development and use. This property is especially important given the critical role of stakeholder involvement in the model development and use process, and has extended to the use of ABMs to aid in Kaizan events [15].

The Scope of the Challenge

Integrating a new high volume trauma patient population into an existing tertiary hospital can be a very complex process. Gaining insight into how the existing physical configuration of a hospital can influence patient flow can target potential bottlenecks and choke points to inform planning. Some factors to consider includes equipment and technology, the overall layout of the intensive care unit, the patient flow from the ER through the intensive care unit then to other units in the hospital when the ICU needs are over. When UCM decided to become a Level 1 Adult Trauma Center in December 2014, there were several significant constraints on how that decision would manifest: (1) a new emergency department (ED) had already been planned in terms of its overall footprint and general layout; (2) the hospital would not be increasing its number of inpatient beds, yet it consistently ran at 90% bed occupancy; (3) the addition of trauma patients would require new, augmented workflows between previously loosely interacting regions of the hospital. The task, then, was to plan for and reconfigure existing hospital operations in order to account for an influx of a new patient population that would utilize resources across all aspects of the hospital at a level of intensity not previously seen at that scale. Given the timeframe for the opening of the Trauma Center it was not deemed feasible to create the detailed simulation model of the UCM hospital, but some preliminary work was carried out in 2016 that could provide some insight into where potential problem areas would lie.

The Proto-Hospital ABM (HABM): A Thought Experiment Aid for Trauma Center Planning

In December 2014 the University of Chicago Medicine (UCM) committed to becoming a Level 1 (highest level) Trauma Center (TC), the only one in the South Side of Chicago, traditionally an epicenter of urban violence and trauma in Chicago. As noted above this decision came with certain constraints: (1) the footprint of the planned revision of the Emergency Department (ED) would not be altered and (2) there would be no new construction of inpatient care units specifically to address the planned Trauma Center. Therefore, the physical and operational accommodation of the hospital to this new patient population would involve: (1) some reconfiguration of the internal structure of the planned ED, (2) organizational changes of existing work units with the hospital and (3) the addition of one new operating room (OR). It was reasonable to assume that the operational consequences of the decision to become a TC given these constraints would significantly impact the functioning of the hospital. We also recognized that the failure to objectively optimize across these factors could have catastrophic consequences on the operations of institutions aiming to become a TC. Operational viability must be a precondition if a hospital is to serve its community, and should represent a fundamental constraint on the planning for a TC. Traditional data-centric analyses cannot transparently generate the prospective scenarios needed to forecast the consequences of planning decisions. The generation of such scenarios requires the representation of health system population and process dynamics that: (1) allows for the modular representation of system components at varying levels of spatial-temporal granularity and (2) facilitates transparency by incorporating stakeholder involvement and interaction. Therefore, we developed a prototype agent-based modeling framework, the proto-Hospital Agent-based Model (HABM) for hospital operations that could be potentially expanded to the specifics of implementing a trauma center within an existing institution (Fig. 2).

Spatial Architecture of the HABM

The abstracted HABM was spatially sectioned into the emergency department (ED), radiology, operating room, ICU and general care units. Individual patients and healthcare providers are represented as individual computational agents located in and moving among the regions of the hospital. We allocated different hospital regions in this abstract model. These regions were the

- Emergency department: in this region we allocated 40 bays in the ER with 2 resuscitation trauma bays.

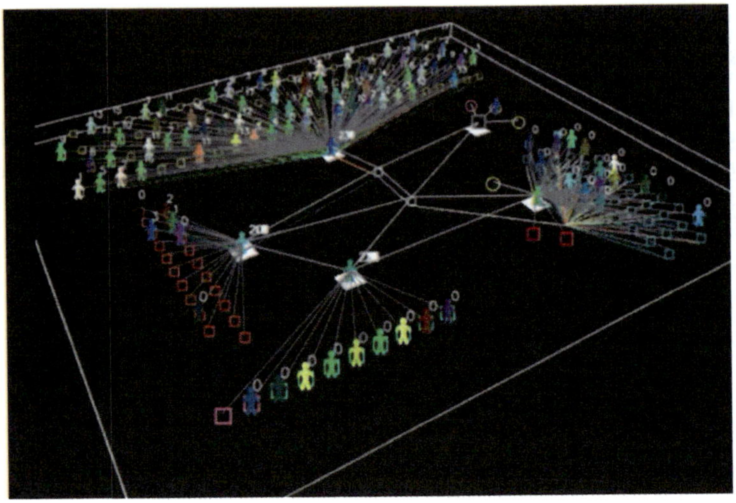

Fig. 2 Screenshot of Proto-HABM. Bed and care unit configuration was modeled as a network, with movement of patients and care providers as agents moving along the edges of the network

- Radiology: this region was constructed to have 1 CT machine in the ER, 2 machines in the main hospital that would be ready at anytime for the admitted trauma patients and lastly 1 interventional radiology suite.
- Operating rooms: we allocated 10 operating rooms that can accommodate trauma surgeries.
- Intensive care Unit: we allocated 20 ICU beds in the simulation
- Floor beds: we allocated 100 floor beds

The overall structure of the HAB, is that of an undirected graph, where nodes represented specific beds within each care area, and atient flow from bed-to-bed and care area-to-care area were represented as edges between nodes representing specific beds. This structure provided the virtual world in which computational *agents* representing patients and healthcare worker could move.

Agents in the HABM

Patient Agents: We recognized that the trauma patient population was a different population that the hospital system was not used to serve. Level 1 trauma center comes with a different level of patient acuity. These patients may have different severity levels of trauma and my require significant resources to coordinate their care. Trauma patients on average have longer hospital stay and have different treatment pathway compared to the average non-trauma patient previously seen at UCM.

Healthcare worker agents: this includes physicians, nursing staff, medical technicians, the environmental staff, support staff including social workers, case management team, administrative staff. Physicians may have different specialties; nurses may also have different skill levels in trauma.

Patient acuity was represented by a weighted stochastic likelihood of adverse events affected by provider response. Providers incorporated capabilities across the delivery spectrum. Economic costs and returns were assigned to the actions of the various agents.

Baseline Assumptions and Simulation Experiments Before and After implementation of the Trauma Center

We first established a baseline proto-HABM representing hospital operations prior to implementation of trauma services, calibrated to economic viability. In the baseline operations in the model, we anticipated our ward occupancy to be about 70% and the intensive care unit occupancy to be about 50%. In our simulations, we estimated our elective surgical cases to utilize about 80% of the hospital beds and that was a hard cap. After developing the baseline simulation system, the next step was the implementation of the trauma population on top of the baseline operations system. We assumed that the implementation of the level 1 trauma system will add significant number of patients to the already established hospital system. As an initial estimate for the total amount of trauma admissions, we estimated about 30% penetrating trauma. Of this 30% penetrating trauma patients, we anticipated 1/3rd of the patients will go to the OR emergently, 1/3rd of the patients will require surgical intervention after 24 hours of observation or go to the OR the following day. With 30% of the level 1 trauma patients being penetrating, we anticipated 70% to be blunt trauma with 1/10 if the patients going to the OR within 24 hours of presentation.

Simulation experiments were the performed with differing trauma populations and resourcing plans to identify process bottlenecks and critical operational tipping points between viable and non-viable scenarios. This was done by increasing the trauma volume, identifying bottleneck points, correcting those bottlenecks (given physical structure constraints) and continuing to increase trauma volumes until the system "broke." The results of these simulations showed the following Process bottlenecks in order of exposure: (1) ED Patient Flow resulting from delays in non-trauma dispositions, (2) ICU beds and (3) effect on Next-Day Surgical Schedule, where delays in non-trauma urgent cases spill over into elective schedule the following day, creating a domino effect of case back-log. Of interest, we also recognized the following factors as not being as significant: (1) Total hospital bed capacity and (2) Emergency access to the operating room.

Conclusion

We recognized that the proto-HABM was a rapidly developed, proof-of-concept project. Despite its abstraction we believed that the proto-HABM generated spatio-temporal dynamics that could account for diurnal, weekly and seasonal variation in patient type and volume. Healthcare agent rules could incorporate both empirical performance data as well as stakeholder conceptions for best-practices and expectations. While remaining a "toy model" the HABM did provide system-level insight and qualitative suggestions to where problem areas might arise, namely that existing ED patient flow, SICU capacity and OR access for emergent-urgent non-trauma patients would be potential bottlenecks to optimizing patient care, and therefore should be targeted for at least close monitoring when the trauma center opened.

References

1. Marshall DA, Burgos-Liz L, Ijzerman MJ, Osgood ND, Padula WV, Higashi MK, et al. Applying dynamic simulation modeling methods in health care delivery research—the SIMULATE checklist: report of the ISPOR simulation modeling emerging good practices task force. Value Health. 2015;18:5–16.
2. Marshall DA, Burgos-Liz L, Ijzerman MJ, Crown W, Padula WV, Wong PK, et al. Selecting a dynamic simulation modeling method for health care delivery research—part 2: report of the ISPOR dynamic simulation modeling emerging good practices task force. Value Health. 2015;18:147–60.
3. Taboada M, Cabrera E, Epelde F, Iglesias ML, Luque E. Using an agent-based simulation for predicting the effects of patients derivation policies in emergency departments. Proc Comput Sci. 2013;18:641–50.
4. Liu Z, Rexachs D, Epelde F, Luque E. A simulation and optimization based method for calibrating agent-based emergency department models under data scarcity. Comput Ind Eng. 2017;103:300–9.
5. Liu Z, Rexachs D, Epelde F, Luque E. An agent-based model for quantitatively analyzing and predicting the complex behavior of emergency departments. J Comput Sci. 2017;21:11–23.
6. Marie Crandall MM, Douglas Sharp MP, Erin Unger M, et al. Trauma deserts: distance from a trauma center, transport times, and mortality from gunshot wounds in Chicago. Am J Public Health. 2013;103(6):1103.
7. Centers for Disease Control and Prevention. Injuries and violence are leading causes of death. Centers for Disease Control and Prevention. Published February 28, 2022. https://www.cdc.gov/injury/wisqars/animated-leading-causes.html. Accessed 12 June 2023.
8. Wandling M, Behrens J, Hsia R, Crandall M. Geographic disparities in access to urban trauma care: defining the problem and identifying a solution for gunshot wound victims in Chicago. https://doi.org/10.1016/j.amjsurg.2016.06.020.
9. Nathens AB, Jurkovich GJ, Cummings P, Rivara FP, Maier RV. The Effect of organized systems of trauma care on motor vehicle crash mortality. https://jamanetwork.com/
10. MacKenzie EJ, Rivara FP, Jurkovich GJ, et al. A national evaluation of the effect of trauma-center care on mortality abstract. Published online 2006. www.nejm.org. Accessed 13 June 2023.
11. Young JS, Meredith JW. Trauma centers a quick guide. 2020; https://doi.org/10.1007/978-3-030-34607-2.

12. User. Guideline for Intensive Care Unit Design Faculty of Critical Care Medicine College of Anaesthesiologists and Intensivists of Sri Lanka Faculty of Critical Care Medicine; 2016.
13. Guidelines for Intensive Care Unit Design; 1995.
14. Abarbanel H, Braha D, Kelso S, et al. Springer Complexity Editorial and Programme Advisory Board. http://www.springer.com/series/5394
15. Klugl F, Bazzan LC. Agent-based modeling and simulation.

Further Reading

Possik J, Asgary A, Solis AO, et al. An agent-based Modeling and virtual reality application using distributed simulation: case of a COVID-19 intensive care unit. IEEE Trans Eng Manag. Published online August 1, 2022. https://doi.org/10.1109/TEM.2022.3195813.

Kaushal A, Zhao Y, Peng Q, Strome T, Weldon E, Zhang M, et al. Evaluation of fast track strategies using agent-based simulation modeling to reduce waiting time in a hospital emergency department. Socio Econ Plan Sci. 2015;50:18–31.

Ferrer J, Salmon M, Temime L. Nosolink: an agent-based approach to link patient flows and staff organization with the circulation of nosocomial pathogens in an intensive care unit. Proc Comput Sci. 2013;18:1485–94.

Mustapha K, Gilli Q, Frayret J-M, Lahrichi N, Karimi E. Agent-based simulation patient model for colon and colorectal cancer care trajectory. Proc Comput Sci. 2016;100:188–97.

Ben-Tovim D, Filar J, Hakendorf P, Qin S, Thompson C, Ward D. Hospital event simulation model: arrivals to discharge–design, development and application. Simul Model Pract Theory. 2016;68:80–94.

Baril C, Gascon V, Miller J, Côté N. Use of a discrete-event simulation in a Kaizen event: a case study in healthcare. Eur J Oper Res. 2016;249:327–39.

Part V
Partnerships

Opening a Modern Trauma Center at UChicago Medicine: Residency Perspective and Partnerships

Jennifer Cone and Andrew J. Benjamin

Program Director Perspective

Incorporating a New Program Line

The incorporation of a completely new and, by all accounts, busy service line is a logistical nightmare for a program director. Before the University even decided to open the trauma center, there were conversations with key stakeholders, including departmental and surgical education leadership. As it was clear that residents would be the main workforce staffing the trauma center, it was important to make sure that the residency could support the mission and help to establish the trauma center.

From a more global program perspective, it was important to both help the trauma center succeed and also ensure a good education experience for the residents. The concerns from the residency standpoint included ensuring adherence to duty hours, ensuring that there was not an inordinate amount of time spent on the trauma service in comparison to the rest of the rotations, appropriate coverage of both trauma and other rotations, and ensuring a good educational environment.

At the time of the opening of the trauma center, University of Chicago had seven categorical positions each year. The vast majority of the residents took two years of professional development time in the lab, so the total complement of available residents was quite large. Having a relatively large program allowed us to better

J. Cone (✉) · A. J. Benjamin
University of Chicago, Department of Surgery, Chicago, IL, USA
e-mail: jcone2@bsd.uchicago.edu; abenjamin2@bsd.uchicago.edu

S. O. Rogers, Jr (ed.), *Creating a Modern Trauma Center*,
https://doi.org/10.1007/978-3-031-66524-0_21

accommodate staffing the trauma service without undue gaps on other services. The entire resident and service schedule for the year was evaluated to decide where to pull residents. Cases and patient volume on each service were considered when deciding which services would lose resident coverage.

Residency Partnerships

While the residency was quite large and could accommodate much of the coverage, we quickly realized that partnerships would be necessary to fill the complement of residents needed. This was achieved twofold: internally and externally. Multiple service lines within within the University had hard or soft residency graduation requirements for rotations on trauma. These services included Emergency Medicine, Orthopedic Surgery, Urology, and Plastic Surgery. Leaders from all involved services met with both General Surgery program leadership as well as Trauma program leadership. Most programs were able to send interns to rotate on trauma. Because Emergency Medicine was able to send multiple residents at a time, each for two months out of their intern year, space was created on the trauma service specifically for their residents. The Orthopedic Surgery, Urology, and Plastic Surgery interns were felt to be equivalent to General Surgery interns and substituted on the schedule as such. Plastic Surgery was additionally able to send their PGY-2 residents for a month rotation, which alleviated some the burden of providing general surgery mid-level resident coverage.

As most of the available coverage was junior resident coverage, we recognized that outside partnerships would be necessary to help fill the complement of senior residents needed to cover the service. To this end, the Section Chief of Trauma reached out to all the residency programs in the city of Chicago as well as friends with leadership in surgical education to enquire about potential partnerships. Swedish Hospital of Seattle agreed to partner with University of Chicago and send 12 months of PGY-4 coverage each year. Both programs came to an agreement on travel and living arrangements for the visiting residents. As with any visiting resident, both GME programs and the ACGME needed to approve of a new rotation location.

Logistics

From a very basic standpoint, we now needed to ensure that residents were appropriately trained to take care of trauma patients. We held ourselves and the residents to incredibly high standards. We wanted to ensure that the residents were getting direct teaching and feedback from the faculty that they would be working with. Furthermore, we wanted to ensure that bad habits learned at other centers were not carried over to University of Chicago. The trauma faculty immediately began hosting and teaching Advanced Trauma Life Support (ATLS) courses for our interns and refresher courses for our senior residents. The faculty also began trauma-oriented didactic lectures during the residents' protected education time.

While the residents at University of Chicago were some of the best trained surgical residents in the country and previously rotated at a different Level 1 trauma center, we also wanted to ensure they felt comfortable with some of the more complex operative exposures. ASSET (Advanced Surgical Skills for Exposure in Trauma) is a course organized by the American College of Surgeons Committee on Trauma hosted by separate site institutions that teaches learners key exposures of surgically challenging anatomic areas. The course is hands-on, using a low learner to cadaver ratio. A brief case and overview is followed by dissection of each anatomic area. The course covers exposure of the brachial artery, femoral artery, superficial femoral artery, iliac artery, cervical and thoracic trachea, cervical and thoracic esophagus, carotid artery, vertebral artery, subclavian artery, heart, pulmonary hilum, thoracic and abdominal aorta, superior vena cava and inferior vena cava, pancreas, duodenum, retrohepatic cava, hepatic veins, kidneys, bladder, etc. It also covers fasciotomies of the upper and lower extremities. Because it is so broad, it is a useful review for all surgeons, not just those going into trauma. Previous data has suggested that participation in the ASSET course increases performance of procedure steps, increased anatomic knowledge, decreases skin to vessel loop placement time, and improves self-confidence [1, 2]. To facilitate sending our residents to this course, we obtained an internal educational grant to fund our residents to take an ASSET course in the first 6 months of their PGY-4 year.

As we did not know how busy the service would be, we initially did not know exactly how many residents to put on the trauma service. As a starting plan, we had two resident teams that were separated into day and night coverage. This was decided, in part, because we needed to ensure appropriate case volume before placing chief residents on service. Each team consisted of a PGY-4 or 5, a PGY-3, and three PGY-1s. Residents worked 12-hour day or night shifts. They were off at least one day per week and given two consecutive days off in a four week period for a total of 6 days off in a four week period.

As the trauma service grew in patient volume, residents in the day/night model were no longer able to safely and efficiently care for patients and maintain their duty hours. We thus transitioned to a q3 model after a year. Three equal resident teams were created comprised of a PGY-4 or 5, a PGY-2 or 3, and two PGY-1s. These teams rotated on a q3 schedule for an entire month, with one of their pre-call days being a day off each week. This model ensured more consistent resident coverage for patient care. The patient list was effectively split into three services and each of the resident teams were tasked with rounding on their patients daily. It also ensured that there was a consistent chief and midlevel resident team on-call every day of the week.

As with the creation of any new service line, flexibility and adaptability is of utmost importance. We found that in our busiest months, residents were frequently at risk of violating duty hours. It was necessary to hire and deploy a team of APNs who could help carry the weight of the patient volume. Further, it was necessary to institute a series of service guidelines to ensure both good patient care and also that residents were adhering to duty hours.

Wellness

The University of Chicago Trauma Center is unique in its high volume of penetrating trauma in a patient population that has been substantially affected by structural racism and racial trauma. We recognized that rotating on our service placed residents at a significant risk of burnout, moral injury, and compassion fatigue. Many residents, but particularly minority residents, were profoundly impacted by their experience repeatedly taking care of our patients. We thus created a trauma wellness curriculum for residents on service to help alleviate the resident burden.

The wellness curriculum was designed using existing frameworks and strategies with the partnership of trauma psychologists, psychiatrists, and trauma surgeons that had expertise in physician wellness and burnout. Our curriculum includes three one-hour sessions, led by mental health professionals over zoom, that take place before the trauma rotation, during the rotation, and after the rotation. Each session focuses on psychoeducation and skill building, as well as building a peer support network. We have found that the majority of participants find the program and curriculum valuable.

Resident Perspective

The Pre-Trauma Center Experience

In the winter of 2018, prior to the opening of the University of Chicago's trauma center in May, the experience of handling trauma cases was markedly different. We were not a trauma center, but occasionally we would receive patient drop offs due to the high volume of gun violence that occurred in the surrounding community. I recall a specific incident vividly: receiving a page for a gunshot wound (GSW) to the chest. At that time, a trauma page was synonymous with impending chaos. Rushing to the trauma bay in the emergency department, we were often met with a sense of unpreparedness—rusty cabinets that were missing crucial supplies like chest tubes or surgical instruments. The lack of a defined trauma center meant there were no streamlined protocols or clearly defined roles. As surgery residents, despite our limited trauma training at other institutions, we were frequently thrust into leadership roles amidst this chaos, because we actually had more experience than anyone, including our attendings.

For this particular patient with a GSW to the chest and hypotensive, the urgency was palpable. In the absence of a streamlined massive transfusion protocol, we had to resort to Lactated Ringers instead of blood. After placing a chest tube and draining over a liter of blood, it was evident he might need urgent surgical intervention. Yet, as we were not a designated trauma center, our immediate course of action was to prepare for his transfer. One thing that I remember the most is the shock and anxiety I would have when I first got those trauma pages.

Increase in Acuity

The inauguration of the trauma center in May 2018 at the University of Chicago marked a pivotal moment, ushering in a transformative era for both surgical training and patient care. This watershed event signified more than just the establishment of new facilities; it represented a fundamental shift in our approach to surgery across disciplines.

Before the trauma center's inception, our surgical training, while comprehensive in many aspects, often lacked in high-acuity trauma exposure. Residents, like myself, were exposed to a range of complex surgeries, from Whipples to liver resections, yet the overall intensity of cases was relatively subdued. The opening of the trauma center, however, introduced us to an entirely different spectrum of clinical experiences. It brought with it a diversity and volume of cases that were not only more complex but also demanded rapid, decisive action. This shift to an increased intensity was particularly significant in an era where national trends indicated a general decline in such experiences for residents [3].

In this new high-stakes environment, the pace and gravity of decision-making reached unprecedented levels. Previously, we might have waited hours for an operating room to become available for emergent cases; now, a Level 1 trauma patient could be rushed into surgery within minutes. This expedited process necessitated an immediate application of knowledge, a departure from our earlier, more deliberate pace. Despite the initial stress and steep learning curve, this rapid environment catalyzed our growth as surgeons. We learned to adapt quickly, make critical decisions on the fly, and handle a range of traumatic injuries with a newfound proficiency.

In "The Coddling of the American Mind," Lukianoff and Haidt discuss how shielding individuals from challenges and discomfort can impede their development and resilience. This concept, while primarily focused on the academic and social environment, resonates profoundly with the transformation experienced in surgical training. The philosophy that "Education should not be intended to make people comfortable, it is meant to make people think" aligns seamlessly with our journey in the trauma center [4].

In the trauma setting, the luxury of comfort and predictability is non-existent. The environment is inherently unpredictable, often stressful, and always demanding. It is a setting where quick decision-making, adaptability, and resilience are not just valued but essential for survival—both for the patient and the surgeon. This aligns with Lukianoff and Haidt's argument that exposure to challenges, and learning to navigate them, is crucial for developing psychological resilience. In our case, it translated into developing surgical resilience and the ability to think critically under pressure.

The trauma center's high-pressure environment served as a real-world application of these principles. Here, we could not avoid the discomfort of high-stakes situations or the emotional turmoil that comes with life-and-death decisions. Instead, we were compelled to confront these challenges head-on. This necessity to face and adapt to difficult situations directly contributed to our growth as surgeons. It fostered a mindset that was not only capable of handling immense pressure but also thrived in it. This transformation is a testament to the belief that true learning and development occur not in the absence of challenges, but in one's ability to confront and overcome them.

Thus, the trauma center's opening, while increasing our clinical and technical capabilities, also played a pivotal role in developing our psychological resilience. It underscored the importance of embracing discomfort as a path to growth, a lesson not only valuable in surgery but in life as a whole.

A Stimulus for Growth

The journey from pre to post-trauma center residency training was marked by profound personal and professional growth, albeit accompanied by significant challenges. In the years preceding the trauma center's establishment, encounters with patient deaths were infrequent, making each case deeply impactful. However, this changed dramatically post-inauguration. The high incidence of gun violence in our community meant that we were now regularly exposed to life-threatening injuries and, unfortunately, a higher rate of mortality. This stark contrast in my initial two-month trauma rotation was eye opening—I witnessed more deaths in this short period than in the previous three years combined.

This frequent confrontation with mortality was a double-edged sword. On one hand, it was a crucial aspect of our training, teaching us to navigate the complex interplay of medical ethics, patient care, and the emotional aspects of death and loss. Surgeons must learn to balance the detachment necessary for clinical decision-making with the empathy required to support patients and their families during critical moments. However, the emotional toll of this exposure was palpable. As residents, we experienced a wide range of responses; while some of us could compartmentalize and move on swiftly, others found themselves needing time to process and decompress after intense cases.

In response to these heightened emotional and psychological demands, our residency program demonstrated exceptional adaptability and responsiveness. A key element of this adaptability was the implementation of the trauma wellness program. This initiative was a proactive step towards addressing the mental health and emotional well-being of residents. It provided structured debriefing sessions, access to mental health professionals, and peer support systems, acknowledging that the challenges we faced were not just physical but also mental and emotional.

Moreover, the program's adaptability extended to the academic and training aspects aspects. The curriculum underwent significant revisions to include more comprehensive trauma care modules and simulation-based training, ensuring that we were equipped not only for the technical challenges of trauma surgery but also for its fast-paced and unpredictable nature. This dynamic approach to medical education underscored the importance of a curriculum that evolves with the changing landscapes of medical needs and healthcare environments.

Through these experiences and the support of the trauma wellness program, we grew not only in our technical skills but also in our capacity to handle the emotional and ethical dimensions of surgery. This period of transformation shaped us into surgeons who were not only technically adept but also emotionally intelligent and ethically grounded—professionals capable of navigating the complexities of trauma care with a well-rounded perspective.

Skill Development and Interdisciplinary Learning

The advent of the trauma center at the University of Chicago heralded a new era in both the development of surgical skills and the fostering of interdisciplinary collaboration among residents. This transition played a pivotal role in broadening our clinical repertoire and deepening our understanding of various medical disciplines.

Prior to the trauma center's opening, certain procedures, such as placing a chest tube for a spontaneous pneumothorax, were typically reserved for residents that are more senior. However, with the increased volume and variety of trauma cases, junior residents, including interns and second-year residents, found themselves actively engaged in these core procedures. This shift not only accelerated our learning curve but also instilled a sense of confidence and autonomy early in our training. The range of cases we encountered expanded significantly, from gunshot wounds to motor vehicle accidents, providing us with frequent opportunities to perform and master complex surgical techniques that were once considered rare.

Furthermore, the trauma center's opening enhanced our interdisciplinary training. Previously, our exposure to specialties like neurosurgery, orthopedics, or urology was mostly theoretical or observational. However, the trauma setting demanded close collaboration with these and other specialties, presenting us with a unique learning platform. This interdisciplinary environment was not just about observing; it was an active learning process where we could absorb the nuances of different specialties, thereby enriching our own surgical knowledge and skills.

This collaborative approach extended beyond the operating room. It fostered improved relationships and friendships across disciplines, leading to valuable teaching opportunities and academic collaborations. Engaging with colleagues from various specialties, we gained insights into the holistic management of trauma patients, understanding how different specialties converge in the treatment process. This not only enhanced our clinical skills but also broadened our perspective on patient care, highlighting the importance of a cohesive, multidisciplinary approach in modern healthcare.

In summary, the transition to a trauma center at the University of Chicago significantly enriched our training experience. It provided unparalleled opportunities for skill development, fostered autonomy in decision-making, and promoted a multidisciplinary approach to patient care. These experiences have been instrumental in preparing us for the complexities of modern surgical practice and have played a crucial role in shaping us into versatile, well-rounded surgeons.

Broader Implications

The transformation witnessed at the University of Chicago's trauma center is not just a localized phenomenon but rather part of a larger narrative unfolding across the nation in the field of trauma surgery and surgical training. Nationally, there has been a notable shift in the operative trauma landscape, characterized by a progressive decline in both the volume and diversity of operative trauma cases encountered by general surgery residents. This trend, marked by a significant reduction in total operative trauma cases over the years, can be attributed to various factors, including the proliferation of trauma centers and advancements in non-operative management techniques [5].

Despite this national trend, the establishment of the trauma center at the University of Chicago has bucked this pattern, enriching the training and experiential landscape for our residents. Our center has become a hub for a wide array of high-acuity cases, providing essential exposure that is critical for the development of advanced surgical skills and effective decision-making abilities. This exposure is particularly vital given the variability in surgical critical care, trauma, and burn rotations across different U.S. residency programs, which can lead to disparities in the clinical experience and knowledge base among trainees [6].

Moreover, the trauma center's emphasis on operative autonomy has been a defining feature of our resident education. This autonomy, more pronounced in acute care surgery cases, is essential for comprehensive surgical training. It fosters a sense of ownership over clinical decisions, sharpens critical thinking skills, and enables mastery over complex surgical interventions in high-pressure environments. Studies have shown that such autonomy, while challenging, does not compromise patient outcomes and is, in fact, integral to the preparation of residents for independent practice [7–9].

In this context, the experience at the University of Chicago serves as a valuable case study in how trauma centers can profoundly impact surgical education. While the general decline in operative trauma experience presents challenges nationally, the hands-on experience and autonomy provided by our center have been invaluable in preparing residents for the complexities of modern surgical practice. These experiences ensure not only the readiness of residents for independent practice but also their adaptability to the evolving demands of healthcare, regardless of the specialty they ultimately pursue [10].

Post-Trauma Center Experience

In the year following the trauma center's inauguration, my journey as a resident underwent a dramatic transformation. Serving as the chief resident in our trauma service, I was deeply entrenched in the intense and demanding world of trauma care. One particularly challenging night, having already performed three emergency department (ED) thoracotomies, presented a critical moment that highlighted my significant growth as a surgeon.

During an operation on one of the patients from the earlier thoracotomies, my pager sounded: another gunshot wound to the chest. I quickly unscrubbed and left my attending to continue the operation, rushing to triage the new patient. In the ED, I was confronted with a critically ill patient, blood pressure plummeting to 60/palp, rapidly progressing into cardiac arrest. Relying on the skills and confidence acquired through my recent experiences, I performed my fourth ED thoracotomy of the night. Successfully cross-clamping the aorta, the patient regained a pulse. We swiftly moved the patient to the operating room, where I managed the situation until my attending arrived. His astonishment at my independent resuscitation and initiation of surgical intervention underscored the autonomy and proficiency I had developed in the trauma center environment. This moment made me reflect on the trauma patient we had transferred before the center's opening. The difference was clear: the pager's alert no longer triggered anxiety but a sense of readiness, even under heightened stakes.

Reflecting on this experience, I realized how significantly my perspective and skills had evolved since the trauma center's opening. The alert of a pager no longer triggered a sense of anxiety but instead a readiness to confront and manage high-stakes scenarios. This shift in mindset was not just about clinical skills; it represented a deeper understanding of trauma care and the confidence to make critical decisions independently.

This transformative experience also had a profound impact on my career trajectory. Prior to the trauma center's opening, my inclination was towards pursuing a fellowship in surgical oncology. However, the immersive and challenging experiences in the trauma service after the center's inauguration steered me towards a different path. I discovered a profound alignment with trauma surgery—a specialty that not only presented complex challenges but also resonated with my professional aspirations and skills. It was through these experiences that I realized trauma surgery was where I could make the most significant impact, both as a surgeon and as a healthcare provider.

References

1. Mackenzie CF, Garofalo E, Shackelford S, et al. Using an individual procedure score before and after the advanced surgical skills exposure for trauma course training to benchmark a hemorrhage-control performance metric. J Surg Educ. 2015;72:1278–89.

2. Kuhls DA, Risucci DA, Bowyer MW, et al. Advanced surgical skills for exposure in trauma. J Trauma Acute Care Surg. 2013;74:664–70.
3. Drake FT, Van Eaton EG, Huntington CR, et al. ACGME case logs: surgery resident experience in operative trauma for two decades. J Trauma Acute Care Surg. 2012;73:1500–6.
4. Lukianoff G, Haidt J. The coddling of the American mind: how good intentions and bad ideas are setting up a generation for failure. Penguin; 2019.
5. Hurtuk M, Reed RL 2nd, Esposito TJ, et al. Trauma surgeons practice what they preach: the NTDB story on solid organ injury management. J Trauma. 2006;61:243–54; discussion 254–5.
6. Napolitano LM, Biester TW, Jurkovich GJ, et al. General surgery resident rotations in surgical critical care, trauma, and burns: what is optimal for residency training? Am J Surg. 2016;212:629–37.
7. Kantor O, Schneider AB, Rojnica M, et al. Implementing a resident acute care surgery service: improving resident education and patient care. Surgery. 2017;161:876–83.
8. Sehat AJ, Oliver JB, Yu Y, et al. Declining surgical resident operative autonomy in acute care surgical cases. J Surg Res. 2023;281:328–34.
9. LeCompte M, Stewart M, Harris T, et al. See one, do one, teach one: a randomized controlled study evaluating the benefit of autonomy in surgical education. Am J Surg. 2019;217:281–7.
10. Hashimoto DA, Bynum WE 4th, Lillemoe KD, et al. See more, do more, teach more: surgical resident autonomy and the transition to independent practice. Acad Med. 2016;91:757–60.

Creating a Surgical Critical Care Fellowship

Toba Bolaji, Mihir Chaudhary, Susan Rowell, and David A. Hampton

Building the Infrastructure

The University of Chicago Medicine's (UCM) Level I trauma center's opening was associated with new educational opportunities for the hospital and its trainees. Understanding a patients' acuity, concepts of triage, damage control resuscitation and surgery and correcting metabolic derangements are critical concepts to a surgical trainee's experience. As the number of annual trauma activations increased, the intensive care units became busier. The opportunity to create a Surgical Critical Care (SCC) Fellowship was apparent.

Training programs are the means by which we develop young physicians. The apprenticeship style model of graduate medical education has been the gold standard for medical training since the early 1900s [1]. Training programs create an educational environment that reinforces standards in patient care and allows for new ones to develop. The additional focus on educating the next generation of surgeons while providing direct clinical care does not result in a deficit to patient outcomes. A systematic review by Van der Leeuwet et al., evaluated the effects of training programs. They concluded that patient care was safe and provided equal quality of care between trainees and faculty [2]. Additionally, higher order training programs can provide a workforce pipeline for recruiting new physicians with a specialized skill set. This investment in young physicians can create a consistent, well-trained workforce. Another benefit of Fellowship programs is the environment they create for research and innovation. This academic environment promotes curiosity and critical thinking. Building these programs require a healthy and dynamic

T. Bolaji (✉) · M. Chaudhary · S. Rowell · D. A. Hampton
Department of Surgery, Section of Trauma and Acute Care Surgery, University of Chicago Medicine, Chicago, IL, USA
e-mail: Oloruntoba.Bolaji@uchicagomedicine.org; Mihir.Chaudhary@uchicagomedicine.org; susan.rowell@bsd.uchicago.edu; dhampton2@bsd.uchicago.edu

S. O. Rogers, Jr (ed.), *Creating a Modern Trauma Center*,
https://doi.org/10.1007/978-3-031-66524-0_22

atmosphere that compels all providers to remain abreast of and challenge the standard of care while striving to create future novel therapies.

To advance the care provided to patients undergoing increasingly complex operations, Critical Care Medicine programs were developed [3]. Subsequently dedicated surgical critical care programs were established to match the intensive care units (ICU) staffing needs. The traditional model of critical care management relied on non-intensivist service lines and consultants. The critical care intensivist model was introduced in the 1990s after ICU based service lines that solely managed and coordinated the care of the critical ill were shown to have better outcomes [3]. Since then, ICUs staffed by intensivists have been associated with decreased ventilator days, decreased ICU and hospital length of stay, and decreased mortality [4, 5].

The UCM has a robust collection of accredited fellowship programs, maintaining over 60 medical and surgical training programs and 12 surgical subspecialty fellowships. The presence of a long-standing, nationally recognized, Anesthesia Critical Care program offered a blueprint to model a Surgical Critical Care (SCC) Fellowship program. The Department of Anesthesiology staff were the primary ICU physicians and understood the University's healthcare system and necessary resources. With the inclusion of the new staff, the ICU care was complemented by the initial and growing cohort of UCM trauma surgeons, all of whom are trained in General Surgery, Acute Care Surgery, and Surgical Critical Care. Additionally new clinical Attendings brought a trauma-informed strategy to managing critical illness and helped to standardize ICU care for the surgical patient.

This multidisciplinary faculty saw the benefit of a Surgical Critical Care fellowship program. To ensure its success, collaboration between the other Surgical and Medical Critical Care fellowship programs—Anesthesia, Medicine, and Neurology—was established. These early discussions developed the foundation for teamwork and allowed the program's foundation to develop. The framework of the program was based on the accrediting surgical critical care program guidelines established by the Accreditation Council for Graduate Medical Education (ACGME). The ACGME is the governing body responsible for all graduate medical programs in the United States. This council dictates the requirements of all medical training programs and provides the rubric for trainees' successful completion of any program. All SCC programs are required to be 12 months in length comprising nine months in a surgical intensive care unit and three months of elective clinical experiences. The SCC Fellowship must have regular educational didactics, and promote Fellow autonomy.

The infrastructure of the program was built by creating processes within the institution that would allow prospective fellows to meet the ACGME's six core competencies:

- ***Professionalism:*** Fellows must demonstrate a commitment to professionalism and an adherence to ethical principles. Our Fellows are given progressive responsibilities to lead residents, students and staff on surgical ICU rounds demonstrating and practicing their leadership, clinical decision-making, and bedside manner.

- ***Patient care and procedural skills***: Fellows must be able to provide patient care that is compassionate, appropriate, and effectively address health problems. Fellows must be able to perform all medical, diagnostic, and surgical procedures considered essential for the area of practice. Through rotations in our ICUs - Surgical, Cardiothoracic, Burn, Medical, Neurological, Pediatric and Neonatal - our fellows develop a comprehensive critical care skill set. Fellows are primarily responsible for leading or supervising all intensive care related procedures.
- ***Medical knowledge:*** Fellows must demonstrate knowledge of established and evolving biomedical, clinical, epidemiological and social-behavioral sciences, as well as the application of this knowledge to patient care. The daily management of a diverse patient population across all our ICUs offers the opportunity for our fellows to demonstrate and exercise their medical knowledge. The Trauma Center's introduction resulted in a large volume of historically marginalized African-American patients from Chicago's South Side. The fellows would be part of the University's efforts to build trust and advocate for these patients including supporting violence prevention experts and the medical legal program.
- ***Practice-based Learning and Improvement***: Fellows must demonstrate the ability to investigate and evaluate their patients' care, to appraise and assimilate scientific evidence, and to continuously improve patient care based on constant self-evaluation and lifelong learning. Through monthly journal clubs and weekly Morbidity and Mortality conferences, our fellows are afforded the opportunity to assess the literature and apply it to patient care in an evidence-based manner. We have developed a weekly multidisciplinary conference where all ICU fellows and faculty come together to discuss interesting cases and topics in critical care from an evidence-based approach.
- ***Interpersonal and communication skills***: Fellows must demonstrate an effective exchange of information and collaboration with patients, their families, and health professionals. The supervised autonomy provided to our Fellows allows them to lead discussions with the team, consultants, patients and families while on rounds. Our Fellows develop competencies in moderating difficult discussions regarding treatment plans, outcomes and end-of-life care.
- ***Systems- based practice:*** Fellows must demonstrate an awareness of and responsiveness to the health care system, including the social determinants of health impact on patient services. The weekly surgical ICU morbidity and mortality conference offers the opportunity to elevate discussions about system processes and socioeconomic limitations for patients.

Building the program through this framework required strategic planning and input from institutional and major stakeholders. Most importantly, the Fellow's contribution to directing their education was integrated into their yearlong curriculum. The creation of an all-encompassing clinical experience is one element of the Fellowship. The appreciation of individual career direction and complementing each learner's ultimate professional goals through a tailored experience is our strength [6].

Philosophy

The program's foundation was built upon a desire to serve Chicago's Southside, a predominately African-American population that has been historically marginalized secondary to inequities in education, health care and professional opportunities. Our mission statement is "to train the next generation of intensive care specialists to provide the highest quality critical care with an emphasis on eradicating healthcare disparities and promoting social justice in medicine". Our program is committed to an empathic and holistic approach to the health care. This in turn requires our Fellows to have a passion to mitigate these healthcare disparities and promote equity [7].

The needs of the Southside community and servicing victims of violent injury make this Fellowship program unique. Our Fellowship experience is not solely centered on bedside care. Fellows are intimately aware of the social vulnerabilities and social determinants of health (SDH) (Economic Stability, Education Access and Quality, Health Care Access and Quality, Neighborhood and Built Environment, Social and Community Context) which affect our patients [7]. While the SDH is beyond the scope of this chapter, these core element directly influence our patient's outcomes and opportunities; their absence or influence often impair our patient's ability to receive appropriate care or attain social advancement. Our Fellows address these issues daily. Our Fellows also work alongside the program's violence recovery team to ensure the environment, which may have contributed to the event that brought a patient to our facility, is identified and instigating factors are mitigated.

Fellowship Selection

Aside from the academic excellence required by all programs, we also prioritize understanding the SDH and a commitment to underprivileged populations. To remove personal biases, all information regarding name, gender, race, and age are removed for each application. The applicant's American Board of Surgery In-Service Examination scores are reviewed. Published manuscripts and conference presentations are screened for content regarding subject matter for Trauma, Acute Care Surgery, or Social Sciences topics. Finally the Curriculum Vitae and Personal Statement are reviewed with attention to key words or phrases such as: "social service", "community", "volunteer", or "international experience". Each applicant is scored on a Likert Scale (2: Interview; 1: Potentially Interview, 0: No interview) in an independent manner by the Program and Assistant Program Director. Those with the highest combined scores are selected for an in-person interview. Web Based interviews are not performed. All Attending Surgeons and Advanced Practice Providers interview the Applicants. Applicants are scored on a second Likert scale (0–5: 0-Not selected to 5-Must Select for Fellowship) by each Interviewer. These scores are averaged to obtain a composite number. Additionally the Interviewer's personalized comments are also recorded. The candidates are numerically ranked and discussed during a ranking meeting where the finally list is created.

The Fellowship of the Future

The future of the fellowship is directed by the continued evolution of general surgery, trauma care, and critical care. As advances in surgical technology and techniques are ever progressing, fellowship training and sub-specialization have become a common pathway for today's general surgery graduates. This has led to a void in general surgery providers and a growing need in emergency surgical care. This resulted in the creation of a new specialty: Acute Care Surgery (ACS). The acute care surgeon can address surgical emergencies and their complex physiologic derangements. The modern acute care surgeon integrates the general surgeon, critical care surgeon, emergency general surgeon and trauma surgeon into one entity. (Kelly et al. 2012) There are five core pillars of acute care surgery. "Surgical rescue" was introduced as the fifth pillar, an additional skillset for the management of procedural complications.

The future of the UCM SCC Fellowship program is limitless. The fellowship's growth includes an expansion to a two-year program, incorporating trauma care and emergency general surgery into the second year. While the first year remains predominantly critical care focused, it will continue to include elective time for learning skills such as: airway management, echocardiography/bedside ultrasound, experiences in surgical rescue, as well as international rotations. We continue to promote social science and basic science scholarship opportunities for our fellows. Alongside these education and research endeavors, we hope to establish the national standard in advocacy efforts for vulnerable communities.

References

1. Camison L, et al. The history of surgical education in the United States: past, present, and future. Ann Surg Open. 2022;3(1):e148.
2. van der Leeuw RM, et al. A systematic review of the effects of residency training on patient outcomes. BMC Med. 2012;10:65.
3. Hanson CW 3rd, et al. Effects of an organized critical care service on outcomes and resource utilization: a cohort study. Crit Care Med. 1999;27(2):270–4.
4. Frankel HL, et al. The role and value of surgical critical care, an essential component of Acute Care Surgery, in the Affordable Care Act: a report from the Critical Care Committee and Board of Managers of the American Association for the Surgery of Trauma. J Trauma Acute Care Surg. 2012;73(1):20–6.
5. Williams M, et al. In-hospital fellow coverage reduces communication errors in the surgical intensive care unit. J Crit Care. 2014;29(3):445–9.
6. Herr KD, et al. Creating and sustaining a successful fellowship program: challenges and solutions. Curr Probl Diagn Radiol. 2017;46(2):95–9.

7. University of Chicago (Ed.). Adult Surgical Critical Care Fellowship. Department of Surgery | The University of Chicago; n.d. https://surgery.uchicago.edu/education/adult-surgical-critical-care-fellowship

Building a Trauma Fellowship

Lea Hoefer and Priya S. Prakash

Surgical Training in the Twenty-First Century

Building a trauma center with long-term vision meant not only recruiting top talent, setting up efficient systems, and providing excellent trauma care 24/7; but also meant commitment to training the trauma surgeons of the future. Going beyond integrating existing surgical, anesthesia and emergency medicine residencies into the functions of the new trauma center, we sought to establish a dedicated fellowship to train surgeons in the developing discipline of Trauma and Acute Care Surgery, with a focus on operative trauma surgery.

Changes over the last several decades in the structure and content of general surgical training have meant that fewer graduating surgical residents enter straight into practice as 'general surgeons' than in the past. Most will now go on to complete fellowships in a surgical subspecialty [1]. Declines in resident autonomy in surgical cases may be in part responsible for this as many residents feel less ready for independent practice [2, 3]. Other factors that may play into this shift include increased compensation available through specialization, earlier exposure to subspecialists, mentorship, and lifestyle factors [1]. This trend towards specialization had threatened to worsen the shortage of general surgeons, as most graduates would go on to perform a smaller number of procedures rather than a broad swath of general surgery services [4]. Additionally, the early nineties saw a decline in general surgery graduates who identified as willing to provide care to the injured [5].

In the midst of this transition to increased specialization, the field of Acute Care Surgery has arisen as an answer to the dearth of general surgeons and trauma providers. The last twenty years have seen the rise of Acute Care Surgery as a specialty that

L. Hoefer · P. S. Prakash (✉)
University of Chicago Department of Surgery, Chicago, IL, USA
e-mail: lea.hoefer@uchicagomedicine.org; pprakash@bsd.uchicago.edu

S. O. Rogers, Jr (ed.), *Creating a Modern Trauma Center*,
https://doi.org/10.1007/978-3-031-66524-0_23

has stepped in to fill this gap and defined itself as encompassing surgical critical care, trauma surgery, and emergency general surgery. As the specialty began to define itself, multiple models were discussed amongst those who were most committed to the preservation of trauma care in surgery. Many were concerned that trauma and critical care alone would not be enough to sustain a robust surgical practice due the increasingly non operative nature of trauma care and the risk for surgical skill deterioration [6]. The inclusion of general surgery practice, and specifically emergency general surgery, filled out the operative practices at centers with lower volumes of operative trauma and cemented the future of Acute Care Surgery as a robust specialty [7, 8]. While the term "acute care surgery" is sometimes used to refer to what is in actuality emergency general surgery, in this chapter, we will specifically discuss Acute Care Surgery (ACS) and ACS training as a paradigm encompassing trauma surgery, surgical critical care (SCC), and emergency general surgery (EGS).

Creating a Robust Experience

One of the main priorities in starting a Trauma fellowship at the University of Chicago was to create a program that would truly train trauma surgeons of the future. This meant training surgeons who are equipped to care for the sickest patients in a variety of situations, with a focus on being able to handle the most complicated traumatic operative emergencies. In his 2017 Scudder Oration at the Clinical Congress of the American College of Surgeons, Dr. LD Britt stated "…there is little doubt that Dr. Halsted was referring to an acute care surgeon when he stated, "Every important hospital should have on its resident staff of surgeons at least one who is well and able to deal with any emergency that may arise."" [9]. Anticipating the high volume of operative trauma that our center would see, there was little doubt early on that fellows trained at our institution would have the opportunity to develop the surgical skills to meet the profile described by Dr. Halsted long ago.

Having treated over 25,000 injured patients, with gunshot wounds being the leading mechanism of injury, the University of Chicago has been uniquely suited to provide fellows with a robust operative experience that remains centered around our own trauma surgery service. Trauma surgeons at the University of Chicago have developed a practice where the trauma surgeon is truly a specialist in their field and can handle a wide variety of operative case. Our surgeons routinely perform operations including abdominal visceral and solid organ trauma, extremity and abdominal vascular repairs, both video-assisted and open thoracic and cardiac surgery, and neck explorations.

The benefit of focusing the fellow operative experience on our trauma service and not on off-service rotations is that fellows receive intensive education in trauma-specific pathology and management. While other surgical specialists have a wealth of knowledge and experience in their respective fields, many deal with disease processes and pathophysiology that differ significantly from those encountered on the trauma service itself. Receiving operative training primarily in trauma surgery allows fellows to develop a knowledge and skill base particularly well suited to managing patients with complex and multi-system traumatic injuries. Fellows learn the principles of damage control surgery, yet are also capable of performing complex dissections and definitive repairs. Trauma faculty have the opportunity to pass on experience and wisdom gained from years of performing trauma operations and provide role modeling and mentorship for the next generation.

Another core component of developing a robust trauma surgery and critical care fellowship was creating a comprehensive surgical critical care training experience. The range of specialty intensive care units (ICUs) at our institution provided an opportunity to expose fellows to experts in cardiothoracic physiology, neurocritical care and neurotrauma, and surgical critical care. Rotations in these subspecialty ICUs allows fellows to gain experience in managing extra corporeal membrane oxygenation (ECMO), blunt and penetrating neurologic trauma, and a wide range of complex pre and post-operative surgical pathophysiology.

Alongside developing operative and clinical skills, a key training experience for trauma fellows is leading a multi-disciplinary trauma team. In our center, that meant creating opportunities for trauma fellows to lead a multidisciplinary team of surgical and emergency medicine trainees and advanced practice providers, collaborate with subspecialty surgeons, and work closely with non-physician staff and clinicians in providing wrap-around trauma care. As discussed in another chapter, integrating longitudinal violence recovery services into trauma care was an immediate priority of our trauma center. Collaborating with violence recovery specialists provides fellows with the opportunity to develop holistic trauma-informed care practices that will elevate their surgical and clinical care of injured patients.

Lastly, the development of our fellowship training paradigms has gone hand in hand with the development of our research program. Starting trauma focused laboratories, developing extensive clinical databases, and participating in multicenter studies and clinical trials is key to providing fellows with the opportunity to contribute to the trauma literature and engage with the academic community. Fellows also have the opportunity to engage in academic development outside of our section by participating in Medical Center or University-wide programs focused on areas such as clinical ethics, community engagement, and surgical education. We feel that supporting trauma fellows in producing research that can be discussed and disseminated at a national level is key to not only their professional development, but also their development as future surgeon-scientists who can advance the field of trauma and critical care.

Tenants of Long-Term Success

In order to ensure the long-term success of the fellowship, it was important to include input from institutional Graduate Medical Education (GME) and Department of Surgery (DOS) residency leadership. Although trauma surgery is not currently certified as an accredited fellowship by the Accreditation Fellowship for Graduate

Medical Education (ACGME), we felt it was important to engrain their frameworks for training into the development of our program.

The ACGME provides standards that ensure that graduate medical education provides a rigorous and standardized training experience, and that the trainees have a safe and effective learning environment. Wanting to engrain these values into our fellowship, we built in ACGME standards such as setting work hour limits for fellows, designating specific faculty education coordinators, providing fellows with ongoing feedback and evaluation, and ensuring that they were integrated into existing training programs in a manner that supported the educational experiences of all levels of trainees.

We also sought to support the long-term success of our program not just by meeting educational standards such as those set by the ACGME, but also by actively supporting fellows in thriving as people both outside the hospital and in. We did this not just by meeting basic requirements such as safe, comfortable call room spaces and enforcing work hour restrictions, but also by ensuring fellows felt empowered by flexible training schedules to take time for important life events such as parental or family leave time.

Recruiting the Next Generation

The evidence is clear that recruiting a diverse population of trainees benefits patients by increasing innovation and discovery, improving communication, and improving clinical outcomes [10–12]. At our institution, we ensure that all faculty involved in interviewing undergo implicit bias training prior to being involved in interviewing and our program centers fair evaluation processes in our recruitment process. Fellows have the opportunity to continue to participate in our department's work to center diversity and equity in all aspects of our work by continuing to participate in the Diversity, Equity, and Inclusion steering committee, subcommittees, or their programming.

As our center and training programs continue to evolve, we have the opportunity to extend the impact of trauma training into residency, medical school, and beyond. Bringing a level one trauma center to the University of Chicago not only drastically changed the experience of the general surgical and subspecialty surgical residents, but changed the type of residents which were recruited to our program. Anecdotally, the existence of a high-volume level one trauma center at our institution has attracted high-performing medical students from across the country with a strong interest in trauma and critical care.

As our center has grown and developed, we have begun to provide opportunities for residents to engage in trauma focused research during their academic development years. This longitudinal research time has provided residents with opportunities for publication, podium presentations at national trauma conferences, and exposure to the field that—along with their robust operative trauma experience during their clinical years—well prepares them to apply for competitive fellowships in trauma and surgical critical care, both at our own institution and across the country. Our trauma center has also drawn medical, pre-medical, and even high school students to participate in research, clinical shadowing, and clinical care when appropriate, thus creating a pipeline of clinical exposure and trauma surgeon development that starts at the early stages of higher education.

Continuing to Elevate the Trauma Training Experience

While creating a brand-new trauma center gave our institution the opportunity to develop a Trauma and Acute Care Surgery fellowship from inception, the changing landscape of healthcare means that continuous improvement and reassessment is critical to maintaining a high-level training experience. We continue to explore training paradigms and opportunities to enhance their training. While our center provides a robust operative trauma experience with some of the most complex patients, tertiary academic centers are often limited in their exposure to 'bread and butter' emergency general surgery patients. Like many institutions, we continue to explore ways we can leverage our partnerships with community partners to train fellows who can practice in any environment and are prepared to handle any case independently.

Continuous evaluation of training program effectiveness and outcomes is important to ensure that we remain at the forefront of acute care surgery education. Just as ACS as a specialty has evolved and continued to change over the last two decades, as our understanding of surgical science, injury epidemiology, and clinical care continues to refine, we will need to continue to adjust our practices to truly continue to train the surgeons of the future.

References

1. Borman KR, Vick LR, Biester TW, Mitchell ME. Changing demographics of residents choosing fellowships: longterm data from the American Board of Surgery. J Am Coll Surg. 2008;206(5):782–8; discussion 8–9
2. Thelen AE, Marcotte KM, Diaz S, Gates R, Chen X, George BC, Krumm AE. Variation in competence of graduating general surgery trainees. J Surg Educ. 2024;81(1):17–24.
3. Oliver JB, McFarlane JL, Kunac A, Anjaria DJ. Declining resident surgical autonomy and improving surgical outcomes: correlation does not equal causality. J Surg Educ. 2023;80(3):434–41.
4. Stitzenberg KB, Sheldon GF. Progressive specialization within general surgery: adding to the complexity of workforce planning. J Am Coll Surg. 2005;201(6):925–32.
5. Richardson JD, Miller FB. Will future surgeons be interested in trauma care? Results of a resident survey. J Trauma. 1992;32(2):229–33; discussion 33–5
6. Richardson JD, Spain DA, Livingston DH. Trauma and acute care surgery: the evolution of a specialty. J Trauma Acute Care Surg. 2022;92(2):242–9.

7. Richardson JD, Miller FB, Polk HC. Can we improve the surgical manpower for providing trauma care? A model for success. J Trauma. 1993;34(6):773–4.
8. Spain DA. A review of "Will Future Surgeons Be Interested in Trauma Care? Results of a Resident Survey" (1992). Am Surg. 2021;87(2):191–4.
9. Britt LD. Trauma: still the cornerstone of acute care surgery specialty. J Am Coll Surg. 2018;226(3):211–22.
10. Wallis CJD, Jerath A, Aminoltejari K, Kaneshwaran K, Salles A, Coburn N, Wright FC, Gotlib Conn L, Klaassen Z, Luckenbaugh AN, et al. Surgeon sex and long-term postoperative outcomes among patients undergoing common surgeries. JAMA Surg. 2023;158(11):1185–94.
11. Valenzuela F, Romero Arenas MA. Underrepresented in surgery: (lack of) diversity in academic surgery faculty. J Surg Res. 2020;254:170–4.
12. West MA, Hwang S, Maier RV, Ahuja N, Angelos P, Bass BL, Brasel KJ, Chen H, Davis KA, Eberlein TJ, et al. Ensuring equity, diversity, and inclusion in academic surgery: an American surgical association white paper. Ann Surg. 2018;268(3):403–7.

Military Civilian Partnership at the University of Chicago Trauma Center

Nicholas Jaszczak, Timothy P. Plackett, and Kenneth L. Wilson

Main Body of Chapter

Violence and war are a great burden for society. We see this sad burden in both the military and civilian environments. Unintentional injury is the leading cause of death in the United States for all people from the age of 1 through 44 [1]. Although in most civilian settings, the traumatic injury mechanism tends to be different from those seen in the military, certain areas of Chicago see levels of gun violence that mimic a war zone. A tragic reality is that the risk of firearm-related death and injury among young adult males in some areas of Chicago has been shown to be higher than during wartime service in Iraq and Afghanistan [2]. Regardless of whether a traumatic injury occurs in a military or civilian setting, our goals of preserving life and minimizing morbidity are the same. Throughout history some of the biggest advances in reaching these goals have come during periods of conflict as the experience in treating a high volume of casualties has led to innovations in care.

The recent prolonged wars in Iraq and Afghanistan have exhibited several of these advancements that arise from the horrors of war and violence. The decades of war have led to an increased focus on the rapid control of hemorrhage through the use of tourniquets, early evacuation to definitive surgical care, and a focus on blood product based damage control resuscitation. The spread of these innovations has saved lives in both the military and civilian world. As these conflicts have come to

N. Jaszczak (✉) · T. P. Plackett · K. L. Wilson
Department of Surgery, Section of Trauma and Acute Care Surgery, University of Chicago, Chicago, IL, USA
e-mail: njaszczak@bsd.uchicago.edu; tplackett@bsd.uchicago.edu; Kwilson9@bsd.uchicago.edu

S. O. Rogers, Jr (ed.), *Creating a Modern Trauma Center*,
https://doi.org/10.1007/978-3-031-66524-0_24

a close, it remains important to continue to make advances in trauma care for the benefit of future patients.

With this clear common purpose in mind, collaborations between military and civilian trauma care are currently expanding. The military civilian partnership at The University of Chicago is one of eight collaborations with academic civilian trauma centers initiated by the Army Surgeon General. The Army Medical Department Military Civilian Trauma Team Training (AMCT3) program was developed with the mission to ensure medical skills sustainment of critical wartime specialties with an emphasis on ensuring the readiness of those personnel serving on 24 active duty Forward Resuscitative and Surgical Detachments (FRSD). The collaboration at the University of Chicago was aligned with the 759th FRSD which was an unprecedented alignment of an FRSD to a civilian training platform. Four members of the FRSD are stationed full time with a goal of expanding to include shorter term rotation of other team members. In 2021 the AMCT3 program at The University of Chicago was initiated with 2 active duty surgeons. These surgeons were soon joined by an emergency medicine physician, a certified registered nurse anesthetist (CRNA), two nurses and a physician assistant (PA). In this chapter we will review the long history of military and civilian collaboration in our country, discuss significant events in expanding these relationships, review the benefits to both sides of the partnership, and discuss the experience at the University of Chicago.

Although there has been a recent growing interest in military civilian collaboration, this is not a new concept. Over a century ago as our nation faced the challenge of caring for the large scale casualties from World War I, military and civilian collaboration was instrumental in meeting the needs of the injured. As the war in Europe grew, the Army knew its medical resources were not enough. The Surgeon General of the Army, Major General William C. Gorgas told Congress in January 1916 that it had less than 5 physicians per 1000 men [3]. Civilian surgeon Dr. George Crile who had volunteered in the Spanish-American War and at an American hospital outside of Paris early in the war advocated that major US civilian hospitals contribute to the war effort [4]. The American Red Cross joined this project and collaborated with the US military to form base hospitals organized from the staff at major academic institutions. These civilian center affiliated base hospitals formed the backbone of the hospital service in France [5]. Although a variety of factors over time eventually led to a different organization of medical care, the positive impact of these collaborations must not be forgotten.

In modern times we have also recently seen the benefit of the collaboration of military and civilian medical care in the response to COVID-19. The pandemic presented challenges to our civilian health care system that were addressed with significant support from the US military. The Department of Defense led multiagency governmental vaccination development and logistics (Operation Warp Speed), embedded medical teams in US hospitals and auxiliary care sites and administered vaccines at Community Vaccination Centers at the request of the Federal Emergency Management Agency [6].

Unfortunately, our country has also had to learn the lessons of what can happen when there hasn't been adequate collaboration between military and civilian trauma care. Following Operation Desert Storm in the early 1990's, Donald Trunkey reviewed the Army's medical capability for the conflict. Dr. Trunkey's article on Lessons Learned highlighted deficiencies in preparation for the wartime mission including a need to maintain currency in trauma care through training in a contemporary civilian trauma center [7]. In response to this critique, Congress passed legislation in 1996 requiring the Department of Defense to conduct a demonstration project of trauma training in a civilian hospital [8]. In 1998 a Forward Surgical Team was sent for 1 month of training at Ben Taub General Hospital. Although this collaboration subsequently ended, it encouraged the development of other collaborations. In 2000 the US Army established a training program at Ryder Trauma Center in Miami. The US Navy established a program at Los Angeles County/University of Southern California Trauma Center. The US Air Force established programs at University of Maryland Shock Trauma Center, St. Louis University, and the University of Cincinnati Trauma Center.

While these partnerships were able to build connections between military and civilian trauma care, there was still a need for further collaboration. In 2014 the Military Health System entered into a strategic partnership with the American College of Surgeons (MHSSPACS) with the goal of exchanging information in surgical quality, education and training, trauma systems and research. Then in 2016, a landmark report from the National Academies of Sciences, Engineering and Medicine advocated for a national trauma care system integrating military and civilian trauma systems to achieve zero preventable deaths after injury. The recommendations in this report stimulated legislative action. In the National Defense Authorization Act for Fiscal Year 2017, Section 708 Congress mandated the Department of Defense to establish partnerships with civilian academic medical centers to maintain critical wartime medical readiness skills and competencies. This subsequently was made into law through the Mission Zero Act passed as part of the Pandemic and All-Hazards Preparedness and Advancing Innovation Act of 2019. A framework guiding these collaborations was published by the American College of Surgeons in 2020 called The Blue Book: Military-Civilian Partnerships for Trauma Training, Sustainment, and Readiness. Multiple military and civilian partnerships have developed since this time including the partnership at the University of Chicago.

Recent literature continues to support the ongoing necessity of these partnerships. In a comprehensive analysis of combat casualties over the past 80 years Cannon confirmed a long suspected "peacetime effect" on mortality with higher observed to expected mortality ratios after periods of relative peace [9]. The vital importance of maintaining currency in trauma care at all times is now widely recognized although a single best method of maintaining this currency is not agreed upon. One aspect of currency in trauma surgery is surgical caseload. The surgical volume at Army hospitals has been shown to be significantly lower than at civilian hospitals [10]. As surgical volume is only one aspect of maintaining readiness, attempts have been made to better delineate what determines readiness for trauma care. With the goal of promoting readiness of military surgeons, the MHSSPACS developed the Knowledge, Skills, and Abilities (KSA) Clinical Readiness Program (CRP). The

KSA metric developed from this program provides a means to quantify deficits in clinical readiness. An analysis using this metric showed that KSA metric points and procedural volume at military hospitals has been decreasing since 2015 whereas these have been increasing in civilian hospitals [11]. All of this suggests that exposure to trauma relevant care at military hospitals alone is not enough. Collaboration with civilian partners therefore benefits the military community.

At the same time, partnership with the military benefits the needs of the civilian community. The opening of an adult trauma center at the University of Chicago in 2018 brought much needed trauma care to the South Side of Chicago. The area surrounding the hospital experiences a high level of gun violence and had previously been considered a trauma desert without rapid access to a level one trauma center [12]. Upon opening, the trauma volume quickly exceeded expectations. In the first year, it treated 2988 adult trauma cases with an initial staff of 7 trauma surgeons. The volume of patients seen increased annually and by 2021 the volume was up to 4772 adult trauma cases. The additional staffing provided through the military partnership helped the hospital meet the needs of the community. Additionally, knowledge shared from military deployment experience to colleagues, fellows, residents and students has enhanced the training at this academic institution.

Implementation of the military civilian partnership at the University of Chicago has been aided by several factors. First, the Trauma Medical Director has extensive military experience as a US Army Reserve Surgeon. The vision for the flow of patients in the trauma bay has been shaped by his extensive deployment experience with an overall goal of having the trauma bay function like a combat based forward surgical team. The University of Chicago has a long history of collaboration with the government dating back to World War II when scientists working on the Manhattan Project developed the world's first controlled self-sustaining nuclear reaction under the University of Chicago's football field stands. Current collaboration with the military at the University is encouraged by the Office of the Provost's Office for Military-Affiliated Communities.

The collaboration at the University of Chicago launched in 2021 initially with trauma surgery. The surgeons were brought into a trauma and acute care surgery section that covers three different services: trauma, surgical critical care, and acute care surgery. While the trauma service is exclusively covered by the trauma surgeons, institutional responsibility for surgical critical care is shared with anesthesia critical care, and the acute care surgery institutional coverage is shared with general surgery. This results in approximately 75% of time being dedicated to trauma, 15% to acute care surgery, and 10% to surgical critical care. During onboarding, the new trauma surgeon spends time on all three service lines with senior faculty available to provide mentorship as needed. The very first week of service is generally a full week of running the trauma service during the daytime and is taken paired with a senior partner. All subsequent shifts were taken independently. This onboarding process lasts approximately 2 months.

Both the university and the military have benefitted from the care provided through this partnership. A review of cases performed by military surgeons at the University of Chicago in their first year illustrates that the experience has been robust. One AMCT3 surgeon performed 444 trauma evaluations and resuscitations. This resulted in 185 operative procedures, including 80 laparotomies, 15 thoracotomies, 15 vascular exposures, and 20 vascular repairs and/or shunt placements. The other AMCT3 surgeon performed 424 trauma evaluations and resuscitations. This resulted in 194 operative procedures, including 92 laparotomies, 15 thoracotomies, 25 vascular exposures, and 17 vascular repairs and/or shunt placements. Particularly relevant is the number of vascular cases performed, as deploying surgeons have typically self-reported low the levels of confidence with these procedures [13]. The relatively high volumes of vascular trauma cases have left both surgeons comfortable performing these procedures to the extent that one was recently deployed to fill the vascular surgeon position during a deployment. From the University of Chicago perspective, the work of these two surgeons covers approximately 16% of the clinical coverage for this trauma and acute care surgery section. They also provide formal lectures and bedside teaching on daily rounds with the fellows, residents and medical students. Both surgeons have been recognized with teaching excellence awards and have expanded the knowledge of the next generation of surgeons.

In addition to the trauma surgeons, other disciplines have also become a part of the partnership. The Army team also includes an emergency medicine physician, a certified registered nurse anesthetist, a critical care nurse, an emergency room nurse and a physician assistant. All of these providers have been able to maintain currency in acute trauma care through their work at this busy trauma center while providing great care to the patients in this community. Future goals of the program at the University of Chicago are to expand it to provide training for US Army reserve members in the region as the initial experience has been so successful.

The success of this partnership is a great example of the benefits of collaboration between military and civilian trauma care. The common goals of improving trauma care make this seem like an intuitively obvious necessity for the nation. Lessons learned in both the military and civilian environment benefit health care in the other. Collaboration now also has the potential to make it easier to coordinate healthcare when sudden catastrophic events overwhelm resources in a certain area whether that be a large scale foreign conflict or local natural disaster. Expansion of military-civilian trauma care partnerships like this over time show great promise for the benefit to all.

References

1. 10 Leading Causes of Death, United States 2020. https://wisqars.cdc.gov/data/lcd/home
2. Del Pozo. Comparing risks of firearm-related death and injury among young adult males in selected us cities with wartime service in Iraq and Afghanistan. JAMA Network Open. 5(12):32248132.
3. Ryan. Walter B. Cannon's World War I experience: treatment of traumatic shock then and now. Adv Physiol Educ. 2018;42:267–76.
4. Marble. Professional doctors but amateur soldiers: the US Army's affiliated hospitals program, 1915–1955. War Society. 2008;27(1):39–58.

5. AMEDD Center of History & Heritage: Development of Red Cross Medical Department Units. https://achh.army.mil/history/book-wwi-volisgo-gen02
6. Goralnick. Improving care during peacetime war and disasters: a call for agile military civilian strategic alliances. Ann Surg. 2022;276:3657–e658.
7. Trunkey. Lessons learned. Arch Surg. 1993;128:261–4.
8. Schreiber. Military trauma training performed in a civilian trauma center. J Surg Res. 2002;104:8–14.
9. Cannon. Comprehensive analysis of combat casualty outcomes in US service members from the beginning of World War II to the end of Operation Enduring Freedom. J Trauma. 2020;89(supplement 2):s8–s15.
10. Edwards. Army general surgery's crisis of conscience. J Am Coll Surg. 2018;226(6):1190–4.
11. Dalton. Analysis of surgical volume in military medical treatment facilities and clinical combat readiness of US military surgeons. JAMA Surg. 2022;157(1):43–50.
12. Crandall. Trauma deserts: distance from a trauma center, transport times, and mortality from gunshot wounds in Chicago. Am J Public Health. 2013;103(6):1103–9.
13. Tyler. Combat readiness for the modern military surgeon: data from a decade of combat operations. J Trauma Acute Care Surg. 2012;73:s64–70.

The Making of a Medical-Legal Partnership in a Level I Trauma Center: Recovery Legal Care

Tanya L. Zakrison, Rhea Pillai, Nisha Sen-Gupta, Julia Chavez, Ernestina Perez, Carly Loughran, Isaac Green, Christine Goggins, Kimora Custon, Franklin Cosey-Gay, Carlos Robles, and Elizabeth Tung

Background to the Structural Determinants of Health

Firearm violence is an urgent public health crisis in the United States (US). **More than 652,000 people** in the US died from firearm injuries between 1999 and 2018 [1]. Compounded by the pandemic and its many effects, 2020 became the deadliest year for gun crime in recent history. The trend continues in 2021 with more than 26,000 gun violence deaths occurring to-date [2]. Firearm homicide, in particular, is the third leading cause of death among persons aged 10 to 24 years and is **the leading cause of death among Black men (<45 years of age)** [3]. This disproportional racial impact that this preventable homicide has on individuals and communities of color has been identified as an urgent human rights crisis [4]. Even those who recover from firearm injury face significant barriers to support for adequate recovery [5].

Absent a serious consideration of the macro-level context in which this crisis of firearm violence persists, especially regarding the ubiquitous role that the Social Determinants of Health (SDOH) play in society, solutions cannot be generated. The SDOH are "conditions in the places where people live, learn, work, and play that

T. L. Zakrison (✉) · R. Pillai · N. Sen-Gupta · J. Chavez · E. Perez · C. Loughran · I. Green
C. Goggins · K. Custon · F. Cosey-Gay · C. Robles · E. Tung
Section of Trauma & Acute Care Surgery, Department of Surgery, University of Chicago, Chicago, IL, USA
e-mail: tzakrison@bsd.uchicago.edu; rheapillai@uchicago.edu; Nisha.Sen-Gupta@bsd.uchicago.edu; juliachavez@uchicago.edu; Ernestina.Perez@uchicagomedicine.org; cjl78@georgetown.edu; igreen@legalaidchicago.org; Kimora.Custon@uchicagomedicine.org; fgay@uchicago.edu; FranklinN.Cosey-Gay@uchicagomedicine.org; Carlos.Robles@uchicagomedicine.org; etung2@bsd.uchicago.edu

S. O. Rogers, Jr (ed.), *Creating a Modern Trauma Center*,
https://doi.org/10.1007/978-3-031-66524-0_25

Fig. 1 The SDOH

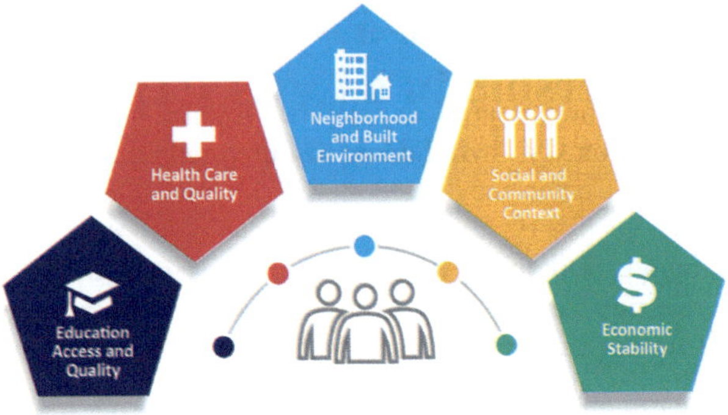

affect a wide range of health and quality-of life-risks and outcomes" [6]. These range from ensuring access to economic stability, quality education and health care, ensuring a safe neighborhood and social and community networks (Fig. 1).

The absence of adequate SDOH increases the risk of community-level firearm violence. In particular, the rich-poor gap, lack of economic opportunity and public welfare spending have demonstrated robust associations with firearm homicide rates [7]. The SDOH have also been recognized by patients and providers alike as being a root cause of firearm injury and mortality [8]. Historic and structural racism has increasingly been recognized to be a major contributor to the community-level firearm violence that persists in urban centers throughout the US [9]. For example, historic redlining of communities of color can be traced directly to census tract metropolitan areas with the highest rate of contemporary firearm violence [10–12]. In fact, the SDOH are often considered in parallel to the *Structural* Determinants of Health which examine "all social and political mechanisms that generate…stratification and social class divisions in society and that define individual socioeconomic position within hierarchies of power, prestige and access to resources" [13].

According to the conceptual framework established by the World Health Organization's Commission on the Social Determinants of Health (CSDH), these structural determinants of health interact through intermediary determinants which are themselves considered SDOH. To address the inequities in the SDOH, the CSDH recommends:

1. targeted programs for disadvantaged populations.
2. closing health gaps between worse-off and better-off groups.
3. addressing the social health gradient across the whole population.

Addressing both the Structural and SDOH (SSDOH) have been recognized as crucial in both the prevention and recovery of firearm injury, especially in the pediatric population [14, 15].

Trauma centers have been recognized as hospitals with specialized human and material resources that are best organized to care for moderately to severely injured trauma patients, affording them the best chance for survival [16]. This remains true when treating victims of firearm violence, including pediatric age groups [17]. In the US, trauma centers stand on the front lines of the interpersonal firearm violence epidemic. With injury re-injury rates as high as 65%, injury prevention advocates are exploring ways to close this revolving door to decrease violent injury, similar to the methods that have been used effectively to reduce the incidence of cardiovascular disease and cancer [18]. While trauma center designation is achieved through political and geographic pathways at the state level, harmonization of trauma quality of care occurs through the American College of Surgery's Committee on Trauma (ACS-COT) trauma center verification, review and consultation program [19]. In order to obtain ACS-COT verification credential, trauma centers *must* have an organized and effective approach to injury prevention and must prioritize those efforts based on local trauma registry and epidemiologic data [20]. This includes for the prevention of firearm violence. With trauma centers across the US increasing from 1154 in 2002 to over 1675 only 8 years later, the potential for nation-wide firearm injury prevention is significant [21, 22].

Given the widespread nature of firearm violence in the US, injury prevention programs affiliated with US trauma centers have been established as Hospital-Based Violence Intervention Programs (HVIPs). HVIPs are multidisciplinary, 4-step programs that identify patients at risk of repeat violent injury and link them with hospital and community-based resources aimed to address underlying risk factors for violence. The ACS-COT even provides information for trauma centers to establish their own HVIPs for injury prevention [18]. This injury prevention work is supported by society statements namely from the Eastern Association for the Surgery of Trauma (EAST) which is the largest trauma organization in the US [23]. Specifically for firearm violence, they call for "violence and injury prevention programs that address conflict resolution" with the "Recognition of the other factors that affect these issues including structural violence [the avoidable impairment of fundamental human needs [24]], domestic violence, and mental health." [25] While HVIPs focused on holistic care ranging from the individual to the SDOH, one of the key recommendations for HVIPs is the concept of the "teachable moment", immediately after the trauma patient is stabilized, "during which time a potential client is more likely to be amenable to change given that he/she just went through a major life event." [26] This historic HVIP focus on individual, attitudinal and behavioral change is pervasive in some centers while guidance on impacting the SDOH lacking [27]. HVIPs are often under-funded and under-resourced and thus face challenges in addressing the SDOH, even when mandated to do so [18].

Community-level violence that disproportionately affects young Black men is related to the interaction of structural, local, and individual factors including institutional racism, mass incarceration, poverty, neighborhood disadvantage, as well as social and individual trauma [28]. These specific factors may or may not be addressed in a standardized fashion in HVIPs as no core set of outcomes yet exist [29]. Given that the trauma re-injury rate for Black male survivors of firearm violence has been reported to be as high as 65% due to repeat violent victimization, re-focusing national HVIPs specifically on addressing the SSDOH, instead of individual behavior modification, remains a matter of public health urgency [30, 31].

Without addressing barriers to economic empowerment including income, housing, education, criminal records and family stability, true empowerment for legitimate violence prevention remains elusive. One novel approach for support of patients detrimentally affected by SDOH inequity is by providing individual, family and community support through medical-legal partnerships (MLP). MLPs connect medical and surgical providers with attorneys to advocate for the health care and collective human rights of patients by addressing their SSDOH [32–34]. While there is a significant research gap on the impact of MLP in trauma, the only study in the US to investigate this demonstrated that trauma-specific medical-legal needs were very prevalent with 73% of trauma patients having at least one medical-legal need addressing the SSDOH, with an average of 2.5 medical-legal needs per person [35]. We surveyed a consecutive, convenience sample of 61 trauma patients, close to 83% of our sample were young Black men with 73% presenting to clinic after gunshot wounds. Our own local data of post-discharge needs of trauma patients has also demonstrated that legal needs represent the second most important self-reported need, after financial needs. We are not aware of any trauma center with an MLP to connect legal supports to the SSDOH for patients affected by community-level firearm violence.

In 2018, the University of Chicago established a new Level I Trauma Center (UCMTC) after a hiatus of 30 years [36]. It is the only Level I Trauma Center located on the South Side of Chicago, located in one of the most violence-plagued and poverty-stricken counties in the country [37]. The South Side has a population of over 625,000 (23% of the population of Chicago), Reflecting our community demographics, 77% of trauma patients admitted to the UCMTC are African American (AA), 12% Latinx, with gunshot wound our most common mechanism of injury. Trauma admissions per year surpass 5000 with a 40% rate of penetrating trauma. According to the University of Chicago Medicine's Community Health Needs Assessment (2018–2019), 53% of the UCMTC service population live in poverty (including 43% of children) with 1 in 2 households at risk of food insecurity [38]. Building trauma resiliency with a focus on violence recovery and reducing health inequities by addressing the SSDOH (access to food, care and employment) have been highlighted as the top 2 of 3 most urgent health priorities facing our South Side communities. The combination inequity in the SSDOH and violence from firearm injury and premature death from chronic illness is so extreme that AA Chicagoans lose more than 9–15 years off their lives, with the racial health gap widening [39].

The UCMTC HVIP, called the Violence Recovery Program (VRP), was established through Michelle Obama's Urban Health Initiative at the University of Chicago, beginning when the trauma center opened. This program provides patients affected by intentional, interpersonal violence and their families with wraparound care for recovery from traumatic injuries. VRP care at UCMTC also begins at the bedside of the trauma patient during the teachable moment. Services include case management, crisis intervention, psychological first aid, re-injury risk assessment, safe discharge planning, community-based service referrals, and help with navigating external health care and social services. Despite excellent individual care, these support systems still face challenges because they cannot fully address the SSDOH as there are currently no legal or financial supports provided through this service.

The Medical-Legal Trauma Partnership

One such strategy that has demonstrated impact in various medical contexts has been the creation of MLPs. These partnerships integrate the expertise of attorneys and legal advocates into healthcare systems, with the goal of addressing structural inequities—particularly the stark inequities in access to justice—that underlie many health inequities. Leveraging legal assistance can address a broad number of HHLNs, including benefits from the Department of Human Services (Food Stamps, Medicaid), employment and military benefits (Social Security and the Department of Veterans Affairs), Crime Victims Compensation (CVC), criminal record expungement, consumer debt, housing, employment, immigration, and child support obligations. For patients affected by violent injury, who are at uniquely high risk of adverse involvement with the justice system, this type of legal advocacy is critical for overcoming the challenges that impede basic pursuits of health and safety.

The potential public health impact of an HVIP-MLP cannot be understanded with regards to improvement in mental health, allostatic stress, and potential reduction in burnout for our Violence Recovery Specialists (VRS) and long-term metrics such as trauma re-injury, length of stay, ED re-admission and more. This has the potential to improve clinical practice across the country by integrating and incorporating an MLP-framework into all HVIPs to 'normalize' the screening and addressing of the SSDOH in trauma care. HVIP services across the country would change, especially on a state and ACS-level. Concepts would change with need for legal support for all trauma patients affected by firearm violence to address the SSDOH. Preventative interventions would be improved for families to protect against future victimization.

HVIP-MLP models may indeed be helpful for patients, families and communities affected by trauma. In fact, these models could be helpful for our entire approach to HVIPs in terms of standardizing interventions across the country to measure effectiveness. The HVIP-MLP model could also potentially support HVIP professionals across the country, who tend to work long hours, may be contractually paid, without benefits, are disproportionately people of color, and most of whom have personal experiences of trauma [40]. This would offset the burden that they face in addressing the overwhelming need of out violently-injured survivors of firearm injury, their families and communities. Given the barriers to the for-profit healthcare system of the US, with roots in white supremacy to historically deny Black, Brown and poor communities from access to care, trauma is often the only portal of entry and interface with the healthcare system for many disenfranchised communities [41–43]. Connecting trauma care to an HVIP-MLP would provide disenfranchised communities with access to multidisciplinary care to address the SSDOH for individuals and families that may not otherwise be able to access the healthcare system.

HVIP-MLP implementation has the potential to change the concepts, methods, technologies, treatments, services, or preventative interventions that drive this field through the following mechanism: HVIP services across the country would change, especially on a state and ACS-level. Concepts would change with need for legal support. Preventative interventions would be improved for families to protect against future victimization. The scientific rationale and need for a clinical trial to test our HVIP-MLP intervention is well supported by preliminary data demonstrating local and national need in trauma patients affected by violence, and information in the literature that shows a myriad of positive outcomes ranging from improved mental health, stress and chronic illness scores, less hospital usage and return visits to the ED, to improved access to the SDOH such as more secure housing, protections for utilities usage, increased access to financial resources and lower health care costs [44].

Recovery Legal Care: The Role of MLPs in Supporting Survivors of Intentional Violence—The Legal Perspective

In this section, we explore the value of implementing an MLP into a trauma center. We will first discuss the MLP model and how legal interventions can be used to address the social determinants of health; then we will discuss the novel HVIP-MLP model (Recovery Legal Care) and why collaborating with an HVIP program can enhance the impact of an MLP, particularly for patients who are survivors of intentional violence. Finally, we will discuss the Recovery Legal Care Program (RLC) [45] and the systems we put in place to bring lawyers onto the trauma team.

Medical-Legal Partnerships

MLPs embed lawyers into the healthcare workforce to address unmet civil legal needs of vulnerable patients [46]. MLPs are a critical component of modern medical centers, enabling the provision of comprehensive care aimed at addressing the broader social determinants of health through legal interventions. The emergence of over 450 MLPs across the US demonstrates the growing acceptance that social dynamics outside the hospital walls impact health outcomes, and holistic patient care demands a root-cause approach. MLPs have often been tailored to help address the unique needs of specific patient populations [46].

Prior research for an MLP-style intervention is rigorous with improvements in patient care ranging from a decrease in readmission to the ED, improvement in self-reported perceived stress, improved medical outcomes in chronic illness such as asthma, diabetes and sickle-cell disease, better adherence to medication-taking, improvement in mental health, more stably housed with better access to utilities, access to greater financial resources and having clinical services are more frequently reimbursed by public and private payers [44]. The effect of MLPs has been so dramatic for patient health that the American Association of Medical Colleges has supported the creation of several MLPs across the country to address the SSDOH [47]. Despite MLPs existing in 276 health care institutions and 36 states in the country, none work in collaboration with a trauma center or has been integrated into HVIPs to help the most vulnerable patient populations in this country [48].

MLPs can also identify and address major systemic issues. MLPs can help patients identify and close the gap between benefits they are eligible to receive and what benefits they actually receive. Lawyers in the MLP can identify patterns in programs with a broader view than the individual patient and use that information to systemically address issues affecting the broader population around the hospital. These interventions can positively impact the entire service area of the hospital.

The social conditions of poverty can often result in poor health outcomes. Addressing social determinants of health can be a win-win for trauma centers, leading to both improved outcomes and reduced healthcare spending for high-need, high-use patients. Patients who come through a MLP often face a variety of medical-legal needs categories, reflected in the acronym I-HELP: Income, Housing, Education/Employment, Legal Status, and Personal/Family Stability.

Trauma patients have a high prevalence of unmet civil medical-legal needs. No human being deserves or plans to get shot. After experiencing firearm injury many patients find themselves unable to return to work and without the support from legal intervention are left to navigate complex public benefit systems on their own. As mentioned, one study found that the prevalence of at least one medical-legal need among trauma patients was 73% [35].

After experiencing violence many patients are not in the correct headspace to ascertain how to access legal help in a timely fashion. By embedding lawyers into the trauma center, we hope to interface with a population that is underserved at a time when their need is most acute. By going to patients, by appearing at bedside, lawyers can help legally stabilize patients so they can focus on what is most important — recovering from their injuries and decreasing the chances they experience violence, once again, in the future.

HVIP+MLP = Recovery Legal Care

HVIPs provide comprehensive services to survivors of violence. A national survey of legal services offered through HVIPs found that in 2021 no HVIP-MLP partnerships existed with the Health Alliance for Violence Intervention (HAVI) network [46]. RLC combines the interventions of an HVIP with the benefits of an MLP to holistically address the needs of patients [45]. In this way, the RLC program can provide services to patients that are community-integrated, preventive of further harm, interdisciplinary between medical, legal, and social services, and transformative of the lives of patients.

UChicago Medicine's HVIP, the Urban Health Initiative's VRP, is made up of a team of VRS. These specialists, like lawyers, are committed to addressing risk factors for future violent injury and decreasing barriers to long-term positive health outcomes. Unlike attorneys, VRS are experts in psychological first aid and rapport building. Additionally, many VRS are credible messengers from the communities we are serving—meaning that that have firsthand experience of the toll of gun violence. By integrating into an HVIP, lawyers can learn from and piggyback on the trust HVIP specialists have already established with patients and the community. This trust building is incredibly important given the population we are working with and their understandable mistrust of lawyers and the government.

Recovery Legal Care: The Nuts and Bolts of How We Did It

The most important ingredient when building a trauma based MLP is to have partners who are equally committed to building the program. Integrating lawyers into care on site at a trauma center is not easy. There are many systems that must be established for both lawyers and hospitals to feel comfortable sharing sensitive information and space. Some of the biggest barriers to establishing an HVIP-MLP are legal confusion and implementing a Memorandum of Understanding (MOU) or formal partnership agreement [46].

In this section, we discuss the practical aspects of implementing an MLP and harmonizing this with our ongoing HVIP work. We will discuss how patients with HHLNs are identified and enrolled in the program. Identification of a willing legal partner, typically a local Legal Aid organization mandated to care for vulnerable and oppressed communities is a key first step. Involving your organization's legal counsel is important, especially for the establishment of a memorandum of understanding between organizations and the handling of sensitive and confidential patient health information. Other trauma centers who wish to implement a similar program in their medical center can follow these steps as a guideline when creating their own.

Initial Patient Identification

This intervention is considered a critical time intervention, meaning that it is designed to provide support to individuals in the immediate aftermath of their injury, when they will most benefit from an intervention. Thus, our novel MLP closely collaborates with our HVIP, the VRP to identify patients who have recently presented with violent injuries and who may be eligible for legal services. This fusion of the MLP with VRP embodies the HVIP-MLP model which we call RLC.

The VRP team list encompasses all trauma patients with violent injuries regardless of age, residence, or physical status. They share this list with the RLC research staff on a weekly basis, and then the team screens these patients for eligibility criteria via the Electronic Medical Record (EMR). Patients with injuries resulting from interpersonal violence (e.g., firearm injuries, stab wounds, assault/battery) qualify for our care, whereas those hurt in self-inflicted injuries or accidental falls do not meet the intake criteria. Moreover, only patients ages 14 years or older are eligible for the RLC program at this time.

Eligible injuries for RLC services	**Non-qualifying injuries**
Gunshot wound Assault/battery Stabbings Domestic violence Pedestrian in a hit and run	Self-inflicted injuries Vehicular crashes Accidental falls
Eligible characteristics	**Non-eligible characteristics**
Illinois resident Age 14 or older Alert and awake (or if family member present on their behalf) English speaking (or Spanish and translator present)	Out of state resident Under age 14 Minors without guardian presence and consent Intubated, no family around

Although the VRP sees both patients who are inpatient and outpatient, RLC prioritizes inpatient cases. This ensures that our public benefits attorneys can conduct the intake appointment in person, at the bedside. Being able to meet with patients in person contributes to the high compliance and retention rates in the program compared to discussions over the phone. Having civil rights and public benefits attorneys as part of the care team, communicating with patients at the bedside, is a novel approach to trauma care.

First Contact

If a patient meets all the eligibility criteria, they can then be approached by the RLC team for the initial phase of needs screening. This stage is considered the patient's first direct contact with the MLP part of RLC.

Upon entering, we confirm that the patient is awake and medically capable of understanding and responding to questions, in English or in Spanish. Patients who are intubated, sedated, or otherwise presently unable to communicate or grant permission are deferred to be screened later should they regain those capacities. By postponing, but not permanently excluding such patients, we aim to extend our support to all qualifying violent trauma sufferers once they are medically stable. If the patient is a minor, a parent or guardian must be either present in the room or available in real time via telephone to provide consent on behalf of the patient and/or answer the screening questions. For Spanish speaking patients, we use a hospital-approved translator to communicate with the patient. Additionally, we relay this to the legal team to ensure they have the necessary resources to communicate with the patient. These steps are taken to confirm that the patient can consent to participating in the program and understands the questions asked since some questions include legal terminology or uncommon phrases.

A short introduction is provided about who the research screener represents, the RLC program, its mission, and the potential legal services the attorneys can assist with. Because our legal team is licensed only in Illinois, we also verify that patients were injured in and are currently residing in Illinois prior to proceeding to the legal screener.

Flow: Patients Admitted to the UCMTC with Injuries

- VRP has list of patients with violent injuries
- If eligible (Illinois resident, qualifying injury type, etc.)
  - Legal screener conducted

    If I-HELP questions are a "no", then patient = negative screen
    If any part of I-HELP is a "yes", then patient = positive screen

    - Legal Aid Chicago attorneys come to the bedside

Legal Assessment

If the patient is interested and consents to answering the legal screener questions, the research team member then goes through the legal assessment by asking specific questions. If a patient would like to be screened later, we accommodate those requests. The legal screener was developed in the encrypted online software known as REDCap and has multiple sections. The first section helps with obtaining basic but necessary details such as the patient's room number, legal name, demographic information, and contact information. We also record the contact information of the staff member conducting the legal screener. Following this, the next section is a broad question asking if the patient has concerns related to any or multiple of the I-HELP fields: income, employment, housing, legal status, or personal/family stability.

If a patient responds "yes" to any of the questions in the I-HELP section, more questions related to the specific social determinants of health are generated to gain a better understanding of the types and extent of legal needs the patient and/or their family would like assistance with. Once the screener is complete, there may be additional privacy-related authorization paperwork requiring patient signatures. In our case, these signatures are necessary prior to contact by the legal team due to Health Insurance Portability and Accountability Act (HIPAA) privacy rules and hospital policies handling protected health information [49]. Once the screener is complete and authorization is given by the patient, we notify and send the information to the legal team and the necessary hospital department. There is currently a maximum cap of six positive screens that can be obtained per week. This reflects the legal team's caseload, staffing, and the severity or number of a patient's socioeconomic and legal needs as one patient may have multiple HHLNs that need addressing by attorneys.

In our RLC program, Legal Aid Chicago staff attorneys and paralegals come into the hospital and visit patients directly at the bedside—much like the initial legal screening—within 48 to 72 hours upon receiving the patient information for the positive screens. The program uses this novel approach of a "warm hand-off" to minimize barriers to support. Many patients are unhoused, have had their cell phones damaged or confiscated, or no longer have their vehicles, making traveling to the legal office difficult or impossible. By having attorneys visit patients directly, RLC incorporates a trauma-informed perspective, one where there is a collaborative, trusting, and empowering relationship built between the violence recovery, research, legal teams, and the patient. If a patient is discharged prior to the legal team's hospital visit, the patient is contacted via phone, email, or through their emergency contact. From the point of contact onwards, the attorneys work on applying for assistance programs, appeals, and even represent someone in court if they have been unjustly denied benefits.

A patient can have multiple HHLNs, meaning numerous legal cases are opened for just one person or family. The most common concerns are income, employment, and housing; these HHLNs are often interconnected with one another. Case completion can range from weeks, months, to years depending on the severity of a patient's (now client's) situation. By integrating the VRP, research team, and legal providers into one cohesive network, we aim to maximize a patient's socioeconomic and resource support to yield beneficial outcomes.

Guideline for Other Trauma Centers

The end of November in 2023 marked one year of successful screening for RLC at the UCMTC. Other trauma centers who wish to replicate a similar set-up in the future can use the RLC program as a model to guide the creation and development of their own, and curate it to best serve their center's needs. There are many aspects that have been working well in terms of maintaining cohesion between the multiple different facets of the program — medical, research, legal, violence recovery, and administrative sides — to make it run smoothly. There were also aspects that were changed and workshopped throughout the year as the program was being piloted.

Regular Communication

To maintain cohesion between the separate entities that make up RLC, communication plays a key foundational role in the stability of the program. The effort was made to have regular Zoom meetings every two to three weeks to discuss the program's implementation, challenges and troubleshooting as a team. These meetings were designed to address any questions, concerns, quarterly data reviews, or insights people had about the progress of the program which created a more unified front. The important part of an MLP is that everyone in it is an equal member of a non-hierarchical team. Like individual puzzle pieces fitting together, it is essential that instead of viewing the members who make up the program as solely being from different organizations (e.g., medical side vs. legal side), together they all make up one team to see the big picture. Meeting regularly helped maintain this mentality throughout the first year of this MLP which made for effective communication when troubleshooting issues that arose and determining a successful workflow.

Additionally, since the initial funding for RLC was from federal grants, we had the benefit of community member input for RLC though our Community Advisory Board PRAXIS—Practicing Radical Action by eXpanding Inclusive Societies. PRAXIS is comprised of community members, some with a personal history of firearm injury, carceral experiences, activism on the South Side and include medical students from the Pritzker School of Medicine at the University of Chicago, faculty, and staff. PRAXIS has been guiding community-based research endeavors undertaken at UCMTC for the past 4 years now.

Minimizing Patient Burden

Besides ensuring effective communication between team members, another aspect of RLC that is important for broad reproduction is removing any burden to enrolment from patients. When the research side of the team would conduct inpatient legal screenings, it was pivotal that they explain clearly how there would be no financial burden on the patient. After enduring a violent injury and the psychological trauma that comes with it, it is critical to ensure the program is only helping patients but also is not adding to their trauma. For this, and through federal funding from the Department of Justice and the National Institutes of Health, patients enrolled in the RLC program receive legal care at no cost to them or their family members. As opposed to screening patients in the emergency room, capturing data regarding the HHLNs of violently injured inpatients allows our attorneys to act during a critical time intervention window through early bedside contact.

Team Member Care

A successful MLP in a trauma center setting requires that all persons involved are cared for, including both patients and staff members involved in the program's implementation process. Each team member of RLC, including attorneys, was required to undergo trainings and occasional check-ins at the University of Chicago with one particularly assigned city-wide community outreach and social worker skilled in trauma-informed care and support. These training sessions served as a method of easing team members into working specifically with violently injured trauma patients and providing them with resources should questions arise regarding staff-patient interaction. This kind of support also acknowledged the vicarious of secondary trauma that all team members were at risk of developing, given the severity of the trauma witnessed by non-medical personnel, and the accompanying stories of injury and harm. The follow up check-ins are important for building team rapport and creating safe spaces for decompression every few months to combat potential burnout and compassion fatigue. Other trauma centers should highly consider a similar space for their team members to facilitate a global trauma-informed approach that best benefits the patients' inpatient experience. In addition, this is a novel approach to care and resilience that our Legal Aid Chicago attorneys will be able to apply in their workspaces in the future.

Because RLC is the first of its kind — a program designed to provide trauma patients free legal aid at the bedside — its uniqueness meant that there was not an exact predetermined formula to follow. However, by having a consistent line of communication, the team was able to come to innovative solutions quickly when issues arose during the pilot phase after the program's initial launch. To combat these issues that arose, changes were made that directly improved several components of the MLP. Outlined here are some of the changes made for future consideration. These included modifications to the legal screening questions, dates, and times to screen patients, and other similar challenges requiring early modification.

Modifications During Pilot Phase

When developed, the legal screener was validated and revised by multiple team members before the initial launch. Yet, as the legal screener was being piloted by the research side of RLC, certain aspects of the screener were found to be confusing or unclear to the patients. After brainstorming with the rest of the team during the regular Zoom meetings, consensus was drawn on a select few questions to either modify, omit, or add. For example, some low-yield questions that were omitted included asking patients about medical debt and the need to help obtain a government ID or birth certificate. This was because they did not directly relate to the I-HELP social determinants of health needs and did not correlate to a positive screen.

Questions that were modified for clarity were for age, contact preferences, and CVC. Many patients in the age range between 18 and 22, while not legally a minor (thus a legal guardian is not required for participation), were nonetheless asked if they preferred to have a parent involved in the screening. Biological age does not always coincide with emotional age, especially in the setting of a life-threatening injury. Thus, the legal screener was modified in REDCap to verify with participants under the age of 22 years if they felt comfortable speaking alone or preferred to have a guardian present. The wording for contact preferences was reduced to prevent repetition. CVC represents an important reimbursement program (of up to $45,000 in Illinois) in all states for anyone who has experienced violence, including from firearms, and their family members. CVC questions were moved to be a part of the income section of I-HELP instead of as a separate section to ensure no false positives from patients only requesting help with CVC applications.

Questions that were added included prompts that asked patients if they were an Illinois resident to ensure eligibility, room number and the patient's assigned Violence Recovery Specialist for easier identification, demographic characteristics for research analysis purposes, and whether they were in custody or assaulted by the police for legal support. A separate pathway was created for patients and family if they had concerns about criminal charges. Alongside this, questions relating to their housing were added as it was found many patients' concerns denoted in the "other" text box section were regarding the day-to-day safety of their housing or their inability to pay rent which was not on the original version of the legal screener. Significant alterations were not made to preserve the integrity of previously collected and recorded data for the purposes of analysis.

One part of the screening process that required workshopping was identifying the ideal times and days to see patients. It was found that a rotating schedule was more efficient, on both the research and legal sides. Originally, multiple members of the research side would go into the hospital to screen followed a day later by the public benefits attorneys. At times, patients would be discharged prior to warm handoff to our attorneys. To remedy this, a switch was made for the attorneys to arrive earlier in the week to meet for in-patients admitted over the weekend and build better attorney-patient rapport. Instead of multiple people screening different patient rooms at a time, the research screeners went into the hospital separately at staggered times. This allowed them to circle back and see patients who were previously busy in a procedure or not in their room later instead of missing them altogether. Once used to the caseload expectations, our attorneys also started a rotating schedule; each lawyer would take one week instead of splitting the caseload weekly. This allowed for more time to focus on their particular caseload and dedicate more time to the RLC program.

Other barriers that arose throughout the course of the pilot phase were language barriers and unforeseen technology problems. Spanish-speaking patients were able to be included later with the addition of a Spanish speaking research assistant, localizing official hospital translators and interpreters at Legal Aid Chicago. Weekly summary emails were sent between the research and legal sides for more direct communication on which six patients were added to the program along with notes about potential accommodations and clarifications (e.g., Spanish-speaking, intubation, and medical power of attorney, etc.). Additionally, a "master document" was created to better record who was screened, who could not be screened and why, deferrals, patients to re-approach after the six-patient cap, and reasons for declines or negative screens. It would be beneficial for other trauma centers to establish this early on for better integration and record-keeping purposes.

Program Limitations

While we feel that other trauma centers could benefit from our learning curve associated with the RLC program, there are still some limitations to consider. One of the most significant obstacles for RLC has been obtaining authorization from patients for attorneys to access their EMR. Many times, patients may screen positive with our legal screener, but are uncomfortable having to sign authorization forms due to a lack of trust in local and societal institutional. This is still an ongoing issue that is reflective of challenges relating to marginalized populations' historical mistrust in medical institutions. Nonetheless we have been able to receive most authorization forms by explaining in-depth how the consent is required for the legal advocates to have temporary access to their medical record in order to visit them at the bedside. Once the free legal services are completed, then Legal Aid Chicago loses access.

The predominant hardship has been capacity, simply because program capacity is six patients enrolled in RLC per week at this time. This is phenomenal for this new and unique program, but expanding reach would be even better. Additionally, there are seasonal patterns, as demonstrated by higher admission rates during the summer months with warmer weather compared to the winter. The volume fluctuations can make the six-patient maximum difficult when due to capacity, not all patients are screened during a summer week. This contrasts with, at times, an insufficient number of patients screened during a winter week, given discharges directly from the emergency department or as in-patients, prior to screening. The ideal goal is to help all trauma patients with their public benefits and other HHLNs, but at this time, RLC is constrained to a select handful of patients each week.

As the public benefits laws and policies shift with the times, RLC will need to adapt. One such example is the end of federal benefits associated with COVID-19 relief, or new work requirements for the receipt of SNAP or other federal programs, creating new barriers for access. Overall, other trauma centers that wish to implement an effective MLP within their own trauma centers can use RLC as a guide. The main takeaways are to maintain cohesion, communicate regularly between groups, and adopt a trauma-informed and patient-centered approach through regular and timely communication.

How an MLP Benefits the HVIP Team: The Violence Recovery Program Perspective

RLC effectively ensures patients have access to free legal care at the start of their healing journey. The VRP serves many patients and families in different socioeconomic positions. The role of the VRP is to assist violently injured patients and their families. At the same time, they remain in the care of the clinical team at UCMTC and during the post-discharge period. The VRP also provides violently injured patients and families with resources to prevent re-injury, and to ensure all are receiving the support they need. Utilizing psychological first aid and intensive clinical case management to really understand all the social determinants of health patients face is a key objective of this program. Within this, some patients need economic and structural resources; however, they cannot obtain them due to socioeconomic barriers.

Obtaining such resources would be beneficial, but they are not always accessible to patients, which can be an important source of harmful stress. While hospitalized, patients are being treated for their injuries, primarily working to heal physically, emotionally, and mentally. In many cases, patients are also concerned with their lives outside the hospital, especially when discharged. Patients, at times, are unable to work, both short-term and long-term, which can cause a patient to need extensive resources such as disability, rent assistance, and CVC support. Furthermore, some patients may need assistance with emergency relocation, to move away from a dangerous environment. They may need assistance with reaching out to property owners or may be experiencing a public benefits claim denial even though, legally, they are entitled to make an emergency move. These are just a couple of challenges patients face when they are hospitalized after being violently injured. Although patients acknowledge the need for resources, it can seem often unreachable or impossible for patients, especially without the support of the VRP.

VRP advocates often encounter barriers themselves trying to help our patients access these systems. There can be a successful referral by connecting the patient with a resource or organization, but denials and waitlists are barriers patients often face. The collaboration with attorneys and their legal aid organizations has been very effective in working with patients to expedite wait times or appeal denials.

MLP is a highly supportive and helpful resource system, not only for patients but also for the VRP team through the following:

1. Patients who work with RLC are provided with multiple support systems, systems that follow their needs and help them become obtainable.
2. RLC has allowed patients to work one-on-one with on-site attorneys through Legal Aid Chicago, who can further help patients with:

    (a) learning about their legally entitled resources
    (b) following patients long-term
    (c) advocating on behalf of patients and families to connect to resources:

(i) to support health and nutrition
(ii) disability assistance
(iii) CVC
(iv) effective reporting
(v) criminal record expungement
(vi) fighting eviction orders
(vii) employment security

Through the legal screening questionnaire and verbal conversations with patients and their families, RLC can determine what resources patients can receive and, after that, help them become obtainable.

A shared resource patients utilize is CVC. This resource reimburses patients for medical, counseling, relocation, lost wages, funeral expenses, and more, up to $45,000 per individual in the state of Illinois. Family members of victimized individuals also qualify [50]. This program is underutilized with only 6% of eligible persons applying, with a 40% approval rate [51]. Successful applicants have been disproportionately white men whose first language is English, the group facing the lowest rate of victimization in the US [51]. The reimbursement is for losses that have occurred due to their injury. RLC has been successful in assisting our patients with the highest amount of reimbursement funds that we've seen since our founding. These resources are provided to victims of violence and, in some cases, their families as well. VRP works with patients to complete their initial CVC application. Our Legal Aid Chicago legal partners have also enriched the understanding of the application process and requirements to complete the CVC form, which has improved the VRP team's advocacy when assisting patients. Furthermore, Legal Aid Chicago is also excellent at understanding, interpreting, and explaining legal jargon within the CVC form and other public benefit applications and forms. Having their assistance in these matters has greatly increased VRPs capacity to focus on crisis intervention and case management. Therefore, it helps to enforce correctly completed CVC applications, adequate documentation reporting to support applications, and more. RLC assists with the ongoing application and documentation needed for CVC, often a cumbersome process that takes months to years [52]. If or when a patient is denied CVC, RLC can assist with the appeal process. This helps the patient because they know they have a support system to help them in the case of rejection and help to relieve stress. This allows the patient to work with RLC to resolve the issue. This pro is significant as the reimbursement from CVC is a substantial resource to violently injured patients and may provide resources to prevent re-injury.

There is a significant impact in having on-site care for patients. Engaging on-site with patients helps to reduce barriers. Meeting with a patient face-to-face provides trust, lowers communication barriers, and builds clarity. At times, patients in the hospital who are violently injured may be distrusting of strangers. Strangers are individuals with whom patients need to become more familiar, such as staff. Meeting face-to-face patients and their care team can have a conversation and build rapport.

Lastly, in the instance that a patient is in police custody, in-person legal aid support is the most appropriate and ensures patients are receiving legal support while receiving clinical care, even when in custody.

RLC has allowed us to harness the power of the legal field in addition to the power of the social services field to give our patients the different forms of justice they seek. At the start of their admission, patients are familiarized with VRP and have an assigned specialist, when they are skeptical of Legal Screeners, MLP Attorneys, etc. VRP helps to bridge the barrier and supports communication between patients and these teams. Having all teams on site is incredibly beneficial because this allows patients to elaborate their needs to MLP comfortably. In turn, it helps patients receive resources they may need. At times, patients may have another concern that is brought up, and VRP & MLP would work together on the patients' needs to better service them. Lastly, RLC is beneficial on-site because it creates an environment for all care teams (Surgical, VRP, MLP) to communicate a patient's needs effectively. RLC is an essential patient resource; it bridges the gap in care teams and is an added support system for patients to connect them to resources. The VRP's growth has allowed an expansion to capacity and has created specialized services including outpatient VRS that work with patients that discharge straight from the emergency department and RLC that advocates for patients with HHLNs. This allows a richer and deeper collective impact that expands across the medical and legal sectors.

VRP takes the public health approach to addressing all forms of violence. The primary aim is prevention. Engaging with patients after the injury has occurred, is intervention. Moving toward prevention requires understanding the full complexity of the human experience as it pertains to violence. Understanding the culture of violence is the only way to enact effective solutions and to end the vicious cycle and transgenerational transmission of violence that affects human beings over generations. Thus, it is necessary to marry the legal field with the field of violence prevention and intervention. When addressing physical injury, we have found that a patient's stories and experiences are never just about the injury itself. When we hear what led to the injury, we hear so many layered and complex stories. The VRP is not only addressing the violence one individual enacts against another person, but we are also addressing violence that systemic racism causes by creating the dire conditions that are ripe for violence to occur. VRP can address the harm, but to create sustainable change to prevent the harm from occurring again, it's vital to understand and advocate for changes in policy that affect patients and their families. With RLC we are capitalizing on the opportunity to use the legal scope to assess the broken and complicated health and legal systems to determine what medical and legal interventions we need to effectively intervene structurally and prevent re-injury. These strategies on the individual level and at a systems level are essential. RLC allows us to operate at both levels.

Our preliminary research findings have shown that RLC has had success in addressing the HHLNs of patients. Together, Legal Aid Chicago civil rights lawyers with VRS are making a collective impact. Now that we are starting to understand the benefits of RLC, we can teach other HVIPs about the importance of this approach so that they are better informed to help instead of harm. The medical and legal fields have left many communities with so much mistrust. We recognize this reality and work diligently to ensure that our attorneys and violence recovery specialists are working with our patients in a trauma-informed way. Together, we are highlighting the strength, agency, and choice of our patients, and advocating on their behalf, when necessary, using our influence toward our patients' defined pursuit of justice. We believe that our model can be beneficial for other emerging MLPs and HVIPs in the nation.

Evaluating Success

Although results from our pilot MLP are promising, more robust longitudinal measures must be gathered to assess impact of our MLP on long-term patient and family wellbeing. Implementation science is applied in the first phase to assess program feasibility and if it is pragmatic and acceptable to users. A mixed methods approach should be used, to obtain the most comprehensive understanding of program impacts, successes, and barriers.

Quantitative Data

1. **Trauma-Informed Data Collection Practices**:
   - validated assessments on deficit-based measures (variables that define people by their problems i.e. decrease in HHLN, health, quality of life & mental health status, gaps addressing the SDOHs)
   - asset-based framing (variables related to assets and aspirations i.e. future orientation)
   - measures of resiliency and growth (i.e. post-traumatic growth, resiliency, support, autonomy).
2. **Participant & Subject-Matter Expert Feedback:**
   - Trauma-informed behavioral health practitioners
   - Patient and family participants
   - Community Advisory Board
     - measures to be used, how data are to be collected, implementation and analyses
     - Allows us to validate and test surveys: do these questionnaires make sense? Are they appropriate? Why or why not?
     - One example why we want to do this: Well documented problematic issues with validated questionnaires such as ACES among Black populations [53]

3. **Implementation metrics:** [54]
   - Which framework to use?
   - Anticipated vs. actual implementation outcomes
   - Implementation vs. innovation outcomes
   - Implementation vs. innovation determinants
4. **Process measures**:
   - Data collected from:
     - Patients
     - RLC staff
     - VRP staff
     - Research Assistants
     - Legal Aid Chicago Lawyers
   - Will help with understanding replicability, feasibility, implementation process
   - **Program-level data:**
     - How many patients were seen over time (basic engagement data/descriptives)
     - Methods of patient and family engagement
     - Facilitators and barriers to patient and family engagement
     - Amount of time needed to screen a patient
     - Mean/median number of touches/engagement per patient
     - Lost to follow-up numbers and reasons
     - Frequency of HHLN categories
     - HHLN that MLP is unable to address but may arise (criminal justice needs, immigration needs, non-civil legal needs)
   - **Patient-level data:**
     - HHLN
     - SSDOH needs
     - never/ever received public benefits
     - currently receiving public benefits
     - money and benefits won per patient (and total)
     - month(s) per case
     - number of needs per case
     - willingness to participate, ability to participate, barriers to participate
     - program acceptability, program experience and satisfaction
5. **Outcome metrics:**
   - Determined by multiple iterations of the above, with patient, subject matter expert and community feedback.
   - Develop and share codebook for variables captured
     - Categories of impact: health, legal, economic, other

  - Levels of impact: individual, familial, community, healthcare provider, HVIP provider, civil rights attorneys and program providers, various levels of government
- Structural impacts:
  - Legal metrics for policy change: amicus briefs, class action lawsuits, writ of mandamus, advocacy cases, draft model legislation

Qualitative Data

- For feasibility and better understanding of implementation of novel program in a busy trauma center, individual interviews and focus groups with program implementers and stakeholders should be conducted to understand:
  - Different perceptions/perspective on:
    - how this program helps patients, people's understanding of what the program does, usefulness, how has their perception of HHLNs, recovery, and structural violence changed as a result of program implementation?
  - Who should be interviewed?
    - Implementers and stakeholders:
      - Principal Investigator & Co-Investigators
      - Other trauma surgery staff
      - Legal Aid Chicago staff
      - VRP staff
      - Research Assistants
      - Other ED staff who interface with this program
- Patients and families who have received this program should be interviewed
  - How has this program affected their recovery process?
  - What other supports do they wish were offered by programs like this?
  - Perceptions and feelings of trust and distrust of systems
  - Thoughts on how this may affect long-term recovery (if at all)
  - Short-term or long-term impact?
    - Economic impact?
  - Government responsibility to protect citizens from firearm injury
    - Reparations for failure to do so
      - What would these look like to patients and families?
    - Can RLC help with reparations & measure impact?

Preliminary Outcomes

Within the pilot phase, we were able to obtain preliminary data and outcomes from patient enrollment in our RLC program. During the first 6 months of enrolling patients, we approached 136, with 81.6% of patients consenting to screening. From a demographic perspective, our participants were young adults (27 years or older) and identified as male (79.2%) and Black non-Hispanic (88.0%).

With regards to recruitment statistics, an overwhelming majority of participants screened positive for at least one health-harming legal need (77.9%) and nearly 85% had more than 1 health-harming legal need. Income was the primary concern for most participants, at a rate of 93.4%, followed by housing and employment. Additionally, a considerable number of patients reported being unhoused, having a chronic health condition, and/or having young children dependent on them, which can add immense stress mentally, emotionally, and financially.

After patients were enrolled in RLC and connected to legal services, we observed a variety of positive outcomes related to public benefits access. Most individuals were interested in Supplemental Security Income (SSI), SNAP (food stamps), and CVC, which is a reimbursement program for patients and individuals affected by violent crimes. It should also be noted that in some instances, our lawyers opened multiple legal cases just for a single patient or family, given the circumstances and severity of one's situation, demonstrating how difficult it would be for a person with limited legal knowledge to go about this process on their own. The legal team was able to secure these benefits, and others such as record expungement, for most of the patients who expressed concerns with these. Another interesting finding was regarding patients who previously had benefits and were interested in addressing issues they were having (i.e., reduction, denials, or terminations). We discovered that of the small number of participants with preexisting benefits (16%), all reported barriers to access, indicating a real discrepancy between eligibility and actually receiving entitled assistance. This further reflects how crucial a bedside legal assistance program is in improving access to socioeconomic needs.

An example of one of the remarkable outcomes from RLC would be how one patient was able to work with the legal team to secure monthly Medicaid and SNAP benefits they were always entitled to; after connecting with Legal Aid Chicago, this client now received an additional $1005 for Medicaid and an additional $459 for SNAP (food stamps). On top of these significant amounts, this client was entitled to back payments for these same benefits, acquiring $2010 for Medicaid and $918 for SNAP. As we can see, these dollar amounts can make a considerable difference for patients in reducing financial strain and structural disparities.

The main takeaways from implementing this program were that this was highly feasible, as seen by high participation rates despite high acuity, and high acceptability, which in turn led to remarkably high retention rates (91.5%). This is reflective upon the cohesion and dedication of the various groups comprising of the HVIP-MLP, such as the Violence Recovery Program, the research team, and the legal providers. Additionally, Recovery Legal Care can be considered appropriate to patients, given the high positive rates (95.5%) with most individuals reporting at least one health-harming legal need; similarly, all who reported receiving any public benefits in the past reported barriers to access. This data is indicative of challenges ingrained within the system, confirming how challenging it can be for populations affected by violence to access and receive public benefits, adding on to the daily challenges faced by communities that have been historically excluded from basic economic protections and entitlements.

Case Study

Ms. B and her son JB were referred to Recovery Legal Care after JB was shot and subsequently paralyzed. Through the legal screener, JB was found to need a social security administration (SSA) application due to the severity of his injury and needed help with criminal records relief. Ms. B also had specific needs including help maximizing her SSA benefits and housing concerns after the shooting which was near their home residence. One month after the incident, Ms. B and JB faced issues JB's SNAP and medical coverage being abruptly cut off.

With the aid of the Recovery Legal Care program, the following legal outcomes for Ms. B and JB were made.

- Two month after the application, JB was awarded $830/month in SSA.
- MS. B received support to secure home care for her son JB.
- JB has his juvenile criminal record expunged and sealed.

Currently, Legal Aid Chicago is still working with Ms. B and JB to resolve two more cases of theirs: Ms. B's crime victims compensation application to assist with housing needs and JB's SSDI benefits.

Future Sustainability

Because civil legal aid organizations view the partnerships as an innovative approach to advancing justice, [55] health care organizations have been able to draw from a reservoir of free or low-cost legal services. However, to be scaled up more broadly, partnerships need sustainable sources of financing from both the health care and legal sectors. MLPs are important in addressing Health Equity, a reimbursable metric within the Centers for Medicaid & Medicare Services Framework. Similarly, Medicaid vouchers may be provided for legal care and support of patients. This may lay the groundwork of linking equity metrics in healthcare with legal care.

Senior leader engagement will frame MLP activities in the context of institutional goals, priorities, and mission; they will identify resources, raise program profile, and promote sustainable integration. Without buy-in at this level, sustainability and growth are unlikely. Members of this group should play a role in the planning process and consulted before and during the MOU development.

Conclusion

By increasing access to legal and financial support with our novel, interdisciplinary HVIP-MLP, called RLC, we expect to address significant structural and social needs among patients and families, which may have downstream impacts on physical & psychological health. We also anticipate spillover benefits to our VRS, through a reduction in burnout. Given the potential for rapid national expansion, these findings could inform community facing HVIPs and trauma centers across the US. Future work can measure reduction in firearm trauma reinjury after broad trauma center adoption by the American College of Surgeons Committee on Trauma as part of the validation process of Level I, II and III trauma centers across the US.

References

1. WISQARS (Web-based Injury Statistics Query and Reporting System) | Injury Center|CDC [Internet]. 2021 [cited 2022 Apr 9]. Available from: https://www.cdc.gov/injury/wisqars/index.html
2. Gun Violence Archive [Internet]. [cited 2021 Feb 28]. Available from: https://www.gunviolencearchive.org/
3. CDC. Centers for Disease Control and Prevention. 2019 [cited 2022 Apr 9]. From the CDC-Leading Causes of Death-Non-Hispanic Black Males 2017. Available from: https://www.cdc.gov/healthequity/lcod/men/2017/nonhispanic-black/index.htm
4. Amnesty International [Internet]. 2018 [cited 2022 Apr 9]. Amnesty International report declares gun violence in the United States to be a human rights crisis. Available from: https://www.amnesty.org/en/latest/news/2018/09/gun-violence-human-rights-crisis/
5. Amnesty International [Internet]. [cited 2022 Apr 9]. USA: Scars of survival: Gun violence and barriers to reparation in the USA. Available from: https://www.amnesty.org/en/documents/amr51/0566/2019/en/
6. Social Determinants of Health | CDC [Internet]. 2021 [cited 2022 Apr 9]. Available from: https://www.cdc.gov/socialdeterminants/index.htm
7. Kim D. Social determinants of health in relation to firearm-related homicides in the United States: a nationwide multilevel cross-sectional study. PLoS Med. 2019;16(12):e1002978.
8. Halimeh BN, Hughes D, Evans B, Emberson J, Turco L, Zakrison TL, et al. Empowering the affected: informing community-based solutions through interviews with survivors of interpersonal firearm violence-perspectives of survivors of firearm injuries. J Trauma Acute Care Surg. 2021;90(6):980–6.
9. Formica MK. An eye on disparities, health equity, and racism-The case of firearm injuries in urban youth in the United States and globally. Pediatr Clin N Am. 2021;68(2):389–99.
10. Poulson M, Neufeld MY, Dechert T, Allee L, Kenzik KM. Historic redlining, structural racism, and firearm violence: a structural equation modeling approach. Lancet Reg Health Am. 2021;3:100052.
11. Jacoby SF, Dong B, Beard JH, Wiebe DJ, Morrison CN. The enduring impact of historical and structural racism on urban violence in Philadelphia. Soc Sci Med. 1982;2018(199):87–95.
12. The impact of historical racism on modern gun violence: Redlining in the city of Louisville, KY – ScienceDirect [Internet]. [cited 2022 Feb 4]. Available from: https://www.sciencedirect.com/science/article/abs/pii/S0020138320305490
13. A Conceptual Framework for Action on the Social Determinants of Health [Internet]. [cited 2022 Apr 9]. Available from: https://www.who.int/publications-detail-redirect/9789241500852

14. Abdallah HO, Kaufman EJ. Before the bullets fly: the physician's role in preventing firearm injury. Yale J Biol Med. 2021;94(1):147–52.
15. Borthwell RM, Olanrewaju S, Putnam BA, Kim DY, Chong VE. Recovery of pediatric patients after firearm injury: can health systems do more? Am Surg. 2021;87(10):1644–50.
16. MacKenzie EJ, Rivara FP, Jurkovich GJ, Nathens AB, Frey KP, Egleston BL, et al. A national evaluation of the effect of trauma-center care on mortality. N Engl J Med. 2006;354(4):366–78.
17. Swendiman RA, Luks VL, Hatchimonji JS, Nayyar MG, Goldshore MA, Nace GW, et al. Mortality after adolescent firearm injury: effect of Trauma Center designation. J Adolesc Health Off Publ Soc Adolesc Med. 2021;68(5):978–84.
18. Dicker R, MD, Gaines FB, MD, Bonne FS, MD, et al. American College of Surgeons. [cited 2022 Apr 9]. Violence Intervention Programs: A Primer for Developing a Comprehensive Program within Trauma Centers. Available from: http://www.facs.org/quality-programs/trauma/advocacy/ipc/firearm-injury/hvip-primer.
19. American College of Surgeons [Internet]. [cited 2022 Apr 9]. Verification, Review, and Consultation (VRC) Program. Available from: http://www.facs.org/quality-programs/trauma/tqp/center-programs/vrc
20. Prevention Guidelines for ACS Verified Trauma Centers – American Trauma Society [Internet]. [cited 2022 Apr 9]. Available from: https://www.amtrauma.org/page/NPRC_ACS_Prevention/Prevention-Guidelines-for-ACS-Verified-Trauma-Centers.htm
21. MacKenzie EJ, Hoyt DB, Sacra JC, Jurkovich GJ, Carlini AR, Teitelbaum SD, et al. National inventory of hospital trauma centers. JAMA. 2003;289(12):1515–22.
22. Trauma center. In: Wikipedia [Internet]. 2022 [cited 2022 Apr 9]. Available from: https://en.wikipedia.org/w/index.php?title=Trauma_center&oldid=1076960334
23. Trauma TEA for the S of. Home [Internet]. [cited 2022 Apr 9]. Available from: https://www.east.org/
24. Galtung J. Violence, peace, and peace research. J Peace Res. 1969;6(3):167–91.
25. Trauma EA, for the S of. Eastern Association for the Surgery of Trauma firearm injury prevention statement. Trauma Surg Acute Care Open. 2019;4(1):e000294.
26. The HAVI [Internet]. [cited 2022 Apr 9]. The HAVI — What is an HVIP? Available from: https://www.thehavi.org/what-is-an-hvip
27. The HAVI [Internet]. [cited 2022 Apr 9]. The HAVI – The HAVI – Emerging HVIP. Available from: https://www.thehavi.org/emerging-hvip
28. Richardson JB, Wical W, Kottage N, Bullock C. Shook ones: understanding the intersection of nonfatal violent firearm injury, incarceration, and traumatic stress among young black men. Am J Mens Health. 2020 Dec;14(6):1557988320982181.
29. Monopoli WJ, Myers RK, Paskewich BS, Bevans KB, Fein JA. Generating a core set of outcomes for hospital-based violence intervention programs. J Interpers Violence. 2021;36(9–10):4771–86.
30. Cooper C, Eslinger D, Nash D, al-Zawahri J, Stolley P. Repeat victims of violence: report of a large concurrent case-control study. Arch Surg Chic Ill 1960. 2000. 135(7):837–843.
31. Richardson JB, St Vil C, Sharpe T, Wagner M, Cooper C. Risk factors for recurrent violent injury among black men. J Surg Res. 2016;204(1):261–6.
32. Klein MD, Alcamo AM, Beck AF, O'Toole JK, McLinden D, Henize A, et al. Can a video curriculum on the social determinants of health affect residents' practice and families' perceptions of care? Acad Pediatr. 2014;14(2):159–66.
33. Ko NY, Battaglia TA, Gupta-Lawrence R, Schiller J, Gunn C, Festa K, et al. Burden of socio-legal concerns among vulnerable patients seeking cancer care services at an urban safety-net hospital: a cross-sectional survey. BMC Health Serv Res. 2016;14(16):196.
34. Gard LA, Bartell T, Shah AK, Setrini AB, Sheehan K, Miller CH, et al. Interprofessional education in medical-legal partnerships (MLPs) to address social Determinants of health. J Health Care Poor Underserved. 2021;32(4):1720–33.
35. Hall EC, Current JJ, Sava JA, Rosen JE. The case for integrating medical-legal partnerships into trauma care. J Surg Res. 2022;274:153–9.

36. Peregrin T. New adult trauma center on Chicago's South Side will treat violence as a disease. Bull Am Coll Surg. 2017 Jun;102(6):21–7.
37. Mendenhall R. The medicalization of poverty in the lives of low-income black mothers and children. J Law Med Ethics J Am Soc Law Med Ethics. 2018 Sep;46(3):644–50.
38. 5135547. Issuu. [cited 2021 Jun 22]. 2018–2019 Community Health Needs Assessment – UChicago Medicine. Available from: https://issuu.com/communitybenefit-ucm/docs/ucm-2019-chna
39. Chicago Department of Public Health Releases The State of Health for Blacks in Chicago, the first report of its kind focusing exclusively on the health of Black Chicagoans [Internet]. [cited 2022 Apr 9]. Available from: https://www.chicago.gov/content/city/en/depts/cdph/provdrs/healthy_living/news/2021/june/chicago-department-of-public-health-releases-the-state-of-health.html
40. Violence recovery specialist draws on personal experience to help patients and families heal after trauma [Internet]. [cited 2022 Apr 10]. Available from: https://www.uchicagomedicine.org/forefront/community-articles/violence-recovery-specialist-martinez-sutton
41. Cohen W. Medical apartheid: the dark history of medical experimentation on black Americans from colonial times to the present. Int J Appl Psychoanal Stud. 2009;6(4):356–60.
42. LiPuma SH, Robichaud AL. Deliver us from injustice: reforming the U.S. Healthcare System J Bioethical Inq. 2020;17(2):257–70.
43. PenguinRandomhouse.com [Internet]. [cited 2022 Apr 10]. Medical Apartheid by Harriet A. Washington: 9780767915472 | PenguinRandomHouse.com: Books. Available from: https://www.penguinrandomhouse.com/books/185986/medical-apartheid-by-harriet-a-washington/
44. Impact [Internet]. Medical-Legal Partnership. [cited 2022 Mar 30]. Available from: https://medical-legalpartnership.org/impact/
45. Recovery Legal Care—Recovery Legal Care | University of Chicago [Internet]. [cited 2023 Dec 6]. Available from: https://www.recoverylegal.uchicago.edu/
46. Setrini A. Treating poverty: legal tools for health-harming needs. DePaul Law Rev [Internet] 2020 69(3). Available from: https://via.library.depaul.edu/law-review/vol69/iss3/3
47. AAMC [Internet]. [cited 2022 Mar 30]. Evaluating the impact of medical-legal partnerships on health and health inequities. Available from: https://www.aamc.org/what-we-do/mission-areas/medical-research/health-equity/medical-legal-partnerships
48. Healthy Chicago 2025 [Internet]. [cited 2021 Jun 29]. Available from: https://www.chicago.gov/content/city/en/depts/cdph/provdrs/healthy_communities/svcs/healthy-chicago-2025.html
49. Health Insurance Portability and Accountability Act of 1996 (HIPAA) | CDC [Internet]. 2022 [cited 2023 Dec 6]. Available from: https://www.cdc.gov/phlp/publications/topic/hipaa.html
50. Illinois Attorney General – Crime Victim Compensation Program [Internet]. [cited 2021 Aug 16]. Available from: https://ag.state.il.us/victims/cvc.html
51. Reports and Surveys—Alliance for Safety and Justice [Internet]. Trauma, Dignity and Restoration December 2019. [cited 2023 Dec 9]. Available from: https://allianceforsafetyandjustice.org/reports-and-surveys/
52. Chicago Sun-Times [Internet]. 2021 [cited 2023 Dec 9]. Illinois created a program to compensate crime victims. Nearly 50 years later, it's failing. Available from: https://chicago.suntimes.com/2021/7/9/22566035/illinois-crime-victim-compensation-program-delays-failures
53. Giovanelli A, Reynolds AJ. Adverse childhood experiences in a low-income black cohort: The importance of context. Prev Med. 2021;1(148):106557.
54. Damschroder LJ, Reardon CM, Opra Widerquist MA, Lowery J. Conceptualizing outcomes for use with the Consolidated Framework for Implementation Research (CFIR): the CFIR Outcomes Addendum. Implement Sci IS. 2022;17(1):7.
55. Stsepaniuk K. The justice gap problem solving: history and innovation. Campbell Law Rev. 2021;44(1):65.

The Cold Call

Marc D. Horton

I looked up at the clock and counted in my head what time it would be in Chicago. Nine AM seemed an appropriate time to make the call. Since I was a kid, I have always hated asking people for things. My Catholic high school required we sell chocolate bars as a yearly fund raiser and I always did abysmal—requiring my parents, who couldn't afford it by the way, to have to buy what I didn't sell. It was never my favorite time of year. The phone rang a couple of times and an executive assistant answered. "Dr. Selwyn Roger's office."

"Good morning. This is Dr. Marc Horton, from Swedish Medical Center in Seattle. He doesn't know me but I would like to make an appointment for a telephone meeting with Dr. Rogers."

"One moment please," was her response as she placed me on hold. I was going through my calendar again reminding me what dates and times would work and what I would say if perhaps she sounded like I might be dismissed. While I was doing this, the phone suddenly clicked and I was unexpectedly connected.

"Good morning, this is Selwyn Rogers. To whom am I speaking? What can I do for you?" So began my somewhat out of the blue, cold call to someone whom before I had never met. So began the partnership between two programs, two institutions, two cities, and two surgeons who as fate would have it, would become two friends.

The Merriam-Webster dictionary defines partnership as "a relationship usually involving close cooperation between parties having specific and joint rights and responsibilities." Swedish Medical Center is an independent academic medical center that is the cornerstone of a health care delivery system that started over a 100 years ago, serving the people of an ever-growing region. It has trained outstanding surgeons since it opened its doors. It was founded in Seattle in 1910 by Dr. Nils Johanson, MD, a Swedish immigrant surgeon (that is correct, that is why it was

M. D. Horton (✉)
Swedish Medical Center General Surgery Residency Program, Seattle, WA, USA
e-mail: Marc.Horton@swedish.org

S. O. Rogers, Jr (ed.), *Creating a Modern Trauma Center*,
https://doi.org/10.1007/978-3-031-66524-0_26

named Swedish) who went to medical school at the University of Colorado and eventually made his way to the Pacific Northwest. He was not satisfied with the sterility of local Seattle operating rooms so after finding additional local Swedish businessmen investors he purchased an apartment building for $10,000 and Swedish Hospital became an entity. The first baby was born at Swedish that year. Dr. Johanson started his own nursing school at Swedish, which would eventually combine with the University of Washington School of Nursing. In 1920, as was standard at the time, he set up an internship for medical student graduates prior to them going into practice. Though he had previously had a number of apprentice trainees over the years, in an effort to provide more advanced surgical training he later established a surgical residency program that more closely resembled our present structure, sometime prior to 1948. Dr. Johanson also recruited only the best attending surgeons to come to Swedish. One such recruit was Dr. William Hutchinson. After his younger brother Fred succumbed to cancer, he founded the Fred Hutchinson Cancer Research Center. The Fred Hutch Cancer Center (as it is known today) still provides cutting edge cancer research. The Swedish surgery department still performs a high volume of procedures across all the surgical disciplines. Swedish has a longstanding, accredited general surgery residency program that provides our residents with an early, high volume operative experience. Dr. Hutchison trained the late Dr. Clarke Hoffman, MD who trained me. The legacy continues. Our graduates are highly sought after, as they are extremely well-trained general surgeons as well as competitive applicants for further fellowship training and subsequent academic positions elsewhere in the country if they so desire. We originally graduated one chief resident a year. This grew to two, then three and now five per year. Over the past ten years we have had a 100% pass rate on the American Board of Surgery Qualifying and Certifying exams. We have a 100% matching percentage for our residents seeking fellowship training since 2004. I came to Swedish in 1988 and since 1993 I have been either the associate program director or program director of our general surgery residency. I was very fortunate to have Dr. Ryan Martinez, MD join me as the associate program director in 2012. We are fortunate to have an outstanding surgical faculty who are dedicated to excellent surgical outcomes and look upon teaching as being part of being a surgeon. This has been our mantra since Dr. Johanson's time.

The University of Chicago is one of the premier institutions of higher education in the country. It was founded in 1890, followed by the School of Medicine in 1927. It's modern Department of Surgery was founded by Dalla Burton Phemister, MD in 1928 and has continued as a prestigious institution of higher education in the training of future surgeons, presently under the guidance of their program director, Associate Professor of Surgery, Dr. Jennifer Cone, MD and their chair, Professor of Surgery Dr. Jeffrey B. Matthews, MD. The trauma center is directed by Professor of Surgery and Executive Vice President of Community Health Engagement, Dr. Selwyn Rogers, MD.

Among many things, this chapter could have been titled "The Tale of Two Cities." There are similarities between Seattle and Chicago that are noteworthy. Full disclosure—Seattle is my hometown. I was actually supposed to be born at Swedish, but that is a story for another time. That being said, many would agree that Seattle is a great city. The people, music, food, ocean/lakes/streams, mountains, and quick access to Canada are hard to beat. Over its history it has gone through numerous booms and busts, only to continue to come back and land on its feet. Examples include, but are not limited to the fishing industry, the lumber industry, the Olmstead designed park system, the 1897 Klondike gold rush, the shipbuilding boom that peaked in World War I, Boeing (which moved cooperate headquarters to Chicago before eventually moving to Arlington), and more recently—Microsoft, Amazon, and many other tech companies. This local geographic area has been inhabited since the last glacial period (@8000 BC) by indigenous peoples. Experts tell us that in the mid-1850s the indigenous Coast Salish people (Duwamish and Suquamish) were known to inhabit the western bank of the Duwamish River. Chief Seattle was born around 1786 on or near Blake Island and is the city's namesake. In 1889 a fire destroyed the entire central business district. The city was quickly rebuilt using brick this time around. This new construction was 20 feet above the original street level. Tours of Underground Seattle are still available. Seattle was host to the 1962 World's Fair. I remember the excitement of attending as a youngster and the Space Needle still stands as a monumental reminder to the endeavor.

The similarities between the two cities are not lost on me. Chicago played an important role in America's history and has been a dominant midwestern city since the 1880s. It was incorporated in 1837. French exploders, missionaries and fur traders came to the area in the late seventeenth century, finding local Pottawatomie indigenous people there when they arrived. The name Chicago is thought to have come from the Algonquin word shikaakwa meaning stinky onion. Early explorers noted the local lakes and streams to be full of wild garlic and onions. There was also a Chief Chicagou who was an indigenous Michigamean leader. Later Chicago developed into a Midwest center for transportation, railroad, manufacturing, meatpacking, commerce, finance, and higher education, to name a few. In 1871, the Great Chicago Fire destroyed the city's central business district, which was rebuilt. Chicago hosted the 1933 and 1893 World's Fairs. The book about the latter, The Devil in the White City, by former Seattle resident author Erik Larson is a great read.

I have always loved Chicago. It is one of my favorite places to visit. I graduated from Carroll College, a small liberal arts college in Helena, MT. The pre-medical program was directed by my friend and mentor, the late James J. Manion, PhD. With letters of recommendation from Dr. Manion, the majority of Carroll graduates went to one of three medical schools: the University of Chicago, the University of Washington, and Saint Louis University. One of my best friends from Carroll went to the University of Chicago Pritzker School of Medicine before training in Obstetrics and Gynecology at Michael Reese Hospital in Bronzeville. Michael Reese unfortunately closed its doors in 2009. My friend still lives and practices in suburban Chicago. Chicago is the headquarters of the American College of Surgeons (ACS). The ACS Clinical Congress is occasionally there. It always gives me an excuse to visit. I was actually inducted into the College as a Fellow in Chicago years ago and just recently proudly completed my service as a member of the ACS Board of Governors. Even given all this history with Chicago, I would have never dreamt of what would come to fruition so quickly between our two institutions.

As surgical educators and program directors, we have the responsibility to provide residents as broad and deep of an experience as possible, in all aspects of surgical specialties, preparing the following generation of surgeons for all walks of life. At Swedish we are constantly reviewing surgical volumes, written and oral exam scores, and evaluation of clinical skills. We also have the responsibility to provide training in all the new technologies that will eventually be part of everyday practice. We believe in the premise that if you are not getting better, you are getting worse. We are never satisfied with achieving minimum requirements established by governing agencies regarding case volume numbers and other requirements. We strive to lead from the front in all categories of surgical training. Though our desire to increase the number of trauma cases for our residents became an issue, the responsibilities don't end with meeting case volume quotas.

There are other important aspects in the education of new surgeons. There needs to be a better recognition of the causes of the disparity in the delivery of healthcare in our country, whether that be racial or financial. We desperately wanted to promote the racial diversification of our own general surgery residency program. For reasons unclear to me, we have never graduated a Black resident from our program. In the US, according to recent Zippia demographic data, 13.6% of the population is Black. 5.7% of physicians are Black, but only 1.8% of surgeons are Black. We also wanted to better serve the underserved communities in our country, on both the local and national levels. We wanted to increase our residents' awareness of and need for more research in gun violence and gun control legislation, and to increase our residents' experience in caring for the victims of other trauma and gun violence. In the US, civilian firearms outnumber people. There are 120 guns per every 100 people according to the Small Arms Survey. This unfortunately has become evident in many of the communities in our country, including Seattle, where in 2023 the record of homicides in a year was broken. This has certainly become especially pertinent to what is happening on the south side of Chicago. It is not acceptable to become tone deaf to what is going on in Chicago, Seattle or anywhere. We are robbing our communities of young people's potential to be great, to make a difference. We can't become desensitized to this violence. How is it that our military is sending Army surgeons to this same trauma center to keep up their skills because it is the closest experience, we presently have to a wartime theater. We really need to have this sink in.

Harborview Medical Center in Seattle is the only Level I Trauma Center in our 5 state WWAMI (Washington, Wyoming, Alaska, Montana, Idaho) Region. For this reason, it is inundated with a plethora of general surgery residents from nearby programs. Swedish residents rotate there in the emergency room and burn unit as first year residents. They spend 2 months in their second year in the trauma ICU. As third year residents they rotate on a trauma service. In the past they routinely logged the necessary number of trauma surgery cases during that rotation. Over the years we noticed the case volumes for the third year residents to have slowly dwindled, as cases that used to be performed by third year residents began going to higher level residents and fellows. So, while the required American Board of Surgery trauma surgery numbers have not decreased and more blunt trauma patients are managed nonoperatively—the number of penetrating trauma victims in this region has not increased to meet the training demands. I in no way mean to imply that Harborview is not extremely busy, it was just the distribution of cases involving residents that slowly became an issue for us. We initially tried to have our residents go to Harborview in their fourth year, but that proved not to be a viable option. This prompted us to look elsewhere, to make sure our residents would get the best training possible and assure their trauma case numbers would rival the high volumes they achieve in all the other subspecialties. It also started me wanting to better address the non-case volume aspects of a surgical education mentioned previously; diversity, gun violence education, the disparity in healthcare delivery and underscoring our responsibility to care for the underserved.

I wasn't thrilled at the thought of our residents having to go elsewhere for training, but after years of trying it became apparent that was going to be needed. I was especially concerned for residents already part of our program who didn't know they would be going somewhere else to train for a few months. As I looked up and down the left coast, everyone appeared to have the needed full complement of residents. I certainly wasn't interested in our residents going somewhere else to get the same or slightly improved experience. An old Army friend and program director said he had heard the University of Chicago was building a much needed new trauma center on the south side of Chicago. However, since they had already met their cap, they couldn't increase their compliment of University of Chicago surgical residents. He also explained that given prior commitments and the local political milieu, the other nearby Chicago medical schools wouldn't have residents available to help staff this new center. This begged the question; would this new center be looking for resident participation from outside the area? Hence, my cold call to the director of a brand new the trauma center that had not yet opened its doors.

As I already stated, it wasn't just the case volumes I was looking for. As surgeon leaders and educators, it is our responsibility to graduate residents "that look like America." In a move to be intentional regarding the diversification of our residency classes, we developed two additional programs in 2021. With support of our Office of Health Equity, Diversity, and Inclusion, Swedish funded two Diversity Surgery Sub-Internship Scholarships each year for any US medical school fourth year student from an ethnicity underrepresented in surgery, to come and spend a month with us. We also partnered with Meharry Medical College, a Historically Black College/University (HBCU) Medical School in Nashville. We became a regular year round training site. Selected third year Meharry students, come to Swedish for their third year surgical clerkship. We hope these two programs will encourage minority students to inquire about Swedish and apply to our program. We want them to come and see what we are all about; to help us make a difference. Our premise is that this partnership will encourage any students of color who are interested in surgery to come to Swedish and consider it as a place to train.

Though there are some similarities in our family dynamics, Selwyn and I couldn't have been from starting points further away from each other. Selwyn Rogers was born in St. Thomas and grew up on St. Croix in the United States Virgin Islands. He came from a non-medical family. His parents actually didn't go to college.

Regardless he enjoyed school, particularly the sciences and consider being a high school science teacher before being enamored by the idea of being a physician. That mindset resulted in him going to Harvard for medical school and then the Brigham and Woman's Hospital and the Massachusetts General Hospital for surgery residency and fellowship. He gravitated to trauma surgery because he wanted to "take care of the whole patient."

I was born and raised in Seattle, Washington. I did not come from a college educated family. My grandparents were Italian and Irish immigrants. My father was the first of his generation to go to college and he did so on an ROTC scholarship. I was a good student, enjoyed the sciences and eventually considered medicine for a career. I had very important mentors and teachers along the way who directed me appropriately. I graduated from the University of Washington School of Medicine, did my general surgery residency at Swedish Medical Center in Seattle and completed the Executive Development Program from the University of Washington Foster School of Business.

That very first cold call was surprisingly successful. We knew from the beginning that we had something that was going to work for both sides. It was as if we were longstanding colleagues. My conversation with Selwyn was positive and engaging from the onset. This had as much to do with our personalities as it did our common goals and how they complimented each other. The information I had received from my friend regarding the trauma center's need for resident coverage was correct, for all of the reasons that had been outlined. So, there was definitely a need from both sides. The devil would be in the details. We decided the next move was to do some work in tandem. We would investigate what the University of Chicago would need to make this work and we would work with the Accreditation Council for Graduate Medical Education (ACGME) and the American Board of Surgery (ABS) to bring on another training site for our residency program. We flew to Chicago and had a dinner meeting at Prime & Provisions. The next day we toured the construction site of the nearly finished trauma center. Selwyn wanted as senior level residents as we could swing. Due to Chief resident requirements, that made the 4th year our best target. We usually have 5 residents per year, but that can be 4 occasionally. We agreed to each resident spending 2 months of their fourth year, resulting in us supplying resident coverage for 8–10 months per year. Swedish would continue to pay the residents' salary and the University of Chicago would help with travel and pay the residents' rent in Chicago. We would start this relationship when they opened in May 2018. Having shared goals for the institutions, leaders and region propelled us all in the direction of making this happen. Going back on the overarching goals I had to do our part to change the world made this even more special. Since both programs thought it reasonable to date before we got married, we did three one year contracts. A year and a half into that agreement we both went all in and Swedish is contracted to provide fourth year residents to 2033 and hopefully beyond. Also, after the first year, University of Chicago requested we cover a full R4 FTE, which we agreed to. Regardless of how many fourth year residents we have any given year, we always have one in Chicago. Not surprising, we now have a number of our residents pursuing trauma/critical care fellowships after residency.

Hopefully the 2024 Match will assist in diversifying our residency program and we can continue on the road to achieving all of our goals.

Selwyn and I have become friends. We use the term "brothers from a different mother" to describe our relationship. I admire what he has done and is doing. We text back and forth about college football, the World Cup, and our European travels. He has come to Swedish as a Grand Rounds lecturer and received one of our teachers of the year awards from our residents. I am planning a trip back to Chicago to discuss what else we can do to promote our agenda. This is not a "them" problem. This is an "us" problem. We are adamant about making a difference through an intentional partnership. Just talking about injustice, disparity and racism is no longer enough. We have all been called to action and we are doing our best to answer that call. I will often sign emails or texts with him to "keep the faith," but I'm not just saying that to him, I'm saying it to myself as well.

Walt Whitman was an American nineteenth century poet. What I didn't know was that he served as a Civil War healthcare worker. He had no medical training but provided basic physical and psychologic assistance to the soldiers in need, preserving their dignity and individuality. He has also been rumored to have coined the phrase "be curious, not judgmental." I for one think these are words by which to live.

Part VI
Perspective

Faculty Development in an Academic Trauma Center

John C. Alverdy and Jeffrey B. Matthews

Introduction

Trauma surgeons working in an academic medical center will often argue that they are "too busy to be productive," implying that their ability to generate scholarship that is meaningful in the context of academic promotion is limited by their clinical responsibilities. Thus, the term "productive" may mean one thing to the individual faculty member and another to their leaders. For example, to many stakeholders such as department chairs, section chiefs, hospital administrators, etc., clinically busy trauma/critical care surgeons may be considered productive by the long hours of outstanding care they provide to their patients, by their roles as educators in the "trenches", and by their status as role models for professionalism and dedication to their patients. Yet to the individual faculty member, the demands of this level of service may not feel personally rewarding as it seems to conflict with the goal of wider recognition of one's expertise and impact through original scholarship, academic promotion, and more visible leadership roles. Of course, one might argue that being an expert clinician, influential educator, and a role model to students, residents and fellows imparts valuable institutional impact irrespective of whether it is considered strictly "scholarly" in the traditional sense. Yet, the service commitment required to achieve this level of impact is not insubstantial and can lead to disillusionment, burnout and job dissatisfaction, especially when there is misalignment

J. C. Alverdy (✉)
Department of Surgery, University of Chicago, Pritzker School of Medicine, Chicago, IL, USA
e-mail: jalverdy@bsd.uchicago.edu

J. B. Matthews
Department of Surgery, The University of Chicago, Chicago, IL, USA
e-mail: jmatthews@bsd.uchicago.edu

S. O. Rogers, Jr (ed.), *Creating a Modern Trauma Center*,
https://doi.org/10.1007/978-3-031-66524-0_27

between the expectations of the institution and the aspirations of the individual faculty member. Sometimes the misalignment is already evident during contract negotiations. Well-trained applicants may select a particular employment opportunity based on pragmatic factors such as salary, location, medical center prestige, and personal/family/childcare needs rather than the extent of support for their individual academic or professional development. Often, newly-minted surgeons fresh out of long years of training are enthusiastic to establish their clinical credibility and independence by assuming full clinical loads. They may accept a higher initial clinical effort commitment imagining that they will either be able to carve out sufficient time on their own to pursue their scholarly interests or renegotiate for additional it protected time once they already have a "foot in the door.". Perhaps herein lies the challenge. Medical centers and departments of surgery need well-trained high level trauma/acute care surgeons to care for some of the most complex and critically-ill patients in the hospital, and the expertise of these surgeons depends on technical practice and repetitive experience ("reps") that derive from high effort allocation to clinical service. The question then becomes: how does leadership balance the imperative for expert clinical service with the individual's broader career aspirations including their ability to create "scholarship?"

It is important for incoming faculty to understand how leadership expects a department or section to align with the goals, service requirements, educational and research missions of the medical center or university. First, a chief/chair must provide high quality clinical service that is responsive to the needs of patients, families, the local community, and referring physicians, as well as the requirements of the medical center. Second the clinical service must conform to a business model that works within the financial capabilities of the medical center university and other institutional stakeholders. Finally, leadership must ensure that the educational and scholarship missions are properly balanced with the clinical enterprise. The dictum, "no margin no mission" is often used to describe this delicate balance; so does its inverted variation "no mission, no point". The aggregate enterprise must strike a realistic balance among the clinical, research, and educational components of the tripartite mission, but there will assuredly be substantial heterogeneity among faculty members in the individual distribution of "effort" for each domain. The personal expectations of an individual faculty member may not perfectly align with the department's perspective of their role in achieving each element of the institution's mission, and this misalignment can lead to confusion, disillusionment and burnout.

Faculty Development in a Newly Formed Academic Trauma Center at the University of Chicago

The existing structure of the various University of Chicago programs in surgery, their didactic curricula, conferences, research programs and high standards of excellence, lent itself well to formation of the academic enterprise within a newly-founded section of trauma and critical care surgery. Once an outstanding section chief was recruited, the plan was to leverage this framework to allow recruited faculty to meet regularly with the section chief, chair, vice-chair for research to begin to develop their academic ideas and to engage in the multiple ongoing research efforts within the department of surgery and university at large. However, it must be stated that the initial institutional priority was to recruit clinical faculty who would develop the necessary clinical processes and protocols to enable the launch of the adult level 1 trauma center on May 1 2018. This effort took precedence over all other missions, because on that date the University of Chicago Medicine went from treating zero adult trauma patients to being the busiest center in Chicagoland essentially overnight. The number of faculty initially recruited turned out to be too low, because the initial volume of trauma patients was 2× higher than predicted. This inevitably slowed the development of the academic programs and led to some frustration particular by the junior faculty. The heavy clinical service load created a gap between their individual aspirations and the demands of patient care. However, as additional faculty came on board, the faculty could better balance their clinical service obligations with opportunities for academic development. Their efforts to gather preliminary data and to submit grant proposals both within the department and outside of it, were facilitated by regular "research in progress" meetings attended by the chair, the vice-chair of research and numerous senior faculty serving as mentors and coaches. This gave each faculty member the opportunity to present their research ideas, obtain feedback, and secure the release of startup funds. For more senior faculty, and for those who were more interested in community engagement, multiple opportunities for collaboration were available. These included world class collaborators within the Harris School of Public Policy (https://harris.uchicago.edu/about), the Crime lab (https://crimelab.uchicago.edu/), the department of economics, the law school, etc. For example, recent partnerships across institutions and disciplines addressing the medical legal issues faced by trauma patients has resulted in key publications outside the traditional venue of basic biologic research [1].

For those interested in the biology of trauma and clinical trials, multiple mentors, senior funded faculty and independent scientific investigators (PI MD/PhDs with an established research program) were made available for collaboration. For example, interest in the role of TXA (tranexemic acid) as an agent that can affect the outcome of blunt head trauma is being explored by senior investigators in trauma [2].

Most recently the department of surgery recruited a director of health services research and implementation science at the University of Chicago department of surgery. Dr. Ted Skolarus (https://www.uchicagomedicine.org/find-a-physician/physician/ted-skolarus) has been charged with developing the heath services research line of investigator for surgeons interested in this field. He regularly mentors and guides faculty seeking extramural funding (K- level and R-Level NIH funding) in the field of health services and implementation science. This body of research focuses on creating new knowledge in the field of surgery related to the organization and delivery of health care services and their outcomes. Implementation science is concerned with issues that seek to identify barriers to healthcare, following which various evidence-based strategies can be implemented and outcome from surgery modified. As might be imagined, health services research and implementation science is highly relevant to the care of patients suffering from traumatic injury and critical illness.

As a result of recruiting an outstanding team and the availability of world class research services, the trauma service has developed an ongoing database registry to capture all clinical metadata on trauma patients admitted to the University of Chicago Trauma Service via the Center for Research Informatics (https://cri.uchicago.edu/). Multiple investigators are now collecting plasma, swab samples (nasal, rectal, fecal, etc.) and fluid samples (urine, CSF, etc.) which are biobanked and analyzed to pair to the clinical metadata.

Productive Faculty Are a Medical Center's Greatest Asset

Among the many challenges to leadership is hiring faculty that are not only productive, but who also also feel productive, maintain job satisfaction and feel facilitated to pursue their personal career goals. Given that trauma surgeons are highly educated and highly trained, many choose to work in an academic medical center with the goal of developing a career highlighted by academic productivity. Academic productivity now comes in many forms; one can develop into a master clinician/educator or can become an independently funded investigator. Progressive academic departments need to recognize this variability and provide resources, compensation and rewards so that these values are appreciated. The aphorism "allow faculty to do what they love and they will be productive" probably still holds true today. Recruiting and retaining highly productive faculty who enjoy their jobs is not only in the best interest of the academic medical center, it is its greatest asset.

The Promotion Process at the University of Chicago Department of Surgery

The process of recruiting faculty to an academic department of surgery should, in theory, result in faculty that are fundamentally promotable. It is critical that all faculty understand the criteria for promotion and that they regularly meet with leadership to track their progress and make adjustments as needed. At the University of Chicago, there are two academic tracks, the School of Medicine track (SOM) and the research track. Faculty in both tracks can receive tenure, however tenure at the University of Chicago is conferred when an individual's scholarship if determined to be within the top 10–15% of those in the field. Most faculty recruited to the University of Chicago in the department of surgery are recruited into the SOM track, which does not automatically confer tenure. However faculty in the SOM track at the University of Chicago are "tenureable" once their scholarship has reached a point of national visibility commensurate with the criteria set by the committee on appointments and promotions (COAP). There are several examples of faculty who have begun their appointments at the University of Chicago in the SOM track who have achieved tenure subsequent to their initial appointment.

Independent PI (Principal Investigator) Status

Among the many challenges to leadership is the provision of startup funds to the most promising research/investigators in the department with the expectation that they will obtain sustained and continuous extramural funding. With rare exception, investments in research by surgery departments are costly and the return on the investment cannot be viewed with short-sightedness. For example, there is an major opportunity cost when surgical faculty are not engaged in billable services. Also, in today's market of novel and fundable ideas, generating compelling preliminary data to test a scientific premise transformative to a field is a tall order that consumes both time and money. Finally, investments occur in the background of knowing that to successfully compete for R level NIH-type extramural funding, applications have to score in the top 10% of all submitted proposals. In essence, faculty and departments need to be supportive of the efforts of those who are trying to paint their "Mona Lisa" and understand its importance to the overall mission of the medical center.

Scientific Collaborators Independent of the prestige of an institution and the success of a particular basic science laboratory, finding and intellectually engaging with a willing scientific collaborator can be challenging. Scientists that are successful at obtaining funding and publishing in high impact journals are often unwilling to collaborate with junior faculty when they perceive their commitment, engagement, protected time and enthusiasm to be inadequate. Successful scientists are serious scholars who are adept at managing their time and budgets carefully. It is unreasonable to begin a study with a scientific collaborator with the sole purpose that they will simply process and analyze samples; a collaborator must be excited to participate in a given study as it will enhance the own productivity resulting in scholarly publications and an opportunity for grant submission. This requires regular participation, continued intellectual engagement and mutually satisfying contributions that extend and enhance the overall efforts of both laboratories. An intellectual engagement of this type often begins with a scientific question interesting to both parties and the testing of a novel hypothesis that will be of high impact to each party's field. Finding the right collaborator can be a matter of developing the right "chemistry." Serious investigators need to seek out collaborators within their own institutions that are regularly accessible. While website and "connectors" are often discussed as important to pair the needs from one laboratory to another, skillful investigators usually have little trouble identifying those collaborators with whom they develop workable chemistry and fundable productivity.

Mentors and Coaches

Today much is written about matching and pairing junior faculty to more senior faculty member who can act as mentors and coaches [3]. While this is certainly a laudable goal, serving as a mentor or coach requires time and training. Not all senior scientists, be they involved in clinical outcomes, health services or in the basic sciences are good mentors. The idea here is that oversight, collaboration, regular meetings, coaching, review of manuscripts and grants, etc., will improve the promotion process and ultimately the success of junior faculty. While this task is often left to section chiefs and chairs, it should be recognized that the time commitment required to be an effective mentor or coach is significant. Successful senior faculty involved in research often want to be left alone to do their research. Enlisting them as "mentors" is not a matter of simply designating them as such. While the debate is ongoing, grant writers, scientific consultants and other outsourced services, while often available are not necessarily accesible. At the University of Chicago, care has been taken to discuss this aspect of collaboration with faculty and pair them with mentors and coaches who are both willing, available and accessible to serve as effective co-investigators.

Generating Molecular Level Mechanistic Data

While descriptive studies have their place in academic surgery and academic medicine, without formally testing a hypothesis by experiment, their value remains limited. As has been said by a preeminent surgeon-scientist, "seeing is great, but understanding is better [4]." Generating molecular-level mechanistic type data costs both time and money. In the case of basic bench-type research, often transgenic mice must be bred and selective genes knocked out to define the role of a particular molecule or pathway in a disease process. The investment needed to provide compelling molecular level evidence that advances the understanding of a disease process with data that is judged to be transformative to the field is a tall order. As one might imagine, this will require investment, time, resources, collaboration, building of a team and most importantly, risk. In the field of health services research and implementation science, similar preliminary data is needed and can be challenging, time-consuming, costly and risky. Yet without such preliminary data, obtaining extramural funding can be challenging. Even when faculty are successful at obtaining independent extramural funding, they face challenges to which they have no training or experience. These include budget management, providing guidance to surgical resident research fellows to be productive during their two years as fellows and completing the work needed for renewal of their grants. Each of these tasks requires significant "down time" to guide and mentor fellows in the lab, to meet and have lengthy discussions with their collaborators and to satisfy the goal of generating compelling data that is disruptive to their field of investigation. For faculty involved in such work, they often feel anxiety as their capabilities and resources are insufficient to meet the expectation of a review in a high impact journal as well as the reviewers of their applications. More senior level faculty who provide guidance and oversight is needed and the department of surgery at the University of Chicago has designated a vice-chair of research and a section of surgical research to carry out this important service.

Publishing with Purpose

For faculty, there are many reasons that underlie the desire to publish. For some it is to be published, while for others, it is to advance knowledge. Yet for a select few, publications are generated to advance knowledge the field and become a successful independent investigator. Yet it is important to recognize that in an academic department of surgery, the number of publications are often used as a sign of academic productivity. For extramural funding agencies such as the NIH and NSF, publications are often an indication of scholarly productivity and the ability to perform as an independent investigator. Although it is said that clinicians no longer read journals, they read articles, given their wide availability via the internet, it is becoming increasingly clear that the impact factor of the journal where they are published, i.e. reflected by the H index, is being regularly mentioned and used to evaluate the impact of a given body of scholarship. Today, appropriate or not, the H index, reflecting not only the number of publications but also how many times the publication has been cited by others, is being used as an important indicator of publication impact.

Persistence in Submitting Proposals

In order for an academic trauma center to produce sustained scholarship and be recognized for its program in trauma/critical care research, extramural funds, in the form of training grants as well as independent sources to support consumables, is needed as internal funds are not inexorable. There are now various surgical societies from which to draw such support including the American College of Surgeons, the eastern association for the surgery of trauma (EAST), American Association for the Surgery of Trauma (AAST), philanthropic sources such as the Alfred E. Sloan foundation and the Rand corporation and more traditional sources such as the National Institutes of Health (NIH) or National Science Foundation (NSF). Yet for an academic trauma center to be able to recruit and retain faculty interested in pursuing a line of inquiry important to advance the field, centralized resources must be initially available that allow them to generate the preliminary data needed to be competitive for extramural funding. Such centralized resources extend beyond the traditional "start-up" package and should include easily identified collaborators, mentors, a full-time scientific staff (either health services investigators or basic scientists) a grants submission office, a steady line of surgery residents or fellows willing and enabled to dedicate a significant portion of their time to research, etc. These services have been already established at the University of Chicago and are now being extended to incorporate the research efforts in trauma surgery. While the clinical burden in most academic trauma centers is extremely high, the idea that one will assume a significant clinical role and then "see how it goes" to develop a credible and fundable line of inquiry is often a recipe for failure. Time must be protected, resources must be available and the department and section must value the effort put forth by the individual with appropriate "buy-in" to support one's research effort. Leadership must stand firm in its commitment to allow research efforts to thrive as there can be much internal conflict and team resentment and jealousy toward those with protected time or whom such resources are directed. Not much has changed since the time that Francis Moore wrote about such conflicts and resolving them can be quite challenging [5].

For example, there are two important characteristics of the serious scholar that can create resentment among her/his colleagues. As has been written, spending time in "idle curiosity" or considering innovation as "requiring a reality distortion field," might mean that certain faculty appear to be doing nothing while other are working hard to maintain the clinical service line [6]. Yet it is important to consider that becoming a promising investigator in one's clinical field requires more than just high volume publications. It requires generating compelling preliminary data that provide clear mechanistic plausibility to a scientific premise transformative to the field. This is much harder to achieve by descriptive studies alone. It often requires a long-term commitment with publications in high impact, often non-surgical journals whose peer review process is rigorous and requires generating further data and multiple revisions. The data generated from such efforts is then used to convince a grant review panel that the hypothesis proposed is worth testing and the investment will have a high likelihood of advancing knowledge in the field.

Finally, the knowledge that most submitted grant proposals (>90%) will not be successful at obtaining funding, is sobering. Departments and sections of trauma invest both time and money preparing faculty for grant submissions, yet most will not be successful. Some will argue it is a process of persistence, however it is very difficult to determine the likelihood of success as review panels often change and their focus on a given topic can change. Lastly, obtaining successful funding the first time is no guarantee that it will be funded a second time and thus sustainable over the course of one's career. Thus the risk involved in choosing to support one project or investigator over another is substantial and always clear in retrospect. As can be understood, there are many challenges in supporting and successfully producing quality scholarship in an academic trauma center that are probably no different than those in other specialties of surgery.

Practical Steps to Becoming Academically Productive in the Field of Trauma Surgery

Trauma teams have a major advantage relative to other academic surgical practices given that time management can be made more flexible once team dynamics are developed that allow for enough "down time" to collaborate, write and pursue other scholarly works. Perhaps the most important aspect of this advantage lies in the ability of leadership to create trusted teams and a trusted environment. As has been mentioned elsewhere, a team is not a group of people that work together, it is a group of people that trust each other [7]. Therefore, when considering employment in an academic trauma center, team members have to trust each other to provide outstanding continuity of care, proper "hand-offs," back-up call when needed and consultative services that are highly collaborative and understanding of the complexities of caring for a multiply injured patient. Thus the medical center environment itself must be trustworthy in this sense. Once this is established, then faculty can develop a research program with which they share excitement and passion and can then carve out the time with collaborators to successfully achieve their aims. Guidance by the chief of service, vice chair of research and the chair is important so that faculty feel they are empowered to meet not only the expectations of the institution and promotion committee, but also their own sense of scholarly productivity.

It is important for faculty to develop and discuss their plans with leadership so they not only have a roadmap with which to pursue their goals, but also can set expectations for themselves and the section/department. After all, one has chosen to work at an academic medical center to not only provide excellent service, education and to become a role model to others, but also to do something that might advance knowledge in the field. Accomplishing this requires a clear plan that involves understanding one's own passions and also what is feasible and practical given the strengths and limitation of the institution and department.

What About Start-Up Funds, Protected Time and "buy-in" from Other Team Members?

For extremely talented and highly sought after faculty, demanding protected time, start-up funds and "buy-in" from other team member is often challenging. For the majority of incoming faculty, especially for those who are right out of fellowship, securing an academic position that meets their family, location, salary and practice needs takes priority. For clinical surgeons, like all decisions in life, they are made with incomplete information and uncertainty, there being no other. Yet falling back on one's clinical skills and becoming a master clinical surgeon, educator and role model, by default, is not always the road best taken. As in life, there can be many surprises along the way that allow for fulfillment in one's employment that can be unexpected. Yet given the moving target of a medical center's finances, extramural funding, the time commitments to one's family, etc., it is important to be introspective about what can be achieved in a 5–10 year timeframe within a particular academic trauma program and academic environment. Given the long road of education and training to become a trauma surgeon, the delayed gratification and accumulation of debt, obtaining employment that satisfies all needs as an academic trauma surgeon, can dramatically change depending on circumstances. Yet there are practical steps one can take to make sure that the current employment situation is deserving of the extensive time and energy commitment taken at this point.

Planning an Academic Career as a Busy Trauma Surgeon

It is important to understand one's clinical obligations when considering a job opportunity as a trauma/critical care surgeon. In an academic medical center such as the University of Chicago, clinical time can not only be highly consuming, but also emotionally consuming. Understanding your time off, vacation time, post call time off, etc., will help you plan for emotional decompression once a full day of trauma service has passed. It is important not to underestimate the need for this time off, not only for yourself, but for your family/partner. A distracted or emotionally unavailable spouse/mother/father should not be considered "part of the job." At the University of Chicago, we have a vice-chair for faculty wellness who is available to address such issues and provide guidance, resources and referrals for allied healthcare support.

Doing What You Love to Remain Fulfilled and Satisfied

One does not need to aspire to be a "triple threat" in academic medicine to be feel fulfilled and satisfied in their current post. There are many opportunities to contribute to the academic mission besides being a model educator or a basic or clinical scientist. Community engagement efforts such as speaking at churches, synagogues or temples, speaking engagements at high schools, participating in STEM programs, etc., can be fulfilling and are recognized by our promotion process as significant accomplishments. It is important to be able to pursue the things that give your academic career meaning and that are also valued by your institution.

Being Promoted in a Timely and Equitable Manner

At the University of Chicago, the criteria for promotion are broad and intended to be inclusive, equitable and diverse. As each faculty member is involved in efforts that they are excited about and derive pleasure and passion, they should be recognized by the section chief and department as valued accomplishments for promotion. Promotion oversight, promotion committees and the vice-chair for appointments and promotions are tools and positions that should be readily visible and available so all faculty feel that they understand the criteria for promotion and that it is regularly discussed with their section chief. As departments of surgery properly recruit a diverse faculty and populate the medical center with the most outstanding talent available, if they are doing their job appropriately, all faculty should be promoted or at lcast promotable. Our standard time frame for promotion at the University of Chicago is 6 years as assistant and 6 years as associate professor. However, faculty are promoted at the time at which they are ready for promotion and this can come earlier or later than the standard time frame.

Conclusions

The department of surgery at the University of Chicago has been set up to support incoming faculty that chose to develop a line of inquiry that advances knowledge in their respective fieldS. These resources have been incorporated into the newly formed trauma/critical program. We specifically recruit medical students into our residency program who are interested in taking two years off to complete a surgical research fellowship. Some receive their PhDs or MBA during this time, others complete a fellowship in our Ethics program. All in all, trauma/critical care surgeons enter a world class research university with a busy clinical trauma service that can easily accommodate their scholarly aspirations. Since its inception, more of our general surgery residents have chosen to apply to trauma/critical care fellowships than in all prior years. In addition, we are witnessing a growing interest in residents entering trauma-related laboratories with interests in addressing various issues of care for those suffering from traumatic injury and critical illness. These areas of research focus include disparities in health access, social determinants of health, the basic biology of traumatic illness and ethical issues of care.

References

1. Alur R, et al. What medical-legal partnerships can do for trauma patients and trauma care. J Trauma Acute Care Surg. 2023; https://doi.org/10.1097/ta.0000000000004167.
2. Rowell SE, et al. Effect of out-of-hospital tranexamic acid vs placebo on 6-month functional neurologic outcomes in patients with moderate or severe traumatic brain injury. JAMA. 2020;324:961–74. https://doi.org/10.1001/jama.2020.8958.
3. Ladner DP, et al. Transforming the future of surgeon-scientists. Ann Surg. 2024;279:231–9. https://doi.org/10.1097/sla.0000000000006148.
4. Thorp HH, Yaffe MB. Seeing is great, understanding is better. Sci Signal. 2023;16:eadg2868. https://doi.org/10.1126/scisignal.adg2868.
5. Brennan MF, Francis D, Moore MD: 1913–2001.
6. Gertner J. The idea factory: Bell Labs and the great age of American innovation. Penguin Press; 2012.
7. Sinek S. Start with why: how great leaders inspire everyone to take action. London: Penguin Books; 2011.

Surgical Ethics in Trauma

Kylie Callier and Peter Angelos

Introduction

There are many factors inherent to trauma care that contribute to the frequent moral and ethical dilemmas encountered by trauma providers. Proper evaluation and management of trauma patients depends upon the effective coordination of a multidisciplinary team in a complex and sometimes chaotic environment. Instead of the careful deliberation typically used in ethical decision-making, trauma surgeons must weigh risks and benefits and make high-stakes decisions with limited time and information. We will explore the unique ethical challenges that may arise when caring for acutely injured patients. Using our institution's experience on the South Side of Chicago as a framework for discussion, we will address health disparities in trauma care and the professional, ethical, and moral responsibilities of trauma providers to their patients and communities. Lastly, we will describe the public health approach to trauma care and the evolving role of trauma surgeons in advocacy and injury prevention.

Ethical Challenges in Trauma and Trauma Surgery

Clinical ethics is embedded in every type of patient encounter, and clinicians face ethical dilemmas regardless of their field of medicine or type of practice. However, the care of traumatically injured patients presents unique challenges to providers

K. Callier · P. Angelos (✉)
MacLean Center for Clinical Medical Ethics and Department of Surgery, University of Chicago, Chicago, IL, USA
e-mail: kylie.callier@uchicagomedicine.org; pangelos@bsd.uchicago.edu

S. O. Rogers, Jr (ed.), *Creating a Modern Trauma Center*,
https://doi.org/10.1007/978-3-031-66524-0_28

and trainees, many of which do not exist in clinical medicine outside of the trauma bay. The initial trauma assessment and resuscitation requires high-stakes, complex medical decisions to be made within seconds with little to no patient input. There are many well-established guidelines that provide frameworks for navigating different ethical challenges in medicine and surgery. However, these methods imply the ability and time to gather information, organize facts, and deliberate over an ethical solution. Trauma care challenges traditional ethical reasoning and, by its nature, renders many of these methods irrelevant. Not only does trauma care not conform to well-described approaches for structured ethical decision-making, trauma providers may face situations in which even the core principles of medical ethics are called into question.

Central to the practice of ethical medical care are the principles of beneficence, nonmaleficence, respect for autonomy, and justice. Physicians are expected to apply and integrate these principles in their daily practice. Ethical problems are approached by weighing these principles with the relevant circumstances of the case. However, the high acuity and potential for life-threatening injury frequently requires trauma providers to reach decisions about complex ethical issues within seconds to minutes. Furthermore, these fundamental principles do not provide clear-cut solutions. Trauma care and resuscitation requires a balance of what is ethically "correct" and what is medically required. Certain core principles may need to be sacrificed completely to save the patient's life.

Perhaps the most significant divergence from standard surgical ethics lies within patient autonomy. The bioethical principle of autonomy respects the patients' rights to make informed decisions about their medical care based on their values, beliefs, and preferences [1]. In trauma surgery, however, the situation's urgency may limit the extent to which patient autonomy can be practiced. Ensuring that a trauma patient's autonomy is respected while still providing timely and potentially life-saving interventions presents a unique challenge to trauma providers and, at least in some cases, may be an impossible task. The patient may be unconscious, intoxicated, or disoriented and lack the state of mind to participate in their care. Regardless, when a patient arrives in the trauma bay, the assessment begins immediately, and care is provided without hesitation on the basis of presumed consent under the assumption that the patient would want to be saved. Providers are ethically obliged to act in the patient's best interests with little to no knowledge of the patient's desires or advanced directives. Trauma providers may make decisions based on what is in the patient's best medical interests as judged by the providers, which may be viewed as paternalistic by some outside of the field. It is ethically permissible use the best interest standard in treating acutely injured patients, while maintaining the highest degree of respect for the patient's own choices and dignity. The American Medical Association Code of Ethics supports providing the appropriate interventions to meet the patient's medical needs, adding that physicians should always disclose what transpired as soon as appropriate and that interventions may be withdrawn later when the patient's preferences become known [2].

Whenever possible, a surrogate decision-maker should be sought out for patients who cannot communicate their wishes or values as they pertain to procedures and medical treatments such as goals of care or acceptable quality of life. Appropriate surrogate decision-makers may include a family member, close friend, or legally appointed guardian. Similar to the trauma provider, the role of the surrogate is to act and make vital decisions that are in the patient's best interest and collaborate with the trauma team to ensure decisions are made in accordance with the patient's preferences whenever possible. However, the acuity and unpredictability of trauma situations can make such decision-making very challenging. Often, the patient has never explicitly expressed their wishes regarding surgical interventions, medical treatments, or end-of-life care. This is especially true of younger, previously healthy individuals, the very group that constitutes a large portion of trauma patients. Additionally, surrogate decision-makers may be unprepared to be thrust into this decision-making role. Emotions evoked by having an injured loved-one may affect their ability to process information and make decisions. Heightened emotions, time constraints, and difficult topics and decisions to be made are just a few aspects of these discussions that can lead to inadequate communication between families and the trauma team. Trauma physicians must balance compassionate discussion with the need to make high-stakes decisions quickly. While navigating these complex trauma scenarios, trauma teams should emphasize the importance of clear communication, empathy, and respect for the surrogate's role during these challenging circumstances.

Futility and Nonlife-Saving Trauma Care

The concept of futility refers to medical or surgical interventions that are unlikely to benefit the patient or increase survival. If a patient's injuries are deemed not survivable and death is inevitable, the priority of the trauma team should be to provide comfort and alleviate suffering while respecting the dignity of the patient. Invasive procedures causing unnecessary pain or suffering would violate the principle of nonmaleficence (avoiding harm) [1]. Furthermore, organ donor potential should never influence active treatment or resuscitation in the trauma bay. While organ donation is considered a public good, the primary responsibility of the trauma surgeon is the optimal care of the trauma patient. Considering the potential for organ donation conflicts with these duties. It is not until cardiac death, brain death, or imminent death that organ donation should be discussed or pursued. Fortunately, there are clearly defined guidelines and systems in place, such as organ procurement organizations, that remove much of the moral burden from trauma providers in such situations [3].

Ethical dilemmas also arise after stabilization of a critically injured patient is achieved, when treatment objectives may focus on long-term functionality, pain management, and quality of life. Decisions regarding the extent of medical or surgical interventions can be ethically complex, especially when discussing interventions that provide marginal or uncertain benefit to the patient. There may be differing opinions among medical staff, patients, and families regarding what constitutes a meaningful benefit. Physicians may perceive further treatments or procedures as unlikely to achieve the desired outcome, while family members may cling to hope and insist "everything be done". This tension is often compounded by the stress of trauma situations, cultural and personal differences about life and death, and differing interpretations of quality of life, all of which should be taken into consideration when navigating these discussions. Such situations require nuanced, compassionate deliberation between experienced trauma providers and surrogate decision-makers. Moreover, allocating limited resources to non-critical or non-life-saving procedures poses ethical questions about fairness and equity, such as in the scenarios discussed below.

Although it is common to hear medical providers refer to some treatments with a very low likelihood of success as "futile," we recommend avoiding whenever possible. When medical caregivers refer to a treatment as "futile," patients and/or surrogate decision-makers often assume that futility is a medical fact. However, no matter how unlikely to be effective, interventions are only futile relative to a specific goal. Thus, we recommend that rather than referring to treatments as futile, caregivers should instead more accurately state that a treatment is "highly unlikely to meet a specified goal" [4].

Triage and Allocation of Resources

The allocation of resources in trauma care presents ethical dilemmas centered around the core ethical principle of justice (fairness in access to and distribution of resources) and balancing individual and societal needs [1]. In mass casualty situations or when resources such as blood products, intensive care unit beds, or personnel are scarce, trauma providers must make difficult decisions about which patients receive immediate care and where to allocate limited resources. While triage protocols are designed to help guide these decisions, the reality of applying such protocols can lead to ethical conflicts. Ethical principles such as equality, in which each patient is given the same care, and utility, in which the total benefit is maximized across all patients, may be at odds. Furthermore, there may be great tension between the clinician's duty to provide the best possible care for the individual patient and the need to consider the health of the population.

The presence of vulnerable populations exacerbates these challenges. It is imperative to recognize bias and avoid discrimination based on age, race, socioeconomic status, or disability. Care should be delivered impartially, and while protocols are designed to help manage these complex situations, they may have unintended biases leading to unequal distribution of resources and the propagation of disparities in health care of marginalized populations. Triage protocols should be constantly reviewed and adapted to reflect current climates. Transparent, ethical decision-making processes must be used to address potential problems with triage systems. A commitment by trauma providers to fairness and justice is required to ensure that resources are allocated to maximize benefit and minimize harm for the collective population while respecting the dignity and rights of individual patients.

The Trauma Team

A wide range of healthcare professionals comprise the multidisciplinary trauma team that must work cohesively to provide high-quality care during high-pressure situations. Team members include providers from multiple specialties, such as surgery, emergency medicine, anesthesia, nursing, and support staff, all of whom provide care and input during the trauma assessment and resuscitation. The team leader, often the trauma surgeon, is tasked with making decisions and coordinating the team's activities. An ethical leader must lead with compassion and fairness and eliminate potential biases while making decisions and organizing team members to achieve the desired outcome [5]. Team dynamics are crucial in navigating ethical challenges as they arise. In addition to a trauma leader guided by strong ethical principles, recent studies suggest that the cultural diversity of the trauma team may be just as important in providing ethical, patient-centered care [6].

Academic trauma centers offer trainees the opportunity to develop distinct clinical skills necessary for surgical training. However, the setting of trauma care may pose an ethical dilemma when caring for this unique and inherently vulnerable population, as direct supervision of trainees is not always feasible. Attending trauma physicians must allow trainees to develop the technical and clinical judgment skills in stressful situations that are imperative to surgical training, but they also must ensure the best patient outcome. Attending physicians may decrease direct supervision as the trainee demonstrates proficiency in clinical and surgical skills to ensure appropriate, high-quality care for patients while also fostering autonomy and preparing residents for increasing responsibility as they move through training. Training programs should also strive to create an inclusive learning environment that encourages trainees to ask questions and seek help when needed.

However, the field of trauma surgery is unpredictable, and the reality is that situations are possible in which the attending physician and/or senior resident may be caring for other critically ill patients and not immediately available. Academic centers should recognize this possibility and ensure the appropriate staffing for their center to prevent the potential harm caused to patients moral distress to the trauma team. These situations are not limited to the emergent care provided to the patient. Trainees may encounter challenging situations outside of the trauma bay that they lack experience with or are not adequately trained for which also raises ethical concerns. Such situations include engaging in end-of-life discussions with patients and/or families or informing families about the death of a loved one. Some institutions have begun to address the challenge of adequately preparing trainees to engage in such difficult conversations; however, most surgical residents still receive little formal training on these critical aspects of patient care. Preparing surgical trainees for such important and potentially ethically challenging discussions is an important area for improvement for surgical training programs.

Trauma Systems and the Ethical Responsibilities of the Trauma Surgeon

Disparities in Trauma Care

The field of trauma is inexorably influenced by the community or population being served and social determinants of health that cast shadows over the equitable care of trauma patients. When treating trauma patients from disadvantaged communities, a multitude of ethical considerations arise. The outcomes of trauma patients reflect the systemic and individual variables associated with the unequal distribution of health resources as well as access to and quality of medical care. Factors such as ethnicity, type of insurance, and socioeconomic status have all been associated with worse outcomes in trauma patients. These issues demand careful deliberation and compassionate responses from trauma providers.

Cultural competence and preventing the adverse effects of bias and discrimination are crucial in providing equitable care to patients in lower socioeconomic areas and racial and ethnic minorities. Whether implicit or explicit, provider bias can manifest in the quality of care delivered by affecting surgical decisions, management protocols, and/or follow-up strategies. Providers must recognize how certain factors impact a patient's care and remain vigilant about potential unconscious and institutional biases. Factors such as limited health literacy or language barriers can contribute to challenges in education and informed consent of patients or surrogate decision-makers. Understanding and respecting different cultural beliefs and practices can protect the dignity of the patient, improve communication, and foster trust between providers and patients and their families.

Lower socioeconomic populations and communities may be plagued by delays in treatment due to under-resourced or lack of medical facilities or transportation barriers in both rural and urban settings. These populations are frequently situated in "trauma deserts", where high-quality emergency services are scarce or non-existent. Studies using census tract data have shown that Black-majority neighborhoods in large urban areas, including Chicago, are particularly associated with disparities in geographic access to trauma care. Longer prehospital transport times are known to contribute to higher mortality rates, especially in penetrating trauma mechanisms, and these areas have a high rate of penetrating injuries [7]. This raises significant concerns about structural inequality placing the lives of racial minorities at risk [8].

Recognition of the potential causes of disparities in trauma care is essential to implement measures to mitigate these inequities. Ongoing education about the social determinants of health and how to address them in practice should be provided to trauma staff. Research efforts aiming to understand and address the needs of disadvantaged populations should be encouraged. Trauma providers should have a broader role in advocating for improvements in health care systems and policies. This will be discussed further in the next section.

Public Health Approach to Trauma Care and Injury Prevention

Trauma systems have evolved and are constantly changing and adapting to the needs of the communities they serve. Similarly, the approach to trauma care has shifted as traumatic injuries, especially those resulting from violence, are increasingly viewed as a public health issue. It is now widely accepted that trauma care is a complex continuum that begins before an injury occurs and continues beyond recovery. The modern trauma system has been defined as "an organized and comprehensive public health response to injury within a specified geographic area that includes injury prevention, prehospital care, triage and transport, acute medical and surgical care, rehabilitation, education, and research" [9]. This approach to trauma care enforces the concept that trauma is not merely a series of isolated incidents, but a preventable public health issue and, as such, suggests that the role and ethical responsibilities of the trauma surgeon extend far beyond the operating room.

Professional surgical communities have confirmed this role. The American College of Surgeons Committee on Trauma (ASC-COT) describes optimal trauma care as including prevention, access, prehospital care and transportation, acute hospital care, rehabilitation, and research activities [10]. The current guidelines published by ASC-COT that serve as a framework for verification of trauma centers require all centers to have an injury prevention program and demonstrate collaboration with community organizations to support injury prevention efforts [10, 11]. Trauma providers are uniquely positioned at the intersection between health systems and the individual communities and populations in which they serve. Trauma surgeons have professional and ethical obligations beyond the acute setting into the broader context of prevention, education, and continuous improvements to healthcare systems to reduce the incidence and impact of trauma on society and provide accessible and equitable care to all.

Conclusion

There are many challenges to the ethical practice of trauma surgery. The ethical dimensions of rapid-fire decision-making and life-saving interventions demand our utmost respect. The role of the trauma surgeon necessarily extends beyond the technical aspect of treatments and procedures to encompass a deep understanding of the moral and ethical fabric that holds together the trust between patients, surgeons, and society. Surgeons must deftly apply the ethical tenets of autonomy, beneficence, nonmaleficence, and justice as best they can within the constraints of trauma scenarios such as informed consent processes, allocation of scarce resources, and end-of-life decision-making. Doing so requires rigorous and reflective practice and continuous professional development. Furthermore, trauma surgeons have an ethical and professional duty to pursue advocacy and injury prevention on behalf of their patients. Surgical ethics is vital to the evolution of trauma surgery and necessitates a thoughtful approach to the ethical issues surrounding every patient. With appropriate forethought along with compassion and integrity, trauma providers will be able to navigate the ethically challenging scenarios that they face in the unpredictable and ever-changing landscape of caring for traumatically injured patients.

References

1. Beauchamp TL, Childress JF. Principles of biomedical ethics. 8th ed. Oxford University Press; 2013.
2. Chaet DH. AMA code of medical ethics' opinions related to urgent decision making. AMA J Ethics. 2018;20(5):464–6. https://doi.org/10.1001/journalofethics.2018.20.5.coet1-1805.
3. American Medical Association. Guidelines for organ transplantation. In: Code of Medical Ethics. https://www.ama-assn.org/delivering-care/guidelines-organ-transplantation
4. Grossman E, Angelos P. Futility: what Cool Hand Luke can teach the surgical community. World J Surg. 2009;33(7):1338–40. https://doi.org/10.1007/s00268-009-9997-2.
5. Angelos P, Devon K, Ferreres AR, McLeod R, Ellison EC. A crucial moment for reflection on the importance of ethical leadership in academic medicine. Ann Surg. 2021;273(2):e46–9. https://doi.org/10.1097/SLA.0000000000004600.
6. Cobianchi L, Dal Mas F, Massaro M, et al. Diversity and ethics in trauma and acute care surgery teams: results from an international survey. World J Emerg Surg. 2022;17:44. https://doi.org/10.1186/s13017-022-00446-8.
7. Crandall M, Sharp D, Unger E, et al. Trauma deserts: distance from a trauma center, transport times, and mortality from gunshot wounds in Chicago. Am J Public Health. 2013;103(6):1103–9. https://doi.org/10.2105/AJPH.2013.301223.
8. Tung EL, Hampton DA, Kolak M, Rogers SO, Yang JP, Peek ME. Race/ethnicity and geographic access to urban trauma care. JAMA Netw Open. 2019;2(3):e190138. https://doi.org/10.1001/jamanetworkopen.2019.0138.
9. Norton R, Kobusingye O. Injuries. N Engl J Med. 2013;368(18):1723–30. https://doi.org/10.1056/NEJMra1109343.
10. Resources for Optimal Care of the Injured Patient (2022 Standards). Published online 2023. https://www.facs.org/quality-programs/trauma/quality/verification-review-and-consultation-program/standards/
11. Scarlet S. Caring for the wounded: the ethics of trauma surgery. AMA J Ethics. 2018;20(5):421–4. https://doi.org/10.1001/journalofethics.2018.20.5.fred1-1805.

Structural Violence in Trauma Care

Andrew J. Benjamin and Selwyn O. Rogers, Jr

Structural Violence in Trauma Care

Structural violence represents an insidious form of social injustice deeply embedded within societal structures, profoundly influencing individuals' lives and community health in ways that are often not immediately apparent. Originally conceptualized by Johan Galtung, this term broadens the conventional definition of violence [1]. It extends beyond the direct infliction of physical harm to encompass the myriad systematic methods through which social structures inflict harm or place certain individuals at a disadvantage. Due to its often subtle and unnoticed nature, structural violence requires a discerning understanding to recognize its pervasive role in molding the lives and well-being of people and communities.

In the realm of healthcare, and particularly within the context of modern trauma centers, structural violence plays a critical and complex role. Trauma centers, as critical infrastructure in the healthcare system, are designed to provide care for the most severe and life-threatening injuries. They are, by their very nature, a response to acute manifestations of violence and injury. However, the establishment, location, resource allocation, and accessibility of these trauma centers are deeply influenced by underlying currents of structural violence.

The nature of structural violence in healthcare is multifaceted. It includes geographic disparities in the placement of trauma centers, often influenced by

A. J. Benjamin (✉)
University of Chicago Medicine, Section of Trauma and Acute Care Surgery, Chicago, IL, USA
e-mail: abenjamin2@bsd.uchicago.edu

S. O. Rogers, Jr
Department of Surgery, The University of Chicago Medicine, Chicago, IL, USA
e-mail: srogers@bsd.uchicago.edu

S. O. Rogers, Jr (ed.), *Creating a Modern Trauma Center*,
https://doi.org/10.1007/978-3-031-66524-0_29

socio-economic factors rather than purely medical need. This in turn leads to "trauma deserts"in economically disadvantaged areas, where the very communities that might benefit most from immediate trauma care are potentially those least likely to have access [2]. Furthermore, racial and socio-economic disparities influence the quality of care received, with marginalized communities often receiving lower-quality services due to implicit biases, underfunding, and a lack of culturally competent care [3–5].

The causes of structural violence are deeply rooted in historical and ongoing social, economic, and political inequalities. Historical segregation, economic policies, and social norms have led to a concentration of poverty, violence, and health inequities in certain communities [6, 7]. These factors are compounded by broader issues such as racism, sexism, and other forms of discrimination that pervade societal structures, including healthcare systems. The result is a self-perpetuating cycle where the disadvantaged are more likely to experience trauma and less likely to receive adequate care [8].

The impacts of structural violence on individuals and communities are profound. It leads to increased morbidity and mortality, perpetuates cycles of violence and poverty, and undermines the overall well-being of society. In the specific context of trauma centers, the impacts are seen in the unequal outcomes for patients based on their geographic location, race, and socio-economic status. This not only affects the immediate victims of trauma but also has a ripple effect across communities, contributing to broader public health crises and economic strains.

Awakening to Inequity

The University of Chicago, renowned as a leading academic medical center, I now know was once predominantly a symbol of advanced healthcare for the privileged. The lack of a trauma center within a trauma desert was an unintentional form of systemic violence [2]. During the beginning of my surgical residency (which I started in 2013), my focus was primarily on the tertiary care we provided, an approach that often overlooked the broader needs of the surrounding community. It was rare for me to think about what went on only blocks away from the hospital on a near daily basis. Systemic gun violence, at a scale previously unfathomable to me, now regularly interrupts my daily routine with constant notifications on my pager. I would drive from my house to the hospital, oblivious to the fractured communities that surrounded me. This disconnection, I now understand, underlined a wider systemic issue: an academic medical center functioning parallel to, yet disjoint from, the urgencies of its neighbors. My formative years in medicine had painted a picture of privilege, unconsciously aligned with the structural barriers that perpetuated inequity.

The transformation to a trauma center in 2018 marked a pivotal shift, not just in our institution's approach to healthcare, but also in my personal understanding of systemic racism. This change ushered in a new demographic of patients, those who were directly facing the brunt of societal inequities, leaving them vulnerable to poor health outcomes, systemic violence, and even epigenetic changes to their DNA [9–11]. The stark realities of systemic racism—realities that were previously understated within our institution, now had gained sudden prominence.

Through this transition, I personally experienced a profound shift to a more personal and empathetic understanding of systemic racism. It became increasingly clear how closely healthcare delivery is intertwined with racial inequalities, and the significant role that medical institutions can play in bridging these gaps. Engaging with patients on a more personal level, I began to see beyond the stereotypes often perpetuated by media and social media narratives, gaining insight into the authentic experiences and struggles of those in the community.

This journey of witnessing the opening of a trauma center has been a testament to the power of direct patient interactions in reshaping perceptions and fostering empathy. It highlights the importance of genuine, on-the-ground voices in effectively combating systemic racism. The shift in patient care before and after the establishment of the trauma center, the contrasts between media narratives and personal experiences, and the transformative impact of direct patient interaction have been pivotal in understanding and addressing these systemic issues on a personal level. It underscores the vital role of healthcare institutions in not just providing medical care, but also in being proactive agents and frameworks of societal understanding and change.

Beyond the Trauma Bay

Embarking on this new chapter as the University of Chicago evolved into a trauma center, my day-to-day experiences began to starkly differ from my early years in residency. I was now commonly encountering individuals whose lives were deeply entwined with the systemic issues I had previously been oblivious to. Among the many transformative experiences was the case of a 17-year-old gunshot victim on a cold holiday night. While it was memorable, it was also only one of many such interactions that furthered my comprehension of systemic racism since 2018. This incident was not just a medical emergency or an exciting case; it would end up being a window into the realities of the community we served, revealing the depth and complexity of the challenges our patients faced.

It was a typical holiday night on call when the page came: "17-year-old male, GSW to the chest, traumatic arrest". My walk to the trauma bay was automatic, conditioned by countless similar activations since we had become a trauma center. In my earlier years as a resident, emergency department thoracotomies were more common, but we had since grown selective over time. My expectation was grim: pronounce the patient and prepare for the difficult conversation with his family.

Upon arrival, the trauma bay was its usual controlled chaos of activity. The team attached the young man to the monitor and the resident placed an ultrasound probe on the chest, revealing a pericardial effusion and faint cardiac activity. I could hear the words of my mentors as we debriefed all of the previous patients we had done thoracotomies on; "People don't survive gunshot wounds to the heart." Despite my skepticism, we opened his chest. The pericardium was opened, blood evacuated, and an exceptionally large laceration to the right ventricle was stapled closed. The heart was not beating as the blood was pouring in, but on a whim, I decided to administer intra-cardiac epinephrine—a practice we had essentially entirely abandoned knowing that even if the heart began to function, it was likely to only be transient. Remarkably, his heart started beating… and did not stop. We rushed him to the OR and successfully repaired his heart (with a bovine pericardial patch given the size of the injury).

In the days following his weaning from sedation and extubation, I was drawn to his bedside, eager to learn more about this young life we had miraculously saved. The thought that he should not have survived lingered in my mind, and I felt an overwhelming urge to speak with him. Driven by a sense of responsibility, I drove in from home the following week as he recovered in the hospital, hoping to make him realize the extent of his fortune and to inspire him to use this incident as a turning point. This impulse, I now recognize, was rooted in my own biases, a manifestation of stereotyping and unconscious racism. Before I had even spoken to him or seen his face, I had already crafted a narrative about his need for transformation. When I entered his room and found him upright in bed, with his pregnant girlfriend and numerous face tattoos, it only served to confirm my preconceived notions. As I introduced myself and recounted his survival from a gunshot wound to the heart and his death, his lack of astonishment struck me. In fact, he barely acknowledged me. My thoughts drifted to stereotypes many might silently acknowledge but seldom voice: the face tattoos, his pregnant girlfriend, a shooting right before Christmas. This 17-year-old, labeled a "gangbanger" by societal bias, seemed far from a mere child, he was hardened by the streets of Chicago. This moment would later become a retrospective turning point for me, a realization that despite what I had thought was my awareness of racial discourse in our post-George Floyd era, I had yet to fully grasp its nuances given my own internal dialogue. Looking back, I now understand that Reese and I perceived the gravity of the situation differently not because he was an emotionless "gangbanger", but because our upbringings, though geographically close, were worlds apart in experience. It would take a significant degree of engagement over the following months to fully realize and breakdown my own personal biases. Biases that I was hesitant to admit existed in the first place because I thought I was informed on the topic.

Despite the initial cold reception, I resolved to return the next day after completing my work. My subsequent visits were met with similar responses, but undeterred, I persisted throughout the week. Each time I left, I offered my assistance, saying, "Let me know if you need anything." Gradually, he began to open up. As his discharge neared, I sat beside his bed and asked him to share his story. At 17, he was expecting a child and was filled with anticipation about fatherhood. A red tattoo above his right eye caught my attention; it bore a name. Upon inquiry, he revealed it was the name of his best friend, who had been fatally shot last year. They were as close as brothers. He then showed me other names tattooed on his body, each a tribute to a friend lost to gun violence—over twenty in total. These tattoos were more than mere ink; they were poignant symbols of his life's hardships, a narrative I struggled to fully comprehend.

On the eve of his discharge, I visited him one last time. He looked well, his face lit with a smile. In a gesture I had never made before, I offered him my contact number, saying, "We will stay in touch. If you need anything, let me know." In the months that followed, some questioned my decision to maintain this line of communication. However, looking back, I see it not as a mistake, but as one of the more significant and enlightening experiences of my life.

About a week later, I received a frantic call. It was his mother on the line, panic-stricken. Reese had collapsed out on the floor. He had not been eating well due to constant vomiting, "bright green" as his mom described it. I urged her, "Bring him straight to the emergency department. Call an ambulance if you need to." Time ticked away slowly, first 45 minutes, then an hour. My gaze was fixed on the ED waiting room list, convince his cardiac repair had failed. Concern mounting, I called back, "Are you here yet?" Their response unveiled another layer of their struggle to survive on the South Side of Chicago—no car, dependent on a ride from his aunt who lived 45 minutes away. Over the years, I came to realize that such lack of personal transportation was not an isolated incident but a pervasive issue in this part of the city. It made me question: How many patients that I previously perceived as irresponsible for missing trauma clinic appointments, were simply constrained by their circumstances?

Finally, they were en route. By this time, my own heart was racing with anxiety. The moment he arrived; one look was enough to alarm me. He looked to be in extremis—heart racing at 150 beats per minute, his complexion concerningly pale. I immediately found an ultrasound and placed it on his chest, expecting the worst. Surprisingly, it was normal. After administering several liters of fluids, his condition improved noticeably. While my concern diminished, my confusion deepened—the constant bilious vomiting, and inability to even keep down water—did not align with his injuries or our operation. A CT scan revealed an unexpected diagnosis: superior mesenteric artery (SMA) syndrome. It is a condition familiar to every surgeon, often appearing in ABSITE and board exams, yet one that some senior surgeons skeptically claim might not even exist.

I struggled to comprehend. How could a young man, shot in the heart, suddenly develop SMA syndrome? It was only upon truly seeing Reese—beyond his medical history—that the pieces fell into place. I had always viewed him as a slim, yet healthy youth. The truth was far more complex. Reese, living with his overburdened single mother and numerous siblings, including a brother in prison, did things "he knew he shouldn't," to earn money and keep food on the table. When I took a step back and really looked at him, I could easily fit my fingers around his thighs. Inconsistent food availability had led to weight loss over the past months, even before the shooting, and his recent injury must have just pushed him over the edge. In the days following his admission, despite our best efforts, eating was an insurmountable task—unable to even keep down water. We were left with no choice but to insert a naso-jejunal tube fore tube feeding. It would likely take months for him to regain sufficient weight to alleviate the obstruction.

Most patients in Reese's situation would be discharged home with tube feeds, but lacking insurance and adequate home support, he faced another hurdle: an extended hospital stay. This became another phase in my understanding, as I delved deeper into the layers of his life, beginning to unravel the profound impact of his experiences. At 17, Reese's emotional maturity seemed to align more closely with that of a 10-year-old, far from being "hardened" as I had thought when I first met him. As I got to know him better, I learned that he was a senior in high school. However, when I encouraged him to write daily as a form of emotional processing, it became evident that his reading and writing skills were akin to those of a second or third grader. School attendance was a rarity for him due to safety concerns, yet he was routinely passed to the next grade. This was a stark illustration of the inequities within the Chicago public school system, where disparities in local property wealth systemically undermined his chance at a quality education [12, 13].

However, a more alarming issue soon emerged—Reese was addicted to opiates at just seventeen. This reality came into sharper focus as more of his friends and family visited him in the hospital, where many of them revealed they struggled with the same issue. As someone personally touched by the devastation of opiate addition within my own family, witnessing its grip on an entire community was heart-wrenching. The challenges stacked against Reese seemed insurmountable. How could he navigate through this and lead a "normal" life? One of the hardest parts was that, to him, his current life **was** normal. Bridging that gap in understanding, leading him to a healthier lifestyle seemed daunting. Nonetheless, I was committed to providing support,

My years at the hospital, prior to it becoming a trauma center, had been markedly different. In the clinics and on the floors, I interacted with patients coming for their elective operations, discussing topics like their children and interests—subjects that resonated with my own worldview. These conversations flowed effortlessly; their children attended private schools, prestigious universities, and pursued careers as bankers, lawyers, and doctors. Now I was visiting his room each day, looking up words trying to figure out what Reese was saying to me at times, and what things abbreviations like "asl" meant when he texted me. The contrast was stark and eye-opening.

Reese was about to turn eighteen, a milestone he faced with a heavy heart knowing he would spend his birthday in the hospital attached to tube feeds. Curious about his interests, I asked him what he enjoyed. He loved basketball, and Steph Curry was his favorite player. On a whim I looked up the Chicago Bull's schedule, and as fate would have it, they were set to play Golden State, Steph Curry's team, on his birthday. I discussed the idea with my division chief, and he pulled strings to make something incredible happen. By reaching out to Steph Curry's foundation, he was able to secure tickets for the game. Despite his naso-jejunal tube, we arranged a day pass and took him to his first basaketball game, accompanied by his girlfriend and friends. I had been to numerous sporting events, but the sheer wonder and joy in their eyes was something else entirely. It transcended a mere celebration of his birthday; for Reese, it was an act of unconditional kindness, a rarity in his life. His gratitude was overwhelming. With tears in his eyes, he hugged me and confessed that no one had ever done something like this for him. A victim of social disorganization, he had always lived in a transactional society, struggling for basic necessities, both material and emotional [14]. Unlike many, including myself, he had never had the chance to simply be cared for while figuring out life. Getting to know him beyond the stigma and stereotypes, I saw his true nature: a sweet, generous, yet deeply traumatized young man.

In the months that followed, as Reese began to recover and eat independently, his journey continued. He moved away from his neighborhood, sought treatment for his opiate addiction, welcomed the birth of his daughter, and faced unexpected legal challenges due to juvenile warrants. His path was still fraught with hurdles, but he was making steady progress, a testament to the profound impact of systemic racism on individual lives. I observed a newfound calmness and maturity emerging in him. Watching him tenderly care for his daughter, meticulously changing her diapers, feeding, and swaddling her, was a testament to his growth. His decision-making had evolved remarkably from his days on the streets and under the influence of opiates.

Engagement and Empathy: Pathways to Understanding

The transformation of the University of Chicago into a trauma center in 2018 was not just a change in healthcare delivery; it was a pivotal moment in demystifying systemic racism for me. Previously, my comprehension of these systemic issues was largely molded by media narratives. These accounts, often colored by political biases, presented systemic racism in oversimplified or sensational terms, obscuring the intricate and deeply personal experiences of those affected.

The irony of this limited perspective became starkly apparent in the trauma center. Here, systemic racism was not an abstract concept or a tool for political rhetoric. It was a palpable, daily reality affecting real individuals. The patients I met were not mere statistics or theoretical cases; they embodied stories of resilience and struggle, challenging the media's superficial portrayals. They were patients who did not have the means to buy food, missed clinic because they didn't have a car, and couldn't read or write because their schools had failed them. This profound disparity underscored the inadequacy of media in truly capturing the essence of systemic racism. Despite its wide reach, the media often overlooked the genuine voices of those most impacted, instead amplifying more dominant, yet detached perspectives.

In the trauma center, I witnessed the raw, unfiltered realities of systemic racism daily. Daily interactions with patients from diverse backgrounds revealed the true face of this issue - marked by a complex mix of social, economic, and health disparities. These encounters were illuminating and deeply humanizing, challenging my preconceptions and stereotypes.

This firsthand engagement imparted a critical lesson: comprehending and addressing systemic racism transcends media debates and online discussions. It transcends profound rhetorical conversation without action. It demands active listening and learning from the experiences of those enduring its consequences. It is through these personal interactions that we can foster empathy, understanding, and collaboration, laying the groundwork for genuine change.

Reflecting on this journey, I recognize the intertwined nature of the University of Chicago's transformation and my own. The establishment of the trauma center reshaped not only healthcare delivery in our community but also our perceptions of systemic racism. It taught me that true understanding and the fight against systemic racism lie in direct, personal engagement with the communities we serve, but also the power that systemic change from above can have on an individual.

Institutional Awakening: Recognizing Systemic Challenges

This transition was a pivotal moment, not just for me but for the entire institution. As our hospital embraced the trauma needs of the local community, I could see that it also catalyzed a collective awakening among the staff to the harsh realities of systemic racism and violence. Each patient encounter, each story shared, contributed to a cumulative, evolving understanding of these intricate issues. This was not a solitary revelation, but a shared, dynamic evolution by the members of the institution, continually strengthened by our daily interactions.

In this new paradigm, our interactions with patients transcended traditional medical care, fostering a collaborative and empathetic approach that went beyond the typical doctor-patient dynamic. These interactions became dialogues, vital channels to understand the lived experiences of systemic racism, far beyond the often reductive or sensationalist media portrayals. Through these authentic, grassroots interactions, we began to grasp the full impact of systemic racism on health and wellbeing. Daily, I had real, honest discussions with colleagues about what we can do to promote actual change.

Lessons Learned and the Path Forward

My journey at the trauma center has profoundly shaped my perspective on systemic racism and violence. The deeper my involvement with the community, the more acutely I perceived the pervasiveness of these issues and the indispensable role of healthcare institutions in confronting them. This evolution, from my initial days as a resident to my current role as an attending, has been a journey of continuous learning and adaptation.

This experience has underscored the necessity of transcending superficial engagement with systemic issues. Meaningful change demands a deep, personal commitment to understanding the lived experiences of those affected by systemic racism. It calls for healthcare professionals to extend their roles beyond healing, becoming advocates, educators, and allies in combating these entrenched societal challenges.

Reflecting on both my personal and the hospital's professional evolution, it is evident that what started as a medical initiative has evolved into a comprehensive dedication to social justice and health equity. This journey highlights the transformative power of direct community involvement and the crucial need for personal engagement in truly understanding and addressing systemic racism. It highlights what a well thought out systemic change can do to combat a systemic problem.

Looking ahead, the lessons are clear: We must continue to prioritize initiatives that promote direct, meaningful interactions with our communities, valuing these firsthand experiences above detached narratives. Healthcare institutions have a vital role to play, not just as medical providers, but as proactive agents of social change. By fostering empathy, understanding, and action against systemic injustices, we can pave the way towards a more equitable and just society.

References

1. Galtung J. Violence, peace, and peace research. J Peace Res. 1969;6:167–91.
2. Crandall M, Sharp D, Unger E, et al. Trauma deserts: distance from a trauma center, transport times, and mortality from gunshot wounds in Chicago. Am J Public Health. 2013;103:1103–9.
3. Phelos HM, Kass NM, Deeb A-P, et al. Social determinants of health and patient-level mortality prediction after trauma. J Trauma Acute Care Surg. 2022;92:287–95.
4. Herrera-Escobar JP, Uribe-Leitz T, Wang J, et al. The Social Vulnerability Index and long-term outcomes after traumatic injury. Ann Surg. 2022;276:22–9.
5. Spitzer S, Castillo-Angeles M, Thomas A, et al. Social vulnerability index and firearms: how neighborhood health disparities affect trauma outcomes. Surg Pract Sci. 2022;11:100130.
6. Poulson M, Neufeld MY, Dechert T, et al. Historic redlining, structural racism, and firearm violence: a structural equation modeling approach. Lancet Reg Health Am. 2021;3:100052.
7. Poulson MR, Neufeld MY, Barmak L, et al. Redlining, structural racism, and firearm violence in Boston. J Am Coll Surg. 2020;231:e249.
8. Sossenheimer PH, Andersen MJ Jr, Clermont MH, et al. Structural violence and trauma outcomes: an ethical framework for practical solutions. J Am Coll Surg. 2018;227:537–42.
9. Polcari AM, Hoefer LE, Zakrison TL, et al. A novel machine-learning tool to identify community risk for firearm violence: The Firearm Violence Vulnerability Index. J Trauma Acute Care Surg. 2023;95:128–36.
10. Javed Z, Haisum Maqsood M, Yahya T, et al. Race, racism, and cardiovascular health: applying a social determinants of health framework to racial/ethnic disparities in cardiovascular disease. Circ Cardiovasc Qual Outcomes. 2022;15:e007917.
11. Hailu EM, Maddali SR, Snowden JM, et al. Structural racism and adverse maternal health outcomes: a systematic review. Health Place. 2022;78:102923.
12. Jankov P, Caref C. Segregation and inequality in Chicago Public Schools, transformed and intensified under corporate education reform. EPAA. 2017;25:56.
13. Baker BD. America's most financially disadvantaged school districts and how they got that way: how state and local governance causes school funding disparities. Center for American Progress. Available from: http://files.eric.ed.gov/fulltext/ED561094.pdf. 2014. Accessed 13 Dec 2023.
14. Dickson-Gomez J, Pacella M, Broaddus MR, et al. Convention versus deviance: moral agency in adolescent gang members' decision making. Subst Use Misuse. 2017;52:562–73.

The Transformative Impact of the University of Chicago Level 1 Trauma Center Opening on Student and Trainee Experiences

Samuel E. Okum, Darlington Nwaudo, and Selwyn O. Rogers, Jr

A Brief History

For 30 years, the Emergency Department at the University of Chicago Medical Center on Chicago's South Side lacked a key element necessary to provide the highest quality of care to critically-injured patients from surrounding neighborhoods: an operational, adult level-1 trauma center (L1TC) [1]. While the institution made a brief foray into providing trauma care to its greater community through a two-year venture in the late 1980s, it shuttered its formerly-operational trauma center in 1988 due to financial strains from treating thousands of uninsured trauma patients [2]. With the closure of the nearby Michael Reese Hospital L1TC barely a year later, the South Side—a region of Chicago notorious for its firearm injury burden—was left bereft of its own access point to the highest-level of acute care available to critically-wounded patients [1, 3].

Dr. Nwaudo and Mr. Okum contributed equally to this chapter and, as such, are considered co-first authors

S. E. Okum (✉)
Department of Surgery, The University of Chicago Medicine, Chicago, IL, USA

School of Medicine, Johns Hopkins University, Baltimore, MD, USA
e-mail: sokum1@jhu.edu

D. Nwaudo
Department of Surgery, The University of Chicago Medicine, Chicago, IL, USA

Department of Orthopedic Surgery, The University of Chicago Medicine, Chicago, IL, USA
e-mail: Darlington.Nwaudo@uchicagomedicine.org

S. O. Rogers, Jr
Department of Surgery, The University of Chicago Medicine, Chicago, IL, USA
e-mail: srogers@bsd.uchicago.edu

S. O. Rogers, Jr (ed.), *Creating a Modern Trauma Center*,
https://doi.org/10.1007/978-3-031-66524-0_30

In the years following these closures, firearm-related deaths surged in Chicago and across the country, increasing by over 40% nationwide between 2000 and the present [4]. Yet, despite this intensifying crisis of injury and death, the South Side of Chicago remained the most populous urban region in the United States without its own L1TC [1, 5]. As this reality grew increasingly more untenable for South Siders, a grassroots movement was born to demand the return of an L1TC to serve the community [6–9]. Still, the University of Chicago, along with other South Side medical institutions, resisted calls to change the landscape [10, 11].

In August of 2010, this advocacy effort was energized in the wake of the shooting of Damian Turner—a teenage activist and community organizer—some five blocks from the flagship building of the University of Chicago Medical Center [2, 6]. Rather than being rushed there by paramedics, Damian was transported nine miles north to Northwestern Memorial Hospital—the site of the nearest L1TC at that time—succumbing to his injuries enroute [2, 6]. Damian's mother, Sheila Rush, is quoted as saying that "[her] sweet baby could still be alive today if the U. of C. [in reference to the University of Chicago] had a trauma center." [2] Instead, he exsanguinated for 30 minutes on his way to an operating table.

The community saw the cruelty inherent to Damian's untimely death: the geography of their neighborhoods played a deterministic role [2, 6, 9]. Had Damian been shot on the wealthier, whiter North Side of the city, he may have arrived more quickly to one of Chicago's then-four L1TCs to be spared by a timely, life-saving surgical procedure [2, 12].

In large part due to this outrage—and ensuing community advocacy efforts—the University of Chicago announced that their L1TC would reopen [11, 13]. And, on May 1st of 2018, the University of Chicago's L1TC (UCMTC) received its first patient in almost three decades [13]. For the South Side, where dozens—if not hundreds—are shot within a stone's throw of UCMTC's doors annually, this change would be seismic.

The New Trauma Center's Broader Impact on Students and Trainees

Now, five years after the UCMTC re-launched operations, it is abundantly clear that the center's opening has not just served as a life-saving intervention for critically-wounded patients in its community [14, 15]. The center's impact can be observed more broadly on the attitudes and experiences of staff and students affiliated with the University of Chicago Medicine, most profoundly among the generation of students and trainees who arrived at the University during the post-UCMTC era.

The stories of two students, Sam Okum and Darlington "Dar" Nwaudo are particularly pertinent in elucidating the impact of the UCMTC opening on students and trainees at the institution. Both Sam—as an undergraduate—and Dar—as a medical student—arrived at the University in the fall of 2018, just months after UCMTC opened. During their time as U of C. students, both engaged with the center longitudinally through research and clinical endeavors. Now respectively a medical student at Johns Hopkins and an orthopedic surgery resident still at U. of C., Sam and Dar's reflections on their years-long work with UCMTC from its inception until the present provide valuable insight into how the new trauma center has exerted a formative impact on young students and trainees.

Student Reflections During a Paradigm Shift

Sam—even before hearing the story of the new trauma center—was drawn to the prospect of attending the University of Chicago due both to its long tradition of academic excellence and location amongst some of America's most underserved urban neighborhoods. To him, living and studying in such a unique environment would engender opportunities to translate classroom learning to direct community engagement. Raised by a civil rights attorney and, more broadly, among family members who worked at the forefront of the Second Wave Feminist and Civil Rights movements, active engagement in social justice work had always been important to him.

But, as an aspiring physician, doing so within the confines of medical practice was initially a puzzle to Sam. When he arrived on the U. of C. campus as a teenager, he sought to untangle the apparent duality of his ambitions: to productively serve his greater community and to practice academic medicine, a field he then viewed as governed by hierarchy and strict adherence to tradition that frequently fails to seek the perspectives of community stakeholders.

Yet, learning about UCMTC's history and the years-long advocacy effort that underlaid its re-opening served as a catalyst for Sam in understanding how his interests might be interwoven. The trauma center—fundamentally a response to the articulated needs of South Side residents—would serve as an ideal place to gain exposure to a progressive approach to academic medicine, one in which community feedback plays a central role in informing care structure, investments in hospital infrastructure, and research activity.

It has now been over four years since Sam joined the UCMTC research team. In that time, he has worked on a range of projects, from identifying the UCMTC's role in reducing racial discrepancies in ambulance transport times to understanding its impact in eliminating neighborhood disparities in mortality from firearm-related injury. With each new study, additional evidence emerged to support the same conclusion: by finally listening to the communities it serves and mobilizing resources to re-open its L1TC, the University of Chicago Medical Center played a significant role in ameliorating historic disparities in trauma care access and outcomes.

To Sam, though, the most important conclusion that he derives from his work is that academic physicians—through research endeavors among other activities—have substantial power to promote broadscale social change. Since its opening, the UCMTC received a flurry of local and national media attention as evidence surrounding the gravity of its impact emerged. In doing so, the opening has resuscitated a national conversation surrounding how best to provide trauma care services to a population experiencing a surge of firearm-related violence. By challenging decades of "conventional wisdom" held by the Chicago medical establishment that a half dozen, inequitably distributed trauma centers, would be sufficient to provide the highest quality trauma care to *all* Chicagoans, the UCMTC opening underscores how medical stakeholders do not always know how best to care for their communities in a vacuum. Amid this reckoning, University of Chicago students, like Sam and Dar, learned something: there is power in listening with humility and providing good-faith consideration to what their patients' communities have to say.

The Trauma Center as a Harbinger of Cultural Changes

The aforementioned reckoning is emblematic of a broader cultural shift at the University of Chicago that was accelerated, if not precipitated, by the opening of the UCMTC. Sure, community-based health programs have always existed underneath the University of Chicago Medical Center umbrella, the most notable of which being the Urban Health Initiative. Chicago's Pritzker School of Medicine also touts a progressive curriculum that emphasizes the unique considerations of engagement with diverse patient populations and underserved communities. Yet, for decades, material investments made in consultation with community partners were few and far between on campus. According to the founding director of UCMTC, Dr. Selwyn O. Rogers Jr., the UCMTC was the first significant investment in hospital infrastructure on University of Chicago campus that was fundamentally a response to articulated community needs [11]. For an institution that, only a few years ago, was a lightning rod for criticism from South Side activists for paying more lip service to the health disparities plaguing their neighborhoods than taking actionable steps to address them, the UCMTC serves as a brick-and-mortar testament to the institution's pivot to a diametrically more community-informed approach to its provision of healthcare.

One cannot understate the historical significance of the UCMTC as the first exemplification, if not impetus, of the cultural changes currently in motion at the University of Chicago Medical Center. The UCMTC opening is not a singular case, but rather the first of a cohort of new, concrete endeavors on the University of Chicago Medical campus intended to meet the health needs of adjacent South Side neighborhoods. In addition to the UCMTC, a new state-of-the-art cancer center is slated to open on the U. of C. campus in 2027 at a projected cost to the institution of almost one billion dollars [16]. This center, which is expected to serve as a bulwark against the disproportionately high cancer burden in the South Side, is just another example of U. of. C.'s pivot to the community that has coincided with the UCMTC opening. In fact, the institution's strategic vision for 2025 reflects this invigorated commitment to "enhancing the health of [its] local community," wherein the Medical Center intends to be a central participant in "efforts to achieve improved access and care delivery in South/Southeast Chicago." [17]

Crucially, though, the re-centering of community-informed practices to the core of the University of Chicago Medical Center's identity has exerted a reverberating effect on the attitudes and perspectives of the cohort of students and trainees who have engaged with the institution during the post-UCMTC era. As exemplars of this phenomenon, Sam and Dar's stories highlight how students at the U. of. C now understand that community-driven approaches to patient care need not be an adjunct to one's core clinical responsibilities or constitute some sort of "extra-curricular" endeavor. Instead, they can—and should—be foundational to physicians' service to their patients and broader communities.

Changes in the Trainee Experience Post-UCMTC

Beyond his observation of the cultural shift underway at the University of Chicago, Dar's experiences through his almost six years as a U. of C. medical student—and now resident—reflect another dimension of the changes wrought by the UCMTC opening. His own insights, as well as testimony from faculty members at U. of C. and beyond, serve as strong evidence of the tangible improvements in the quality of medical training available at U. of C. after the trauma center opened.

As a teaching hospital, a substantial component of the University of Chicago Medical Center's mission is to prepare trainees for excellence in careers in medicine through immersive learning on patient wards. At the University of Chicago, like many other institutions, residents and fellows therefore serve as the backbone of the provision of patient care and institutional operations. With this in mind, the transition of the University of Chicago Medical Center to operating a high-volume adult L1TC was expected have a significant impact on the trainee experience. Some of the documented changes were anticipated; however, there were many unforseen challenges that resulted in years of adjustments for the various residency programs to fully optimize the training opportunities provided by the trauma center opening.

Six years after the UCMTC opening, trauma is now core to the experience of many residents. During their first year of training, interns from numerous specialties, including orthopedic surgery, emergency medicine, plastic surgery, urology, ENT, general surgery, and neurosurgery spend at least one month on the trauma service. Gaining experience taking care of some of the most acutely ill patients at the hospital from the very beginning of residency shows how central the trauma center has become to the training experience of residents from a diversity of programs.

Hypotheses on the Impact of the UCMTC Opening on Trainees

Before the trauma center opened, prominent chairs and program directors from various subspecialties were asked how they expected the new trauma center to affect their services' operations and, thus, resident training. Their thoughts—which broadly reflect a belief that the UCMTC opening would positively contribute to the trainee experience—are below:

> Caring for injured patients, whether from a car crash or a sports injury or any other cause, is at the heart of orthopaedic practice and is an integral part of what we have always done. We estimate the Level 1 Trauma Center will add about 900 orthopaedic surgeries annually — a roughly 20 percent increase from our current yearly surgical volume. Each of these surgical procedures will be an opportunity for our orthopaedic residents to participate in surgery, so this will be a solid boost to our educational program and will make our residents' experience in trauma among the best in the nation. (Douglas R. Dirschl, MD, Chair, Department of Orthopaedic Surgery and Rehabilitation Medicine [18]).

> Caring for trauma patients requires clinicians to address acute problems, to think on their feet and to operate and/or perform more proficiently. The opening of the Level 1 trauma center will raise the clinical excellence across the continuum of our institution -- in surgery, radiology, nursing, emergency care, and more. It will help us create an even more robust and efficient delivery system. The impact will be positive for our trainees and all involved in the delivery of clinical care. (Mitchell C. Posner, MD, Chief, Section of General Surgery [18])

> There is significant opportunity to understand and prevent trauma whether it's emphasizing driving safety or violence prevention. The potential to positively impact a larger group of patients and their families is humbling. The Level 1 Trauma Center will enhance residency training with greater exposure to serious facial trauma. We will increase the efficiency of our processes, ranging from things such as time from the trauma bay to the OR to discharge planning/length of stay. (Nishant Agrawal, MD, Chief, Section of Otolaryngology—Head and Neck Surgery [18])

> Opening a Level 1 Trauma Center is an extraordinary opportunity for University of Chicago to help better the lives of patients on the South Side. As we track and study the care of trauma patients, we will improve the care of individuals affected by violence and trauma. (David Frim, MD, PhD, Chief, Section of Neurosurgery [18])

> A Level 1 trauma center will bring a higher volume of patients and more complexity in cases to the Section of Plastic and Reconstructive Surgery. We have dedicated craniofacial, maxillofacial and microsurgical (for soft tissue damage) plastic surgeons on our staff, all who will contribute to the care of trauma patients. And we anticipate growth in our program to meet the needs of the individuals affected by trauma. (David W. Chang, MD, Chief, Section of Plastic and Reconstructive Surgery [18])

Adapting to the UCMTC Opening

Despite the collective recognition that the UCMTC opening would provide trainees with more extensive exposure to complex pathology and a higher case volume to buoy their clinical prowess, the opening of the UCMTC initially presented challenges related to the need to restructure care at the University of Chicago Medical Center to support the new center.

The first logistical issue that needed to be addressed was management of the sudden increase in volume wrought by the L1TC. Most stakeholders at the U. of C. anticipated that the new trauma center would bring in more patients, but the challenges that came along with this was underestimated. Not only was there an increased census of new patients, but these patients were more acutely ill and more medically and socially complex than the population that physicians, trainees, and the hospital system were previously accustomed to. From the beginning, most surgical departments needed to form, or revamp dedicated trauma/consult teams to provide the increased workforce needed to take care of these patients.

For the Orthopedic Surgery Department, the solution was designating a PGY2 "night float" resident in the hospital every night to staff new consults and trauma activations. There was also a more senior resident (PGY4 or PGY5) on call each night to support the night float. In the past, this more experienced resident would be able to take call from home and was only required to come into the hospital for emergent overnight surgeries like finger re-plantations or hemodynamically unstable pelvic ring injuries. With the new trauma center, the senior resident often found themselves in the hospital overnight to assist the night float with procedures and preparing patients for the operating room the next morning. Eventually, the Orthopedic Department, like many others, obtained dedicated call rooms in the Center for Care and Discovery building for these residents to have a workspace and the option to sleep in the hospital when needed.

With Growing Pains Came Opportunity

The increased consult volume in the wake of the UCMTC opening resulted in increased operative opportunities for trainees. An example of this on the orthopedic service was the initiation of a dedicated "fracture room" OR that was equipped with all the tools necessary to treat the most complex fracture injuries. Additionally, dedicated scrub nurses and circulators who received specialized training to assist with orthopedic procedures were hired to staff the fracture room around the clock. For residents, this was a major development for their training, since the fracture room setup essentially guaranteed operative orthopedic trauma cases every morning. The overnight residents, meanwhile, gained the valuable experience of working with interdisciplinary teams—including those from the surgical ICU, neuro ICU, and trauma surgery department—to collaboratively treat and resuscitate patients in the middle of the night to optimize them for definitive or temporizing fracture care in the morning.

Six years after the UCMTC opening, it is apparent that the constant influx of trauma patients to the University of Chicago has elevated the overall training quality of U. of C. residents. Traumatic injuries, especially the polytraumatized patient, present with the most complicated injury patterns and the most physiologically challenging clinical situations. As such, U. of C residents are increasingly exposed to injuries that require complex decision-making due to the non-standard presentations of injuries and acut situations, like continuously evolving hemodynamic statuses.

Orthopedic surgery trainees, for example, must now ask questions such as: how do you reduce a dislocated shoulder in a patient with an ipsilateral open elbow fracture? How do you safely identify the neurovascular structures in the open distal radius fracture when standard incision sites and dissection planes have been compromised? How do you position the patient laterally on the OR bed to address an acetabular fracture when they have a cervical spine injury, bilateral chest tubes, and/or are in respiratory distress in the surgical ICU? There are not textbook answers for all these questions. Instead, they require careful collaboration with other subspecialty services, a deep understanding of anatomy, and the technical skills necessary to take care of the polytraumatized patient. The resident experience at the University of Chicago therefore now focuses on imparting a core foundation of problem-solving strategies, providing practice with managing high acuity patients, and working with interdisciplinary teams. This ensures that the residents finish with the proficiencies necessary to take care of any patient in any practice environment in the future.

Bolstering Case Volume for Trainees Amid the COVID-19 Pandemic

Another unanticipated selequela of the UCMTC opening on the resident experience was that it allowed U. of C. to continue providing high level training to residents during the COVID-19 Pandemic. In the spring of 2020, almost all elective cases were put on hold across the country. Even after the hold was removed at U. of C., there was a delay in patients pursuing elective medical and surgical care due to risks and fears of contracting COVID-19 in healthcare settings [19]. However, trauma activations remained high during this time [20] and surgical emergencies continued to be definitively-managed in the operating room. The presence of the trauma center at the University of Chicago allowed many surgical specialties to retain a case volume substantial enough to provide robust training for the residents amid the pandemic. According to Dr. Dirschl, former Department Chair of Orthopedic Surgery and Rehabilitation Medicine, the number of patient transfers to UChicago actually increased during the spring and summer of 2020 [21]. This shows that U. of C. was viewed as an institution with the capability to take care of those in need during the COVID crisis and that the opening of the trauma center was influential in gaining this regional and national reputation. For residents, this lessened the disruption that the pandemic had on their surgical training experience.

Exposure to Trauma-Informed Care

Given the substantial volume of trauma cases that the surgical specialties at U. of C. have absorbed, along with the requirement that interns from all surgery programs rotate on the trauma service, surgical trainees at the U. of C. now gain extensive experience caring for the trauma patient. Additionally, U. of C. surgical residents obtain special training on the provision of trauma-informed care. This training emphasizes understanding the trauma patient's background, recognizing that trauma patients have likely have experienced past emotional/psychological trauma, and delivering care in a way minimizes the potential for re-traumatization. Trauma-informed care also prioritizes working with patients to design a safe discharge plan, which maximizes the potential for physical rehabilitation and minimizes patients' susceptibility to re-injury, especially from interpersonal violence. Given the large patient volume at UCMTC, trainees rotating through the trauma center and surgical floors gain copious exposure to trauma patient care and are provided with ample opportunities to practice the principles of trauma-informed approaches to patient engagement.

Broadening the Reach of New Training Opportunities

The robustness of the training available to residents in the post-UCMTC has transformed the University of Chicago into a Mecca for residency training locally and nationally. For one, the U. of C. trauma service has partnered with the US military to train Army medical staff and physicians to treat critically wounded civilians, thereby imparting skills to treat wounded military personnel in combat zones [22]. Another successful partnership has been with the Swedish Hospital general surgery residency program in Washington State. In an interview discussing the rationale behind the partnership, Dr. Marc Horton, the program director at Swedish, stated that he "wanted Swedish residents to gain a better perspective of the disparities in the delivery of healthcare in our country, both racial and financial" [23]. To Horton, U. of C. was uniquely compelling as a partner institution to accomplish these goals and to "broaden [trainees'] experience [to] make them more complete physicians, surgeons, and people" [23]. The partnership has also positively served UCMTC; visiting residents from Swedish have become integral members of the trauma team, bolstering staffing at UCMTC and allowing the center to take on a higher volume of trauma activations.

The Impact of the UCMTC Opening on Trainee Recruitment

The trauma center opening not only revamped the training environment at U. of C., but, as previously addressed, futher precipitated a culture shift felt across all levels of the institution. These two factors demonstrate how the trauma center has become a recruitment tool for talented trainees interested in clinical opportunities created by the UCMTC opening and the pivot to community-informed care that the opening represented.

Finally, by fostering a culture of advocacy and re-centering community-responsive care at the forefront of the U. of C. mission, the UCMTC opening has attracted residents passionate about taking care of the unique patient population served by U. of C. from both a medical psychosocial perspective. Now, prospective trainees with a calling to address healthcare disparities, serve the historically underserved, and practice community-responsive healthcare are more likely to be drawn to U. of C. for medical training. New, resident-organized initiatives also underscore how a culture of service has taken root among the post-UCMTC generation of trainees. A recently-founded, resident-oriented program called Community Champions has transformed the University's Urban Health Initiative (UHI), the University's community health department, which administers community health initiatives (including a violence prevention and recovery program, neighborhood health fairs, and days of service). Now, through Community Champions, the UHI is at the forefront of preparing the next generation of physicians to participate in a community engagement through a curriculum focused on equipping them with knowledge and skills to create and pursue various community outreach projects during the academic year. Community Champions participants also serve as liaisons for others in their respective specialty/department to become involved with service. Prior outreach events and topics have included health screenings, healthy cooking demonstrations, mental health and suicide prevention interventions, coping with grief seminars, diabetes education, and high school career fairs.

The volume and complexity of patients treated at a L1TC in a major urban area like Chicago conducive to fostering a more challenging training environment. At a medical institution with a L1TC, large censuses of patients with acute needs create a more complicated system of patient management, from longer rounds in the morning, to more medication orders to manage. Additional day-to-day clinical responsibilities in such environments mostly fall on the residents, thus providing additional experience engaging with the complexities of patient management. Anecdotally, the University of Chicago Medical Center's transition to operating a L1TC was compounded with a transition to attracting prospective residents with motivation to take advantage of these additional responsibilities as learning experiences.

In the months after the UCMTC opened, however, residency program directors and department chiefs realized that the additional clinical responsibilities created by the opening were too arduous to be taken care of by the residents alone. The institution has turned to hiring trauma and surgical subspecialty advanced practice providers to assist with inpatient floor management and OR staffing, especially during dedicated resident education sessions. This, too, has created opportunities for residents to gain experience working on teams with multiple levels of providers.

Final Remarks

In the wake of the UCMTC opening, medical training and student experiences have been comprehensively revamped at the University of Chicago Medical Center. Beyond fostering a culture of community-responsive care with reverberant effects on student attitudes and motivations to engage in community-oriented medical practice, the UCMTC opening has bolstered medical training at the institution across multiple domains. Now, U. of C. residents in all surgical subspecialities are afforded with more case hours and exposure to medically complex patients, thereby improving their ability to practice autonomously upon graduation. Furthermore, U. of C. residents now gain the experience necessary to provide their patients with high quality trauma-informed care. They are also more equipped to work collaboratively with interdisciplinary teams to optimize the patient outcomes.

This unparalleled training environment has allowed the university to gain national recognition and become a destination for other hospitals, and even the US Army, to send their trainees to gain expertise in the treatment of traumatic injuries. The invigorated culture of service and community-responsive care, as well as improved clinical training after the UCMTC has served as a recruitment tool for the institution, attracting talented residents with a passion for health disparities work. As an academic institution, the trainee experience has overall benefited from U. of C.'s transition to operating an adult Level I Trauma Center and will help the institution meet its goals of producing humanistic and competent physicians prepared to care for the most complex and severely ill patients.

References

1. Junco ECD, Garibaldi K. Race, gun violence, and equitable access to trauma care. Chicago Tribune. Published June 27, 2018. https://www.chicagotribune.com/2018/06/27/race-gun-violence-and-equitable-access-to-trauma-care/
2. Bushey C. How Chicago activists and their allies forced a reckoning with U of C Medicine. Crain's Chicago Business. Published April 11, 2016. https://www.chicagobusiness.com/section/trauma-protest
3. Tribune C. Michael Reese Quits City's Trauma Network. Chicago Tribune https://www.chicagotribune.com/1989/12/29/michael-reese-quits-city-trauma-network/. Published December 29, 1989.
4. Deaths by Underlying Cause. CDC WONDER Database. https://wonder.cdc.gov/Deaths-by-Underlying-Cause.html. Accessed 2 Oct 2023.
5. Tung EL, Hampton DA, Kolak M, Rogers SO, Yang JP, Peek ME. Race/ethnicity and geographic access to urban trauma care. JAMA Netw Open. 2019;2(3):e190138. https://doi.org/10.1001/jamanetworkopen.2019.0138.
6. Terry D. A death sparks a demand for care. The New York Times. https://www.nytimes.com/2010/10/03/us/03cnchospitals.html. Published October 3, 2010.
7. Sailappan D, Lalljee J. Rallies, Sit-ins, and Padlocks: the History of Trauma Center Activism. Chicago Maroon. https://chicagomaroon.com/25853/news/rallies-sit-ins-padlocks-history-trauma-activism/. Published April 26, 2018. Accessed 3 Apr 2024.

8. Miller S. Community, student activists rally for trauma center. Chicago Maroon. https://chicagomaroon.com/14278/news/community-student-activists-rally-for-trauma-center/. Published November 1, 2011.
9. Tribune C. Youths appeal to U. of C. for formation of trauma center. Chicago Tribune. https://www.chicagotribune.com/2011/08/15/youths-appeal-to-u-of-c-for-formation-of-trauma-center/. Published August 15, 2011.
10. Cao S. Officials defend lack of trauma center, tout UCMC's offerings. Chicago Maroon. Published May 13, 2011. https://chicagomaroon.com/7168/news/officials-defend-lack-of-trauma-center-tout-ucmc-s-offerings/
11. Schorsh K. The inside story of why U of C Medicine changed its mind about a trauma center. Crain's Chicago Business. Published April 11, 2016. https://www.chicagobusiness.com/section/trauma-power
12. Crandall M, Sharp D, Unger E, et al. Trauma deserts: distance from a trauma center, transport times, and mortality from gunshot wounds in Chicago. Am J Public Health. 2013;103(6):1103–9. https://doi.org/10.2105/AJPH.2013.301223.
13. Moore N. After push from activists, Chicago's South Side gets an adult trauma center. NPR. https://www.npr.org/2018/04/28/606716569/chicagos-new-trauma-center. Published April 28, 2018. Accessed 3 Apr 2024.
14. Okum S, Nwaudo D, Rogers S. Association of a new trauma center with geographic disparities in gunshot wound mortality. In: APHA; 2023. https://apha.confex.com/apha/2023/meetingapp.cgi/Paper/542108. Accessed 3 Apr 2024.
15. Abbasi AB, Dumanian J, Okum S, et al. Association of a new trauma center with racial, ethnic, and socioeconomic disparities in access to trauma care. JAMA Surg. 2021;156(1):97–9. https://doi.org/10.1001/jamasurg.2020.4998.
16. Bartosch J. UChicago Medicine breaks ground on state's first freestanding cancer center | University of Chicago News. Published September 19, 2023. https://news.uchicago.edu/story/uchicago-medicine-breaks-ground-states-first-freestanding-cancer-center. Accessed 3 Apr 2024.
17. 2025 Strategic Vision. https://www.uchicagomedicine.org/about-us/2025-vision. Accessed 31 Mar 2024.
18. Rubin, Gretchen. How a trauma center impacts an entire hospital. Published October 6, 2017. https://www.uchicagomedicine.org/forefront/trauma-articles/it-takes-a-village-to-operate-a-trauma-center. Accessed 31 Mar 2024.
19. Ghoshal S, Rigney G, Cheng D, et al. Institutional surgical response and associated volume trends throughout the COVID-19 pandemic and postvaccination recovery period. JAMA Netw Open. 2022;5(8):e2227443. https://doi.org/10.1001/jamanetworkopen.2022.27443.
20. Hahn A, Brown T, Chapman B, et al. How did the COVID-19 pandemic affect trauma volume at an urban level I trauma center? Am Surg. 2022;88(4):758–63. https://doi.org/10.1177/00031348211054075.
21. Chairman's Reflection on COVID-19 Departmental Impact | Department of Orthopaedic Surgery and Rehabilitation Medicine | The University of Chicago. Published July 17, 2020. https://ortho.uchicago.edu/news/chairmans-reflection-covid-19-departmental-impact. Accessed 31 Mar 2024.
22. Bartosch, Jamie. U.S. Army medical staff trains in UChicago Medicine's Simulation Center. https://www.uchicagomedicine.org/forefront/trauma-articles/army-medical-staff-trauma-training-simulation-center. Accessed 31 Mar 2024.
23. Swedish partnership with UChicago Medicine trains young doctors in trauma care. https://blog.swedish.org/swedish-blog/swedish-partnership-with-uchicago-medicine-trains-young-doctors-in-trauma-care. Accessed 31 Mar 2024.

From Mission to Impact: Reflecting on the Trauma Center's Journey

Mark Anderson

When I joined the University of Chicago in the fall of 2022, I spent the first few months observing, listening, and learning, so I could begin to understand what motivates our tremendously talented faculty and staff in the work they do every day. A few months into my term, our institution undertook an important exercise to clarify and articulate these motivations with a formal set of mission, vision, and values statements. These are not meant to be just nice-sounding statements, but the pillars upon which our institutions, the Biological Sciences Division, the Pritzker School of Medicine, and the University of Chicago Medicine, stand. These principles add guidance for our actions, infuse our work with meaning, and drive us to create a better, more equitable future for all.

Since its opening in 2018, the work at our Level 1 adult trauma center has represented the highest ideals of an academic medical center as a force for positive change. As we spoke to thousands of members of our organization and the surrounding community over the course of several months to develop our new guiding principles, it became clear that many of these values were already evident in our trauma center:

- Our **mission**: To pursue globally impactful solutions to seemingly unsolvable challenges, pushes us to think beyond the conventional and tackle the most pressing issues head-on. The trauma center is the hub of our multifaceted response to the urgent and seemingly unsolvable challenges of trauma care.
- Our **vision**: To elevate the human experience with knowledge and healthcare, reminds us that our work has a profound impact on individuals and communities. The trauma center has helped UChicago exemplify this vision by providing not just medical care but a sense of hope and healing to the community it serves.

M. Anderson (✉)
University of Chicago, Biological Sciences Division, Pritzker School of Medicine, Chicago, IL, USA
e-mail: andersonm1@bsd.uchicago.edu

S. O. Rogers, Jr (ed.), *Creating a Modern Trauma Center*,
https://doi.org/10.1007/978-3-031-66524-0_31

- Our **values**—excellence, curiosity, equity, collaboration, and compassion—are the moral compass that guides our actions. The trauma center embraces these values as it seeks innovative ways to address trauma, not merely as a reactive medical facility but as a proactive force for prevention. We hope every step of our growth presents new opportunities to live out our commitment to diversity, workforce development, and partnership with the community.

As we reflect on the trauma center's journey, we see how these principles can become living ideals. They are the foundation upon which the trauma center was established, and they continue to drive its mission of healing, innovation, and community transformation within the rest of the institution.

Pursuing the Good of the South Side Community

The University of Chicago is deeply embedded in Chicago's South Side. While the University's relationship with its surrounding community has at times been contentious throughout its history, today we strive to learn from our community members and rely on them as partners, even as we hope to serve them. The South Side Healthy Community Organization, of which the University of Chicago was a founding member, is an important example of this partnership. It is only by creating many layers of partnerships with our neighbors that we will collaboratively bring about positive change that benefits everyone. We aim to be advocates even where we cannot solve everything, and to build relationships that are grounded in trust, respect, and mutual benefit.

On some days, the constant and urgent stream of trauma care needs makes it difficult to imagine any approach that goes beyond reacting to the wail of ambulance sirens and a crush of incoming patients. But part of our ultimate hope for the South Side includes a shift towards a preventative approach to trauma care. Addressing the root causes of trauma and violence in our community is just as vital, if not more so, than providing healing after the fact.

We envision a future where the focus of our trauma center extends beyond immediate treatment and response to injuries. My friend and colleague Selwyn Rogers, MD, MPH, the founding director of our trauma center, compares this to dealing with an overflowing sink: while our first instinct might be to immediately begin mopping up the water spilling on the floor, the real first step should be to turn off the faucet. As physicians and surgeons, we sometimes focus too much on becoming really good at mopping, without stopping to ask for help with the faucet.

Physicians, public health experts, policy makers and government leaders alike all recognize that the kind of serious injuries requiring trauma care frequently have deeper, systematic causes far afield from the typical practices of medicine and surgery. Rather than focusing solely on the immediate care of patients, we want to engage with the community to help reduce the flow of injuries. This approach delves into the social determinants of health, such as economic disparities and access to preventative care, with the aim of identifying areas where proactive measures can be applied. Extrapolating this approach to its far-off conclusion, the trauma center's most audacious goal is to make itself obsolete.

Our experts aim to deliver patient-centered care and wraparound services while actively engaging community members in the development and implementation of preventive initiatives. Our Violence Recovery Program has engaged more than 8500 patients since it began operation in 2018, providing holistic care to help them and their families deal with the ramifications of traumatic injuries. Physicians, nurses, and other clinical staff not only treat physical wounds but also help provide crisis intervention, psychological first aid, re-injury risk assessment, safe discharge planning, community-based service provider referrals, case management and more.

Violence recovery specialists provide other types of support, including simply listening to patients who are shocked or scared, calling their family and friends, or connecting them with resources like food, mental health counseling, or civil legal support through our partnership with Legal Aid Chicago. The Block Hassenfeld Casdin (BHC) Collaborative for Family Resilience builds on the Violence Recovery Program to focus on the special needs of children and families affected by trauma, by integrating and expanding clinical and community services to help young patients and their families recover from the immediate and long-lasting effects of trauma caused by community violence and domestic or sexual violence.

These are just a few examples of how we are strengthening the ties between the University and the rest of the South Side community through our trauma center, but our true impact in the community extends beyond trauma care. Our commitment to the South Side Healthy Community Organization, which comprises UChicago Medicine and 12 other health providers serving more than 400,000 residents on the South Side, focuses on increasing access to primary and specialty care, preventative and chronic care management, care coordination and community engagement. Our Community Advisory Councils, which are representative groups of volunteer members who live and work in our service areas, including our Hyde Park, Chicago campus and Ingalls Memorial Hospital in the south suburbs, advise us on issues of interest to the broader community. They are essential partners in achieving our institution's goals related to the broader community interests, community benefit, access to care and effective community engagement. Together, we can embrace a vision of trauma care that moves beyond the conventional paradigm of reactive treatment to promote proactive engagement, reducing the incidence of trauma at its source.

The Future of the Trauma Center

Five years after launching our level 1 adult trauma center at UChicago Medicine, it has become the busiest facility of its kind in the city of Chicago. We treated more than 18,800 adult trauma patients in those first five years, in addition to nearly 3000 pediatric trauma patients. Now, we look toward the future with optimism and a sense of responsibility. Our journey has been marked by milestones and achievements, yet our true potential lies ahead.

As stated in our new institutional values, excellence, equity, and compassion will forever remain paramount as we deliver trauma care. We understand that to make a meaningful impact, we must continually strive for the highest standards. To ensure that every patient receives the best care possible, we must nurture the exceptional talents of everyone within our dedicated workforce as well.

The well-being of a healthcare provider team is crucial. Burnout across healthcare professions has spiked in recent years even as the issue has received growing recognition. The intense pace, high-pressure situations, and exposure to disturbing events inherent in trauma care make burnout an especially pressing concern for centers like ours. Just as we want to take a preventative approach to trauma care, we also take a preventative approach to provider health. Instead of providing resources when individuals reach crisis points, our leaders strive to create a supportive culture of resilience that offers work-life balance, space for emotional processing, mental health resources, and strong interpersonal networks.

Moreover, as part of cultivating a healthy workforce, we aim to extend opportunities to young people, embracing the communities in which we reside. By partnering with local educational institutions like Malcolm X Community College, Governor's State University, and Valparaiso University on workforce training programs, we not only contribute to the growth of these young talents toward careers in health care, but also foster diversity within our workforce. This diversity adds richness to our team and better represents the South Side community we serve. In creating these opportunities and fostering a culture of diversity and well-being, we prepare the trauma center for an even more impactful role in the future.

Broader Lessons for Current and Future Trauma Centers

While we ourselves are in a constant learning process, we also hope to use our experiences to guide other trauma centers as they serve their own populations. Although a key theme we have uncovered is the importance of tailoring approaches to the unique needs, characteristics, and culture of each community, there are other high-level insights that can inform best practices nationwide.

The most obvious way to share our trauma care expertise is through direct educational programming. For example, since 2021, we have partnered with the U.S. Army to help train military physicians, nurses and medics ahead of their deployment. By working alongside our experts to treat a wide range of trauma victims, the military medical personnel build skills and gain crisis situation "muscle memory" that will help them save lives in the field.

Zooming out, one of the core lessons we've learned is that trauma encompasses a wide spectrum of incidents, from penetrating injuries like gunshot wounds and stabbing to blunt force traumas incurred from vehicle accidents, falls, and more. This multifaceted nature of trauma challenges us to be versatile in our approach, ready to respond to a diverse range of scenarios with both medical expertise and a deep sensitivity toward psychological and social impacts of these injuries.

Acknowledging complexity is crucial for providing holistic care, and trauma centers must have the capacity to adapt to the unique demands of their communities, with a focus on being prepared for every form of trauma.

Preventing trauma at its roots requires localized strategies and partnerships with the community. This approach has the potential to significantly reduce the burden of trauma on healthcare systems and society as a whole. At the same time, however, we must recognize our limitations as an academic medical center. While we can be deeply engaged with the problems of our community, we cannot—nor should we be—solely responsible for addressing the effects of the endemic poverty and structural inequality that contribute to conditions leading to traumatic injuries. We can certainly make attempts through the kind of partnerships and community engagement I have described above, but I humbly suggest a starting point of first strengthening community at home.

Prior to coming to Chicago, I was the Director of the Department of Medicine at Johns Hopkins University in Baltimore. In 2015, a young man named Freddie Gray died while in the custody of Baltimore police—the ensuing social unrest revealed the pain and deep dissatisfaction many residents of the city felt in the face of police brutality, systemic racism, and institutional inequality. That reckoning forced us to look inward and ask how we as an institution could better understand the community we hoped to serve.

Despite our best intentions, academic medical centers like Johns Hopkins and UChicago that are located in urban areas can feel disconnected from our neighbors. Physicians, with their years of education and training, may not universally relate to the lived experience of the patients they treat or the hospital staff they rely on to do their jobs. During that difficult summer following Mr. Gray's death, we decided to bridge this gap with a simple "know your neighbor" ethos in the workplace—for example, doctors should know nurses; administrators should know facilities personnel; technicians should know support staff. We planned events and encouraged activities to give employees at all levels the opportunity to learn everyone's story. Our belief was that getting to know each other at a more personal level makes you feel part of something bigger, and in a small way, begin to heal some of that pain.

Broadening this "know your neighbor" approach to the area surrounding the medical center and the people who live there enables trauma centers to respond to community needs more effectively. At UChicago, many of our faculty and staff not only work but also live and raise their children in the surrounding South Side neighborhoods, of which we are a part. These neighbors and employees provide UChicago with a valuable window to truly see all of us as part of our community. This sense of proximity and connection should be a model for trauma centers looking to build stronger relationships with the areas they serve.

Yet after five years and counting, we are just beginning the continuous learning process of turning trauma care lessons into actionable guidance and best practices. Each year provides new experiences that should be viewed as opportunities to foster positive change. Our mission, vision, and values combine with the lessons we have learned so far to form an evolving framework for success, providing a path toward collective well-being and resilience in our city.

Future Directions

Selwyn O. Rogers, Jr

At a hyper-local level, the high rate of violence, especially firearm-related violence, has profound impacts on all aspects of community health, including life expectancy gaps between neighborhoods and disparities in health outcomes. The city of Chicago is just one stark example of the structural determinants of health and violence that reverberate throughout urban America.

The University of Chicago Medicine Trauma Center lies in the epicenter of violence on Chicago's South Side. The same factors that drive violence in communities on the South Side such as poverty, racism, lack of economic opportunities, and educational disparities also drive poor health outcomes from asthma, diabetes, cancer, and cardiovascular diseases leading to a thirty-year life expectancy gap between black and brown populations on the South Side and white populations in the loop of Chicago. As we consider these drivers of poor health outcomes, we must identify root causes of health disparities and influence social, political, and systematic determinants (e.g., education, housing, infrastructure, environment, safety and justice, economic development, mental wellness) and develop intersectional approaches to closing the health and opportunity gaps for all people in Chicago.

The University of Chicago Medicine Trauma Center was founded as a result of deep community engagement to address the extreme need for adult trauma care proximate to the South Side of Chicago. Founded in May, 2018, the Trauma Center has thus far cared for and cared about more than 25,000 trauma patients (40% firearm-related injuries) with a less than 5% mortality. The Trauma Center has built foundational trust with the communities that we serve. Furthermore, we have committed to working beyond the walls of the hospital and thinking boldly about systems-level changes that improves the vitality, wellness, and health of

S. O. Rogers, Jr (✉)
Department of Surgery, The University of Chicago Medicine, Chicago, IL, USA
e-mail: srogers@bsd.uchicago.edu

S. O. Rogers, Jr (ed.), *Creating a Modern Trauma Center*,
https://doi.org/10.1007/978-3-031-66524-0_32

communities on the South Side of Chicago. We launched the Violence Recovery Program (VRP), which is an innovative holistic program that aims to reduce the impact of gun violence and decrease recidivism through community-based violence recovery specialists who intervene on socioeconomic drivers of health. The VRP has provided wraparound services for over 7000 patients since its inception. The trailblazing Recovery Legal Care program, supported by NIH and the Department of Justice, assists patients with legal challenges of securing and navigating public benefits, housing, and employment. Research to define the best systems, including rigorous evaluation, informs the design of the appropriate approaches for the context to meet the needs of patients and communities.

As we look forward to the future, we envision the Trauma Center serving as a novel initiative to maximize the potential of all South Siders in a place-based approach at the confluence of research, service delivery, advocacy, and policy. We hope to root the trauma center in authentic partnership with the community. We will aim to deepen our understanding of those affected by community violence and work diligently on prevention. We hope to identify early intervention opportunities and suggest where to allocate city, county, and state resources more effectively. Through partnerships and rigorous evaluation, we hope to develop targeted, community-specific violence reduction and prevention strategies. The findings could inform both public policy decisions and practices at the Trauma Center. Ultimately, the data linkages between VRP and other data warehouses will enhance our understanding of how to address community violence through data-driven, targeted interventions.

We hope that our future work at the Trauma Center will be grounded in the community, where we will foster strong and lasting relationships with community organizations, health care providers, residents, and all learners to strategically improve health and access to quality care in our service area. We hope that we will contribute to create an "all-in" approach to improving vitality, well-being and health across all University of Chicago and University of Chicago Medicine for the communities on the South Side, given the complexity and intersectionability of issues related to investment and revitalization of historically marginalized communities to improve neighborhoods' assets and positive outcomes.

In summary, our audacious goal is that the Trauma Center will serve as a catalyst to mobilize internal and external partnerships to maximize the value of all people throughout the South Side. We aspire be a part of a greater whole committed to decreasing the life expectancy gap, investing in programs that lead to substantive improvements in the quality of life, and quantifiably improving the health and human potential of individuals and communities on the South Side of Chicago and beyond.

Index

S. O. Rogers, Jr (ed.), *Creating a Modern Trauma Center*,
https://doi.org/10.1007/978-3-031-66524-0

GPSR Compliance

The European Union's (EU) General Product Safety Regulation (GPSR) is a set of rules that requires consumer products to be safe and our obligations to ensure this.

If you have any concerns about our products, you can contact us on ProductSafety@springernature.com

In case Publisher is established outside the EU, the EU authorized representative is:

Springer Nature Customer Service Center GmbH
Europaplatz 3
69115 Heidelberg, Germany

Batch number: 09511804

Printed by Printforce, the Netherlands